The Right to Die with Dignity

The Right to Die with Dignity

An Argument in Ethics, Medicine, and Law

RAPHAEL COHEN-ALMAGOR

RUTGERS UNIVERSITY PRESS
New Brunswick, New Jersey, and London

Library of Congress Cataloging-in-Publication Data

Cohen-Almagor, Raphael.
  The right to die with dignity : an argument in ethics, medicine, and law /
Raphael Cohen-Almagor.
      p. cm.
  Includes bibliographical references and index.
  ISBN 0-8135-2986-7 (alk. paper)
  1. Right to die—Moral and ethical aspects—Cross-cultural studies. 2.
Death—Moral and ethical aspects—Cross-cultural studies. 3. Euthanasia—
Moral and ethical aspects—Cross-cultural studies. 4. Right to die—Law and
legislation—Cross-cultural studies. 5. Death—Law and legislation—Cross-
cultural studies. 6. Euthanasia—Law and legislation—Cross-cultural studies.
I. Title

R726.C635 2001
179.7—dc21

                                                          2001019295

British Cataloging-in-Publication data for this book is available from the
British Library

Manufactured in the United States of America

For Dana and Gilad,
whom I love dearly

Contents

Preface

In 1991 I participated in a seminar, "Abortion, Dementia, and Euthanasia," conducted by Ronald Dworkin at Oxford University. Until that time I had not given much thought to these issues, and my research concerns were in very different areas. My doctoral dissertation at Oxford was on the boundaries of liberty and tolerance. Other research interests included political theory, the study of ideologies (National Socialism, Marxism, and Liberalism), and Israeli politics.

Dworkin was in the process of writing *Life's Dominion*, and the students in his class were his guinea pigs. He tried his ideas out on us and listened to our criticisms and objections. It was the most fascinating seminar I have ever attended. My research agenda took an unexpected turn, one that has influenced my life and career. After returning to Israel I embarked on serious research in the field of medical ethics, began to teach seminars on bioethics at the Hebrew University Law School, established a medical ethics think tank at the Van Leer Jerusalem Institute, and joined many national and international professional groups and organizations. This book is the result of nine years of extensive thinking and research. I am still eager to learn and to expand my horizons.

I would like to express gratitude to Ronny Dworkin for introducing me to the field of medical ethics. I am indebted to him for his intellectual inspiration and wisdom. I am also grateful to people who conversed with me about pertinent questions, and/or who read all or part of my writings: Geoffrey Marshall, Isaiah Berlin, David Heyd, Wilfrid

Knapp, Dan Callahan, Bernard Dickens, Avraham Steinberg, Wayne Sumner, John Lantos, Jack Pole, Shimon Glick, Joyce Appleby, Charles Sprung, Carmel Shalev, Robert Streiffer, Moti Halperin, Jan Joerden, Sam Lehman-Wilzig, Fred Lowy, Shlomit Perry, Herb Morris, Ruth Landau, Vardit Ravitzki, Les Rothenberg, Tom Beauchamp, Avner de-Shalit, Gershon Grunfeld, Eike-Henner Kluge, Daniel Sinclair, Peter Singer, and Ashby Sharpe. I have also benefited from communications and discussions with Edmund Pellegrino, Bruce Jennings, Avi Ohry, Antonella Surbone, Amos Shapira, Gershon Growe, Ruth Halperin-Kaddari, John Robertson, Bob Truog, Asa Kasher, Zev Susak, Nachman Wilensky, Leon Sazbon, Ejan Mackaay, John Harris, Keith Andrews, Evert van Leeuwen, Tony Hope, Rebecca Cook, Larry Librach, Martin Tweeddale, Benji Freedman, R. N. MacDonald, Alex Capron, Rosalie Ber, Albert Kirshen, Baruch Modan, Moshe Zemer, Govert den Hartogh, Joe Boyle, Peter A. Singer, Ted Keyserlingk, Saul Smilansky, Vince Cain, Uriel Kitron, Eugene Bereza, James G. Young, and David Kuhl. Their knowledge, experience, and insight were truly enriching and illuminating. I acknowledge with gratitude the invaluable assistance of Randy Wilcox, Martine Bauman, Raymond Plant, Len Doyal, Peggy Battin, Florencia Luna, Margaret Somerville, Diane LeCover, C. van der Meer, Vicki Michel, Dick Pranger, Jocelyn Downie, Henry Perkins, Neil Wenger, and the dedicated librarians at the University of Haifa and at the UCLA School of Law. I also thank my students at the Hebrew University Faculty of Law, the University of Haifa Faculty of Law, and the UCLA School of Law for many inspiring comments and constructive criticisms. It is no coincidence that the preliminary drafts of two of the chapters were written with two excellent students of mine, Merav Shmueli and Monica Hartman.

The completion of this work necessitated research trips to the United States, Australia, Canada, England, and the Netherlands. I am most grateful to the Hebrew University Law Faculty, the University of Haifa Research Authority, the Hastings Center in New York, the British Council, the Fulbright Foundation, the Israel Association for Canadian Studies, and the Canadian government for providing me with grants to carry out the fieldwork.

Early and shorter versions of chapters 1 and 2 were published in *The Journal of Law, Medicine and Ethics* 28 (3) (fall 2000): 267–278, and in *Medicine and Law* 16 (3) (1997): 451–471, respectively. An early and much shorter version of chapter 3 was published in *Theoretical Medicine and Bioethics* 21 (2) (August 2000): 117–137. An early version of chapters 4 and 5, written prior to my research trip to the Netherlands, when I was still supporting active euthanasia, was published in *Israel Law Review* 29 (4) (1995): 677–701. An early version of chapter 6 was published in *Annual Review of Law and Ethics* 4 (1996): 213–232. Versions of chapters 7 and 8 were published in *Issues in Law and Medicine* 17, 1 (2001): 35–68 and *The Journal of Legislation* (2001) respectively. An early version of the conclusions was published in R. Cohen-Almagor (ed.), *Medical Ethics at the Dawn of the 21st Century* (New York: New York Academy of Sciences, 2000), vol. 913 of the *Annals*: 127–149. A Hebrew version of the appendix was published in R. Cohen-Almagor (ed.), *Basic Issues in Israeli Democracy* (Tel Aviv: Sifriat Poalim, 1999), 165–186; a shorter version is forthcoming in *Issues in Law and Medicine* 17, 3 (spring 2002).

The Right to Die
with Dignity

Introduction

In any discussion of death with dignity, the focus of attention is on the right of the patient over his or her body. The main question is whether life should be preserved at any cost. There are two principled opinions: One emphasizes the sanctity of life and sees its maintenance as a substantive intrinsic value. Christian theologians and Jewish halachic thinkers are among those who associate themselves with this opinion. The other emphasizes the autonomy of the patient and his or her right to formulate a decision whether to continue living. This view is espoused by the prevalent liberal thinking. When they use the term *death with dignity*, liberals refer to both the timing of death (people should be allowed, whenever possible, to choose the time of their departure); and the way people die (with the help of medical professionals, people should be able to control the process of dying, maintaining their autonomy and dignity, and maintaining their self-respect).

The notion of autonomy involves people's ability to reflect upon their own beliefs and actions, and the ability to form ideas about them, so as to decide how to lead their lives. The term *autonomy* is derived from the Greek *autos* (self) and *nomos* (rule, governance, or law). By deciding among conflicting trends, we consolidate our opinions more fully and rank our own values. Obviously, in order to be able to exercise autonomy, we need a range of options to choose from; some may be of personal significance, and others may not. Having options enables us to sustain activities that we regard as worth pursuing, and to decide what is worthwhile and what is not; often we must examine diverse alternatives. As Joseph Raz asserts, a person who has never had any significant choice, or was not aware of it, or has never exercised choice in significant matters but simply drifted through life, is not an autonomous person.[1] Choosing the best option or thinking correctly is not a requirement for autonomy so long as we assess the alternatives carefully. The emphasis is not on deciding on the best options or on holding true opinions, but rather on the way in which we come to hold our convictions and make our decisions.

Those who support the sanctity-of-life approach hold that we are not authorized to decide whether or not to forgo living. Conservative thinkers, mainly religious individuals, are among the supporters of this claim. They are joined by secular thinkers who see intrinsic value in biological life, and fear the slippery-slope syndrome that may lead to the termination of life even when patients wish to continue living. Those who support the autonomy-based approach do not conceive of life itself as intrinsically valuable. Life allows us to attain certain goals. When people reach the conclusion that life no longer has meaning for them, they should have the right to opt for death.

Both viewpoints are motivated by the desire to maintain and protect human dignity. While the advocates of the sanctity-of-life model hold that preferring death to life in certain cases harms human dignity, the advocates of the autonomy model say that the consideration of human dignity might lead us to think at times that life is no longer an attractive option. A theme that is frequently reiterated in this discussion is quality of life. The lack of some standard of quality legitimizes, even necessitates, so it is claimed, allowing patients the option of forgoing life if they so wish. Life in itself is not as important as what we do with it. Life in earnest is important, not just the mechanical processes that define life in the superficial meaning of the term. That our hearts are beating and that we can breathe are not sufficient reasons to maintain life.

This is not to say that quality of life constitutes a single criterion by which we judge a person's deeds. Criminal law does not address the quality of life. Different penalties do not exist for murderers on the basis of the victims' quality of life before the murder. We would be appalled if a murderer argued in his or her defense that the victim was a useless creature, led a dull life, and was miserable; therefore, no great loss had occurred. Similarly, we would be deeply disturbed if a physician claimed that there was little point in investing resources in a particular patient because he was seventy-five years old, and his prospects of leading a valuable life were slim.

This book is written from a liberal perspective. Preference is given to the autonomy of the patient, seeing the sanctity-of-life model as justified in moral terms provided it does not resort to paternalism. The sanctity-of-life model cannot be justified when it is imposed on patients who do not conceive of their current life situation as inherently valuable, and hence are willing to entertain the thought of ending their lives. The view that holds that we should always preserve life no matter what patients want, and that patients who opt to die are not able to comprehend their own interests in a fully rational manner, and that therefore we know what is good for these patients better than they do, is morally unjustifiable. This view is morally unjustifiable because it ignores the desires of the patients and does not acknowledge that the preservation of dignity may be valued more than the preservation of life by some patients. We must strive to reconcile the duty of keeping people alive with their right to keep their dignity intact, which may also be considered as an intrinsic value.

The opposition to the sanctity-of-life model asserts that the stance based on a belief in the intrinsic value of life raises a moral dilemma: A person suffers a great pain and wants to die. Those who believe that life is intrinsically valuable object to taking action on the person's desire. But their objection ignores the autonomy of the agent concerned. Can life be intrinsically valuable independent of the interests of the individual? Do these persons (or the state) have the right to impose their will over the will of the individual? Alternatively, it may be argued that people have a right to die because their dignity has an intrinsic value.

The objection to the sanctity-of-life model is accompanied by support for the respect-for-others argument. This argument is derived from the Kantian deontological school that accords all people equal respect. Respect for a person calls for conceiving of the other as an end rather than as a means to something. As Immanuel Kant explained, persons are ends in themselves, entities that are not to be used merely as means, so a limit is imposed on all arbitrary use of such beings, who are thus objects of respect. Persons are, therefore, not merely subjective ends, whose existence as an effect of our actions has a value for us, but such beings are objective ends; that is, they exist as ends in themselves. Such an end, Kant maintained, "is one for which there can be substituted no other end to which such beings should serve merely as means, for otherwise nothing at all of absolute value would be found anywhere."[2]

According to Kant, to respect a person is to treat him or her as a human being, as an autonomous being who is acting upon recognition of the moral law. The assumption is that beings are moral, and Kant's demand is that people act in accordance with the categorical imperative.

In formulating his concept of the categorical imperative, Kant recognizes that each person has an inviolable dignity, which is the reason for respecting persons. The categorical imperative refers to the will itself, not to anything that may be achieved by the causality of the will. Morality, according to Kant, cannot be regarded as a set of rules that prescribe the means necessary for the achievement of a given end, whether the end be general happiness, human perfection, self-realization, or anything else. Moral rules must be obeyed without consideration of the consequences that will follow from doing or refraining from doing something. Moral rules guide our actions and are observed as a precondition for compatibility with actions of other people.[3]

Kant does not speak of the process of decision-making. In contrast, I wish to emphasize the process involved in reaching a decision. In this process we exercise our faculties, using concepts, categories, principles, norms, and to some degree (whether we like it or even if we cannot help it) our emotions. We construct and deconstruct realities, converse and exchange ideas, listen to the advice of others, and share our opinions with people we appreciate. At least on matters of importance, we strive to reach what we perceive as the right decision. As long as people accept the two basic principles that underlie a liberal society—respecting others and not harming others—we accord others respect when we respect their right to make decisions, because they are their own decisions, regardless of our opinions. We simply assume that each person holds his or her own course of life as intrinsically valuable, at least for himself or herself, and in most cases we respect the individual's reasoning.[4] We should give equal consideration to the interests of others and should grant equal respect to the others' life projects so long as these do not deliberately undermine the interests of others by interfering in a disrespectful manner. As John Rawls asserts, "the public culture of a democratic society" is committed to seeking forms of social cooperation that can be pursued on a basis of mutual respect between free and equal persons.[5]

Kant's reasoning should be supplemented by an emphasis on the notion of concern. We not only respect people but also care for them. Kant bases his reasoning on logic, attempting to exclude emotional concerns, but we need to acknowledge that acts are often dictated by emotions. Human nature enables us to rationalize, but often we are controlled by emotional drives. Thus it is not sufficient to speak only of respect. Ronald Dworkin regards political morality as resting entirely on the single fundamental "background right" to human dignity, and to equal respect and concern. By background rights, Dworkin means rights that provide a justification for political decisions by society in the abstract, without connecting them to any specific political institution. Dworkin's claim implies that some rights are better viewed as universal, as applicable to every political framework, because they are essentially derived from the conception of people as human beings.[6] Although this right may be morally applicable to any society, Dworkin would agree that it is not necessarily morally convincing. That is, it may not necessarily be one that every society would wish to adopt. Indeed, the respect-for-others argument can be said to underlie a liberal democratic society specifically, and not just any society.

The notion of concern implies the value of well-being: We ought to show equal concern for each individual's good, to acknowledge that human beings are not only rational creators but also emotional creatures. Treating people with concern means treating them with empathy, viewing people as human beings who may be furious and frustrated, who are capable of smiling and crying, of careful decision making and impulsive reactions. Concern does not demand that we give equal weight, in a utilitarian fashion, to the welfare of a stranger and to the welfare of our children.[7] Instead, it means giving equal weight to a person's life and autonomy.

Scholars who endorse the idea of life as intrinsically valuable adhere to the reasoning that favors dignity but apply different contents. Their view is that keeping people's dignity requires keeping them alive. Nothing is done by the medical staff to keep a patient alive that may impair the person's dignity. Some situations present grave difficulties, but in this model physicians and nurses give their foremost concern to keeping the dignity of gravely ill people. They take care of them; they clean them; they treat the bodies of people who do not communicate with their caregivers as the bodies of human beings. It may be true that such gravely ill patients would not like to see themselves in these situations, in which they are not able to control their natural needs, but once they find themselves in such circumstances they want to continue living. Physicians acknowledge that the introduction of tubes causes discomfort and may be painful to conscious patients. Any interference with the wholeness of the human body may be conceived as infringement of dignity. But as long as patients are not conceived of as a means to something, and the prevailing view regards patients as objective ends, the attitude toward patients can be said to respect their dignity. This view conceives the patient's existence as an end in itself. Keeping the dignity of patients requires that no other object can be substituted for such an end.

The debate revolves around the importance assigned to a person's independent decision-making. Those who endorse the respect-for-others argument as opposed to the sanctity-of-life model understand this argument in more specific terms that relate primarily to the autonomy of gravely ill patients. The defense of personal liberties is founded on the assertion that we ought to respect others as autonomous human beings who exercise self-determination in order to live according to their own life plans; we respect persons as beings who have a capacity to progress and are able to develop their inherent faculties as they choose. In turn we respect them in order to help them realize what they want to be. Each individual is conceived as a source of claims against others—that is, respect for human beings involves the presupposition that others should be allowed to make their own decisions, based on their conception of what is good and just. Treating patients with respect means treating them as human beings who are capable of forming and acting on intelligent conceptions of how their lives should be lived. Respecting a person involves giving credit to the other's ability for self-direction, acknowledging the other's competence to exercise discretion in deciding between available options. Accordingly, each person is viewed as speaking from an individual point of view, having perceived individual interests. We may be asked to give our opinions, or decide to express our views anyway; nevertheless, in many instances we recognize the other's right to make choices. This notion of autonomy is crucial in our considerations. The medical profession is required to respect the wishes of certain incurably ill patients.

The opening chapter deals with some of the concepts and terms frequently mentioned in the debate on mercy killings and death with dignity. In the field of medical ethics, some of the concepts and terms convey a clear meaning. An ethicist could easily discern the viewpoint of a colleague by looking at the language the colleague uses. Thus, for instance, someone who declares an association with the pro-life movement is clearly, generally speaking, against the practice of abortion. Conversely, someone who declares an association with the pro-choice movement is clearly, generally speaking, in favor of a woman's right to choose the fate of her pregnancy.

Similarly, with the end-of-life debate, many phrases have a clearly partisan meaning. *Life as intrinsic value*; *sanctity of life*; *doctors as hangmen*; *doctors playing God*: People who speak in this language would surely be opposed to active euthanasia. Other terms that are often used are *brain death*; *persistent vegetative state patients* (or simply *vegetables*); and *terminal patients*. These terms developed over time into medical concepts. People who use them would most probably argue that there is no sense in maintaining life-sustaining treatment for such patients, that this treatment is futile. I argue that this terminology carries negative implications for patient care.

Some of the concepts and terms used are imprecise, and careful reading is needed to ascertain the intentions of a particular writer. These concepts and terms might be used by advocates of opposite points of view, each justifying his or her position by resorting to the same language. For instance, someone who speaks of double effect, or of death with dignity, might be an advocate of active euthanasia, mercy killings, and physician-assisted suicide, or this person might side with those who argue against this practice. Some of the concepts and terms might be transient; that is, they once had a dubious meaning, increasingly became loaded terms, and today are associated with one or the other of the established schools of thought. This is the case with the term *quality of life*. The concept was first used by ethicists holding various viewpoints on the spectrum of ideas, but increasingly became associated with advocates of active euthanasia, and is contrasted with the notion of sanctity of life. Because of the extensive use of the phrase *death with dignity* by advocates of active euthanasia, this phrase may also become transient and may come to be more clearly associated with the movement for active euthanasia.

Much of this book is devoted to discussing patients in prolonged unawareness, a condition sometimes known as a persistent vegetative state (PVS). The rationale for focusing attention on patients in this unfortunate situation is the following: I am trying to prescribe guidelines and formulas for dealing with large classes of patients. I believe that patients in prolonged unawareness constitute one of the most tragic and morally challenging types of patients.[8] Because patients in prolonged unawareness suffer the most severe form of brain damage that may be associated with long-term survival and often require artificial forms of feeding as well as very costly medical care, this group raises major policy questions for long-term care.

Raanan Gillon argues that PVS patients constitute the most definitive account of empty life, and says that their situation resembles an untuned radio: It is on, but you do not get any program.[9] If it were possible to say something meaningful with regard to these patients, the guidelines and principles prescribed would inevitably be suitable for other patients whose situations are not so grave. In other words, the conditions for maintaining patients in prolonged unawareness are prima facie applicable for all other patients. Of course, each case should be considered individually in accordance with the guidelines, but because patients in PVS (as will be explained in chapter 1, for ethical reasons I prefer the term PCU, *post-coma unawareness*) are in a most tragic situation, it is plausible to argue that what is true for them in the positive way of maintaining life would be true for other patients, both incompetent and competent. Later I make a circumscribed plea for physician-assisted suicide when competent patients are concerned.

Fueling this argument is modern technology, which enables comatose individuals to remain alive in circumstances that at least some of them previously dreaded. Due to the rapid treatment of persons with brain injuries, well-equipped medical centers, early diagnosis by scanning techniques, advanced surgical methods, and highly developed intensive care units (including intensive care ambulances) and postoperative care, modern technology has increased the number of survivors following the acute phase of trauma, strokes, and heart failure. Many of these survivors remain in a state of prolonged unawareness. These patients or their families, as well as medical experts, are often expected to decide whether technology should be utilized to keep gravely ill people alive, or whether death should be allowed or even encouraged. Physicians confront a delicate situation in which their duty to act for the welfare of patients might contradict their own duty to respect patients' liberty. Society is required to formulate guidelines for deciding when to allow seriously afflicted people to die, if they so desire, or whether it would be in their best interest. Courts and ethics committees are asked to lay down criteria to assist physicians in making such judgments, as well as to determine what role families should play in deliberating the future of unconscious patients. Consideration is given to whether or not patients gave prior consent for cessation of treatment when they reach a designated stage of illness, and whether they now understand the explanations of medical matters given to them by physicians.

PCU patients may remain in this situation for long periods of time. These patients have periods of wakefulness and physiological sleep/wake cycles, but at no time are they aware of themselves or their environment. Neurologically, being awake but unaware is the result of a functioning brain stem and the total loss of cerebral cortical functioning. No voluntary action or behavior of any kind is present. These patients might be able, for example, to breathe without the help of a machine, but they are unconscious and obviously uncommunicative.

Injuries inflicted on the brain cerebrum are not the same as injuries inflicted on the brain stem. Legal medicine declares a person whose function of the brain stem and the cerebrum are both absent a dead person. This is not the case when the brain cerebrum is damaged. The brain stem controls basic reflexes, including breathing, heart activity, the sleep/wake cycle, reflexive activity in the upper and lower extremities, some swallowing motions, and eye movements.[10] The brain cerebrum controls sensations, voluntary movements, and conscious activities. Unlike patients whose brain stem is injured, PCU patients may show some progress, and the possibility of awakening is present.

All the chapters in this book relate in one way or another to PCU patients. Chapter 2 deals more extensively with various forms of unconsciousness and suggests some guiding principles. The innovations of this discussion of PCU patients are twofold: First, it contests the term *persistent vegetative state*, arguing that it is unethical—no one would like to be described as a vegetable—offering instead the term *post-coma unawareness* (PCU). Second, unlike many scholars and ethicists (if it is appropriate to call them ethicists) who dismiss the lives of PCU patients too easily, I urge hospitals as a policy not to cease treatment of posttraumatic PCU patients younger than fifty years old within a period of less than two years. The two-year waiting period should be regarded as the minimum period of evaluation before hopes for patients' rehabilitation and return to some form of cognition are abandoned. This study provides data and human stories from the Israeli experience as well as from England, Canada, the United States, and other countries to substantiate this argument.

Chapter 3 provides a detailed examination of the two contrasting models of thinking. It considers the sanctity-of-life approach (the extreme version of the model of life as intrinsically valuable) and the quality-of-life approach (the extreme version of the autonomy model) and examines their flaws. It is argued that in recent years, there has been an increase in the number of requests for termination of life by patients and their relatives. Under certain conditions, the patient may prefer death to a life devoid of quality. The discussion involves two main issues: One is preliminary and deals with the ability to evaluate life; the second focuses on criteria used to distinguish between life thought to have quality and life that is considered to be devoid of quality.

The pertinent religious and secular views are presented, as is the argument in favor of a balance between the sanctity of life and the quality of life. Indeed, such a balance exists in practice. Doctors and laypersons think carefully about quality-of-life considerations and differentiate between lives with and without quality. In this context, the most basic components of a life of quality are examined: consciousness, lack of pain and suffering, and human dignity. The question is whether the absence of any of these components justifies physician-assisted suicide. The chapter also considers the implications of assuming that some lives are not worth living, raising a warning against "sliding down the slippery slope," and describes the difficulties involved in attempting to set criteria for evaluating life.

The fourth chapter delineates the common distinction between active and passive euthanasia, and discusses some of the legal measures that have been invoked in the United States, the United Kingdom, the Netherlands, Canada, Switzerland, and Australia. In turn, through an analysis of some of the themes discussed by Ronald Dworkin in *Life's Dominion,* chapter 5 ponders patient interests. In certain instances, patients' autonomy would be retained and their dignity better served if they were helped to die. The right to life is here conceived as a discretionary rather than a mandatory right.[11] In this connection, a caveat is made regarding advance directives and living wills. A patient may have stated that if her physical and mental condition deteriorated beyond recognition, she would prefer to die. Upon reaching an advanced stage of atrophy, however, she shows signs of happiness when she sees her relatives, or expresses some interest in, say, flowers, food, or her friends; it may therefore be concluded that the patient finds some value in her present unfortunate condition. Therefore, we must ignore prior instructions to the contrary and allow the continuation of her life.[12] People have the right to change their minds, and we should not deny them that right. It is always better to err on the side of life. If it is not possible to determine the patient's past and present desires, and there are no signs that the patient wishes to continue living, then the decision should be made by the medical team in cooperation and consultation with those who are close to the patient: blood relatives, friends, and other loved ones.

Chapter 6 offers a new concept to substitute for the traditional concept of the family. Blood relatives are not necessarily the most important people for the patient. Rather we should focus on the patient's loved ones, those who support the patient during the most difficult times. This consideration is especially noteworthy in regard to AIDS patients, but it is true for other patients as well. A further distinction is made between an implicit and an explicit desire to die, between formal and speculative autonomy. Formal autonomy is evident when the patient actually has made a decision. Speculative autonomy is what the patient would have decided if he or she had the chance to make a decision. Three American court decisions are then examined: *Saikewicz, Spring,* and *Gray.* The first case, *Saikewicz,* concerns a patient who had no family or other loved ones. This fact had a significant bearing on the court's ruling not to provide him with treatment. The second case, *Spring,* involves a patient whose family wanted to withhold treatment from him. We should be cautious in cases like this one, when the best interests of the patient's loved ones seem to come at the expense of the best interests of the patient. The third case, *Gray,* serves as an example of a situation in which the best interests of the patient coincide with the best interests of her loved ones. Attention should be given to the question of whether the patient's loved ones demonstrate a unanimous position in regard to the destiny of the patient.

Any discussion about death with dignity would be incomplete without an examination of the Dutch experience, which, to a large extent, influences the debate on euthanasia and physician-assisted suicide around the globe, especially with regard to whether euthanasia should be legitimized or legalized. Chapter 7 provides a critical analysis of the developments in the Netherlands and analyzes the pros and cons of the Dutch situation. My research involved twenty-eight interviews conducted in the Netherlands during the summer of 1999 with some of the leading figures who are involved in the decision-making process and take an active part in the ongoing debate. Among the interviewees is Henk Leenen, the father of the legal debate on euthanasia, who took an active part in drafting the relevant laws, and the authors of the 1990 and 1995 comprehensive research reports: Paul van der Maas and Gerrit van der Wal. The Dutch guidelines are insufficient, because they do not provide adequate control over the practice of euthanasia; also, the entire policy should be revised and made more coherent and more comprehensive.

As a result of my independent research, I now advocate voluntary physician-assisted suicide but not active euthanasia. The Dutch do not pay much notice to the distinction between the two, although the distinction is valid. Physician-assisted suicide gives patients control until the very last moment of their lives, prevents possible abuse, and assures that they sincerely and independently opt for death. In most cases, patients are able to perform the final act that terminates their lives. In the rare instances of complete paralysis or severe breathing difficulties, when the patient is absolutely unable to activate the lethal needle, only then may the doctor perform the final merciful act.

Chapter 8 examines a more positive experience of dealing with death with dignity. In 1994, the state of Oregon enacted its Death with Dignity Act, resulting in the unprecedented legalization of physician-assisted suicide in one state of the United States. Under the act (Measure No. 16), adult Oregon residents can obtain lethal medications if they have been diagnosed with a terminal disease found likely by two physicians to cause death within six months. The patient's choice must be informed and voluntary.[13]

The chapter analyzes recent developments in Oregon. It discusses the history of the act from its passage in 1994 to 2001, evaluates the strengths and weaknesses of the act, and analyzes the Oregon Health Division's report on the consequences of the act during 1998–2000, the first three years that it was in effect. Several improvements to the act are proposed, including modification of the act to include self-administered lethal injections in situations in which oral medications cannot be taken, the distribution of anonymous questionnaires to patients and their families, additional reporting by pharmacists, the establishment of a small committee of experts to review application of physician-assisted suicide, and mandatory psychological consultations for patients considering physician-assisted suicide. Despite its weaknesses, the Oregon act is a significant step toward establishing the important right of a patient to autonomy and to choice in deciding end-of-life issues. Removing its flaws will help ensure that the act achieves its commendable purpose, to ensure that capable, adult, terminally ill Oregon residents have the right to end their lives in a humane and dignified manner. Adoption of these suggestions will serve three primary purposes. First, it will help ensure that patients are not motivated by depression to choose physician-assisted suicide (PAS). For this purpose, physicians should be assisted by psychiatrists, who serve as advisors. Second, it will enable researchers to distinguish between the perceptions of patients and physicians, which will provide the requisite information for a more informed public debate on the controversial issue of PAS and will create a more knowledgeable, empathetic culture surrounding the terminally ill and their families. Finally, it will help ensure that patients for whom oral medication is ineffective will also have the ability to choose PAS.

The conclusions draw on various ethical, medical, and legal considerations as well as on what has transpired in the Netherlands and Oregon. In some cases not only passive euthanasia but also physician-assisted suicide may be allowed. People should have the ability to control the time and place of their death. In this spirit, six prominent philosophers have referred to an individual death as "the final act of life's drama."[14]

The thesis is that people, as autonomous moral agents, deserve to be treated with dignity, which requires respecting their choices and life decisions. If a person decides that life is no longer worth living, we should respect that decision. If the person needs help, the medical profession should be there to help. At the same time, a voice of caution is raised against mercy killing, criticizing Dr. Jack Kevorkian. If physicians were allowed to assist gravely ill patients to die, pressure might be exerted on old and weak patients without close family relationships.[15] The delicate framework of trust between patients and physicians might crack and practically be replaced by a completely different set of norms. Patients would no longer believe that physicians and nurses would do their best to help them stay alive. Explicitly or implicitly, physicians and nurses might communicate that they expected special gratitude for assisting patients to live. Patients might feel obliged to seek assistance to die to avoid imposing further burdens on their families as well as on medical staff. The right to die might be interpreted as an obligation to die. There is also the fear that the right to die, accorded to patients who are able to decide, might at some point be expanded to justify ending the lives of patients who are not able to decide for themselves. Moreover, we can assume that the incentive for seeking better ways to heal those patients would be reduced.

Therefore, each case should be judged on its own merits, and we should refrain from drawing sweeping conclusions that relate to categories of patients. We may try to prescribe detailed guidelines of conduct (as I do in chapter 2 with regard to incompetent patients in PCU, and in the conclusions with regard to competent patients). Finally, the guidelines should be judged and evaluated in relation to each patient under consideration. The fear of sliding down the slippery-slope from merciful behavior to a disregard for human dignity is, indeed, tangible. Using real-life situations as illustrations, the chapter grapples with the arguments against mercy killings and physician-assisted suicide, prescribing some cautionary measures and safety valves.

One of the examples discussed is the *Eyal* case, which was decided in Israel in 1990.[16] Eyal was a competent amyotrophic lateral sclerosis (ALS) patient who expressed his wish not to be connected to a ventilator. In instances such as the *Eyal* case, patients' autonomy should be preserved, and their dignity is better served by helping them to die. It is not always true that to keep people alive is to treat them as ends, serving their best interests. In some situations, like this one, we show respect for people and their dignity when we help them to cease living. Some patients feel it is humiliating to have to depend on others to perform fundamental human functions, such as eating, taking care of personal hygiene, and natural needs. Some may want to die because they feel exhausted in every meaning of the term. They have satisfied their desires in life; their suffering causes them to lose their zeal for living; and they feel that they constitute a burden on their loved ones and on society in general. They lack self-esteem and are no longer able to view themselves in any satisfactory way. My justification for helping such patients fulfill their requests rests on the assumption that they freely and genuinely express their will to die and that they persist in expressing that desire. The situation, of course, is different in the case of patients in post-coma unawareness, malformed children, or the senile, who are unable to express their wishes. The chapter concludes by offering guidelines for physician-assisted suicide for competent patients who suffer from an incurable and irreversible disease, and who make free, voluntary, persistent, and enduring requests for assisted suicide. The formulation of the guidelines was inspired by the experiences of the Netherlands, Oregon, and the Australian Northern Territory.

The appendix attempts to strengthen the argument for the individual's basic right to health care. The discussion deviates some-what from the core issue of the right to die with dignity, but it is impossible to deal with death and dying without addressing the economics involved, which have at least some direct bearing on the fate of patients (in the United States, this qualification is unnecessary, as economics does have a direct bearing on patients' fate). Scarcity of health care resources might sway doctors to compromise the best interests of their patients. It is pertinent to discuss which policy (or policies) should be promoted and which policies should be rejected while we strive to maintain patients' dignity. Ethically, economic considerations should be excluded from the grounds for ending the patient's life. Attention is paid to three basic concepts: duty, ability, and rights. The following questions are addressed: Does the state have a duty to provide optimal medical care for every citizen? Can the state afford to do so? Do citizens have a right to demand such a commitment?

The cost of health care in the Western world, specifically the United States, Canada, the United Kingdom, and Israel, is examined. Then, recognizing that decisions are influenced by the reality of scarce resources, I examine various approaches to resource allocation, suggesting what I conceive of as a just approach for democracies. I criticize the various versions of the utilitarian approach, while accepting the insurance-based plan as the guiding rationale, supplemented with components of the contract approach. I focus attention on the writings of Daniel Callahan, a preeminent advocate of the age-rationing approach. I believe that Callahan's approach is too cold and detached and that age should not serve as the decisive criterion. My criticism of this criterion stems from two different lines of reasoning: the medical and the moral-contractual. I close by considering the Oregon Health Plan, arguing that it is important, through open public exchange, to raise the question of the extent to which citizens are willing to take part in financing expensive medicine. The state should devise several insurance alternatives appropriate to citizens' ability and willingness to pay for health care services.

The scope of this book is limited to liberal societies. Its rationale is grounded in the Kantian liberal tradition, placing concern for the individual at the center of the argument. All people must acknowledge the equal moral status of others and must treat each person as an end and never as a means to something. But we need to distinguish between the "ought" and the "is." Illiberal societies do not place emphasis on the individual and may apply rules and codes of behavior that are different from those underlying liberal democracies—that is, respect and concern for others, and not harming others. I believe that there are some basic universal needs that all people wish to secure, such as food, clothing, and shelter. But we cannot speak of universal values that underlie all societies in practice. Thus my concern is with liberal democracies that perceive human beings as ends and that respect autonomy and variety. The arguments are relevant to other countries, but because nondemocratic countries do not accept basic liberal principles, the discussion would fall on deaf ears.

1 Language and Reality at the End of Life

Humans are social beings. We communicate with one another, converse, exchange ideas and different points of view via language/s and signs. Language constructs, affects, and changes reality, facilitating communication, promoting understanding, helping to erect bridges between cultures.

Every profession has its concepts, phrases, and keywords that are important to help categorize phenomena, save time, and provide a framework for working together. Medicine is no exception. Here, too, we find some important concepts and terms that deserve probing and analysis. The question may be asked whether these concepts and terms are designed first and foremost to serve the professionals or the clients, the physicians or the patients. They primarily serve physicians, at times at the expense of patients' best interests. The implications resulting from physicians' language may be harmful to patients, and some of the terms they use are offensive and degrading. The concepts adopted from other spheres, as well as the concepts that were developed during the last decades, generate, for patients, an unhealthy atmosphere that may lead to undesirable actions at the end of the patients' lives.

In response to the changing reality, a reality that is very much influenced by advances in technology, during the second half of the twentieth century people in the medical profession adopted the concepts of dignity, quality of life, and double effect, and they developed a new set of terminology to handle the new challenges to the profession. Terms like *futility, terminal, vegetative state,* and *brain death* have become indispensable in the medical setting. Over time, these terms have developed into medical concepts. Because phenomenology is important—language does play a critical role in the shaping and reshaping of our existence—it is important to reflect on the language that we use to describe our experiences, especially that concerning life and death. Demeaning concepts and offensive terminology carry negative implications for patient care.

Death with Dignity

Death with dignity is one of the most complicated and fascinating subjects in medical ethics. The term *dignity* is derived from the Latin noun *dignitas,* which means: (a) worthiness, merit; (b) greatness, authority; and (c) value, excellence. The noun is cognate with the adjective *dignus* (worthy), from the Sanskrit root *dic* and the Greek root *deik,* which have the sense of bringing to light, showing, or pointing out.[1]

The concept of dignity refers to a worth or value that flows from an inner source. It is not bestowed from the outside but rather is intrinsic to the person. As Lawrence P. Ulrich notes, a painting may have value, but it does not have dignity. The value is placed upon it by members of the artistic community in light of the skill of the artist and the aesthetic priorities of the community. The value does not derive from the painting itself. Human beings, on the other hand, can be said to possess dignity as an inner source of their sense of worth. If this were not the case, they would simply be the bearers of instrumental value like all other objects in the world. Instead, human beings are set apart and treated in special ways.[2]

Unlike Leon R. Kass, I do not conceive of dignity as an "aristocratic term of distinction."[3] On the contrary: We all have a right to dignity. Dignity is something that must be accorded to every person from birth—some say, from the moment of conception. We are endowed with dignity and have the right to be treated with dignity. Furthermore, the term *dignity* involves not only objective but also subjective notions. It is the source from which human rights are derived, and it also refers to our own feelings about ourselves.[4] To have dignity, means to look at oneself with self-respect, with some sort of satisfaction. We feel human, not degraded. The term *subjective concept of the self* refers to how we conceive of our life, our achievements, and our place in the world. The subjective evaluation is affected by our individual self-respect, relative to the abilities we believe we possess, and relative to our peers and surroundings.

More specifically, with reference to the role of physicians, preserving dignity means helping patients to feel valuable. The physical move from the familiarity of the home to an unfamiliar hospital entails the transformation from a person to a patient. Sometimes the patient is seen by physicians as a mere case, stripped of personality, representing an interesting disease to be studied, a valuable tool for advancing their research.[5] Hospitals and the medical staff are supposed to care for the patients, but sometimes, especially in research hospitals, it seems that the reverse is the case: The assumption is that patients are in hospitals for the benefit of the medical staff. The shift from a person to a patient to a mere case betrays human dignity. The preservation of dignity involves, among other things, listening to patients' complaints; helping them cure their diseases, or at least assisting them in controlling pain; responding to their distress and anxieties, making an effort to relieve them; demonstrating sensitivity to the physical indignities that occur in severe illnesses; and maintaining patients' sense that they are adult human beings and not infants, case studies, or worse, bodies that occupy beds and consume resources. Patients can feel vulnerable because their self-respect is undermined by their deteriorating condition. In order to maintain patients' dignity, physicians as well as patients' families must help patients retain at least some of their self-respect. The aim is to secure dignified living in severe health conditions.

There may come a point when the belief in the importance of human dignity may lead to the conclusion that physician-assisted suicide should be considered an option. Most people find some meaning in their lives even when they are severely impaired, bedridden, limited in movement, and in constant need of help. In the past eight years I have conducted research in some three dozen hospitals and research centers in Israel, the United States, Canada, England, and the Netherlands. I have spoken with doctors who work in intensive care units, chronic care departments, and wards for patients defined as "terminal." According to the doctors' testimonials, most of their patients (90 to 99 percent) hang on to life (for specific data, see chapter 5). A very small number of people actually consider the option of shortening their lives. An independent, active, and energetic person with desires and ambitions, who becomes in her own eyes dependent upon others, who reaches the conclusion that her life has become a burden to herself and the people she loves, might lose her sense of humanity as well as her self-respect, and this might lead her to lose interest in life and to choose death.

Quality of Life

Many supporters of physician-assisted suicide and euthanasia advance the quality-of-life argument. The phrase *quality of life* has many positive connotations when it is used in a general social context. For instance, we speak of improving the quality of citizens' lives by various means, including diverting public transportation away from crowded neighborhoods, and making efforts to decrease air pollution. Citizens seek to promote their quality of life by purchasing newer and bigger houses, cultivating their gardens, going abroad, and engaging in leisure activities. People use the phrase to describe the ways they promote their comfort, maintain or raise their social status, and achieve tranquillity. Likewise, in medicine, the phrase has positive connotations—for example, in rehabilitation, cosmetic treatments, psychiatry, and psychology. When they deal with end-of-life issues, however, ethicists who support euthanasia apply quality-of-life considerations in a negative sense more often than in a positive one; they do not seek to improve the patient's life but to end it.[6] They refer to certain patients and categories of patients, arguing that their lives lack a significant measure of quality and therefore should not be maintained (see chapter 3). It is not surprising that the supporters of the sanctity-of-life concept distrust the motivations of those who speak of quality of life, regarding quality and life in this context as contradictory and competing concepts. This attitude often serves to justify the termination of life. Furthermore, even supporters of euthanasia and of granting patients the right to decide their own destiny, whether to continue or to terminate life, express suspicion regarding this concept, which during the last thirty years has developed into a concept in medical ethics.

My discussion of this concept is normative. The matter is subjective, in that our quality of life is determined by personal life circumstances and by the way we view them. There is a place to consider the quality of a particular life, but the decision as to whether this consideration constitutes a justification for termination of that life should be left to the patient (see chapter 3). It is important to distinguish between situations in which the justification for terminating life is voiced by the patients themselves, and situations in which other parties—doctors, nurses, hospital managers, ethicists, relatives—postulate justifications for terminating patients' lives. Whenever possible, each individual should decide what constitutes a life of quality, and at what point it becomes empty of quality or value to the extent that death becomes an appealing alternative. No one else should conclude for a patient that her life is meaningless when she finds some value in it, just as no one else should demand that the patient prolong life at all costs when she asks to be helped to die. My objection to paternalism on this issue is absolute.[7] Unfortunately not all people agree with me.

Chapter 2 and the appendix examine the economic considerations that influence this discussion. Some ethicists and policy-makers are willing to sacrifice certain groups of patients whose lives are regarded as lacking substantive quality, and whose care is too costly.

The decision whether to preserve a life or to terminate it should remain in the hands of the patient who is able to express such an opinion. The liberal state should help preserve life, but should not insist on prolonging the lives of patients who feel that such an action would undermine their dignity. The issue is far more complex when patients are unable to express an intelligible and autonomous opinion because they are young, mentally challenged, or unconscious. Such patients are lacking autonomy and the ability to determine their own destiny (see chapter 4).

It is important to examine whether a patient has stated an opinion about extending life after autonomy is lost. If the patient had stated that she was not interested in prolonging life under such conditions, her view should be respected. In the event, however, that the patient stated previously that upon reaching a certain future state of illness she would prefer to die, but when she actually reaches such a state, she shows signs of preferring to continue living, we must respect her present choice (see chapter 5).

Patients in a Persistent Vegetative State

There are those who focus on the right to die with dignity and would like living wills and prior instructions to be an option offered to all patients, not only those diagnosed as "terminal," whose end is nearing, but also to patients in a persistent vegetative state. The use of *terminal* has undesirable consequences, and the connotations of the term PVS are demeaning.

The term PVS is used in reference to patients who are in a twilight zone between life and death. In referring to these patients, I prefer the terms *prolonged unawareness* and *post-coma unawareness*.[8] The logic for using these terms has both medical and ethical considerations. In medicine the term *prolonged unawareness* has replaced *prolonged coma*, because coma (acute sleeplike state of unarousability) is commonly defined today in terms of three elements: closed eyes, no utterance of meaningful sounds, and no adequate motor reaction to external stimuli. If any one of these elements is missing, *coma* should be rejected in favor of *unawareness*. PCU patients, unlike patients in a coma, have sleep/wake cycles.[9] To further clarify the distinction between coma and PCU, it should be noted that a serious injury to the brain stem causes deep, irreversible coma because the brain stem regulates awareness, whereas in cases of PCU the damage is in the cerebral hemisphere, and the possibility for awakening remains.

In these instances, scholars sometimes refer to the state of prolonged unawareness as vegetative. There is an ethical logic behind the adoption of the term PCU. PVS was coined by B. Jennett and F. Plum to describe a set of clinical features associated with profound brain damage.[10] They wanted to identify an irrecoverable and permanent state, and they called the syndrome persistent because they did not have the data to verify an irreversible state.[11] Upon introducing the term in 1972, they commented that it was the most neutral term, with no derogatory connotations. *To vegetate* is defined in the *Oxford English Dictionary* as "to live a merely physical life, devoid of intellectual activity or social intercourse," and *vegetative* is used to describe "an organic body capable of growth and development but devoid of sensation and thought." The term suggests even to the layperson a limited and primitive responsiveness to external stimuli, whereas for the doctor it further means that there is relative preservation of autonomic regulation of the internal milieu.[12]

Nevertheless, the term *vegetative* dehumanizes patients and therefore is offensive to their dignity and to that of their loved ones. It implies that these patients are like vegetables, that they are inferior, subhuman beings and perhaps unworthy of human treatment. From *vegetative*, it is very easy to slip into using the term *vegetables*, as many doctors and even leading authorities in the field do.[13] No one would like to be treated like a carrot or a potato, nor would anyone like the idea that a loved one is being treated as such. Because language is, to a great extent, a reality-building instrument, a warning should be raised against the use of discriminatory and demeaning terms that could cause medical personnel to disrespect patients. We should strive to describe the condition without offending patients or their loved ones. We should not immorally strip patients of their human characteristics and value.

Thus, while the term *persistent vegetative state* is a biased, even degrading one, the terms *prolonged unawareness* and PCU are more neutral. Obviously there are costs involved in changing a medical term, but the major task is to acknowledge that it was a poor choice in the first place, because it is unethical and offensive, and because of the dire consequences that might result from treating patients in such a fashion. After all, there is not much point in spending scarce and costly resources on mere vegetables. On the other hand, *prolonged unawareness* and PCU are terms without inherent biases that describe a certain state of living. The terminology to be used in this matter is crucial: If human life and the dignity of the patient are our first and foremost consideration, then we should select neutral terms that describe the situation without offending the people concerned (see chapter 2).

"Terminal" Patients

The word *terminal* is also problematic, and it probably does not serve the best interests of patients. When we diagnose patients as terminal, it may seem that we are counting their days and are possibly even discouraging them from fighting for their lives. The task of doctors is to help patients live when they want to continue living, not to hold a clock over their heads and count their days. Moreover, in some cases doctors make mistakes. All of us, doctors and laypersons, must acknowledge that our knowledge is limited and that we are vulnerable to error. From my extensive discussions with doctors, I learned of many cases of incorrect assessment. Patients who were told that they had three to six months to live continued living many months after the predicted period. The will to live, which is immeasurable, is difficult to comprehend by rational faculties and to assess in the light of available, often limited medical knowledge. People often surprise themselves by extending their abilities to endure suffering and pain. It is impossible to rationally comprehend our ability to extend our tolerance for suffering. This ability is heightened when people find themselves facing a life-and-death situation. Most prefer to fight until their very last breath. When patients are labeled "terminal," doctors send them several simultaneous negative messages: not only that death is near, but also that the medical staff are giving up, and that the patients' loved ones should begin the mourning period while the patients are still alive. The patients may fear that doctors might not do their best to fight for life. When patients' destiny is in the hands of doctors who seem to have given up, the patients may stop looking to their caregivers for assistance. Hope is an important component of life, and loss of hope diminishes the will to fight for life. This is not to say that doctors should lie. They must report the medical situation accurately to patients and to their loved ones, and not raise false hopes. But they should not smother the power of life by categorizing patients in terms that may weaken their will to live.

Furthermore, there is a difference between discussions among medical staff, and discussions that involve patients and their loved ones. A closed consultation between doctors, nurses, social workers, psychologists, and other caregivers in which *terminal* might be used (in the same manner that other medical terms, not known or clear to laymen, are used) is not the same as an open discussion with patients and their loved ones. Some think that it is important to change the terms within medical circles as well, because what we say affects how we think. Sensitivity to human life should be the guide for doctors in choosing their terminology. Patients who prove doctors' assessments wrong, showing that miracles do indeed happen, need incredible emotional fortitude to continue their struggle. They must gather all their inner strength, often with the help of their friends and relatives and preferably with the emotional support of those professionals in charge of maintaining their lives. Patients should not be labeled "terminal," because not even the most knowledgeable expert should play the role of a prophet.[14]

In *Lee v. Oregon* the court said that even for physicians who specialize in treating a terminal disease, no precise definition of *terminal* is medically or legally possible, because the time of death is known with certainty only in hindsight. As the Ninth Circuit noted (in *Compassion in Dying*, 49 F. 3d, 1995, 590), the terminally ill category is "inherently unstable."[15]

Instead of using the word *terminal*, it is preferable to speak of an incurable condition of the patient, when the doctors think on the basis of available medical literature that the patient is on the verge of death without hope of recovery. Long and detailed explanations are preferable to concise and brutal terms that might hinder the will to live.

Futility

The Latin word *futilis* referred to actions or instruments that were inherently leaky and therefore ill suited for achieving desired ends. The implication was that the use of leaky means would always be in vain, as the leak was an intrinsic defect that would make failure inevitable.[16] According to Lawrence J. Schneiderman and Nancy S. Jecker, the idea of medical futility implies that any effort to provide a benefit to a patient is highly likely to fail and that rare exceptions cannot be systematically produced.[17] Futile treatment can include a treatment that does not produce positive effects—for instance, using plaster to treat cancer, or chemotherapy for a patient with Parkinson's disease. Similarly, tube feeding or intravenous fluids could be futile treatments for patients who are no longer able to assimilate the nourishment or fluids. Furthermore, ineffective efforts to provide nutrition and hydration may directly cause suffering that offers no counterbalancing benefit for the patient. For a patient with severe congestive heart failure, intravenous feeding cannot be tolerated, because the fluid would be too much for the weakened heart. For a patient with a severe clotting deficiency and a nearly total body burn, gaining access to the central veins is likely to cause hemorrhage or infection, nasogastric tube placement may be quite painful, and there may be no skin to which to suture the stomach tube.[18]

It is also futile to provide a radical treatment whose side effects outweigh the good resulting from the treatment. If the side effects are too severe, the patient is better off without this treatment altogether.

Finally, it is futile to treat one disease when the patient is suffering from another life-threatening disease. It is futile to treat gangrene in the leg or to perform an amputation on a cancer patient if the patient is likely to die from the cancer in a few days.

Much of the debate about futility is taking place in the United States. The general context is the need to set limits on health care expenditures. Concerns about costs often underlie attitudes about futility in clinical settings and in public policy discussions. Some doctors argued in the past that loyalty to their patients required that every potentially beneficial treatment be offered, that it was impossible to put a price on life, that even when the chance of success was only one in a million, doctors would still be ethically obligated to provide it. These doctors have suddenly changed their minds and instead now argue that it is unethical to provide such treatments. When reimbursement incentives changed and doctors began to lose money instead of making money from providing certain treatments, these doctors suddenly discovered an ancient ethical obligation to refrain from providing those treatments.[19] Consequently the debate shifted away from definitions of futility to discussions of rationed care. Some researchers believed that it would be easier to achieve a consensus about rationing and that it expressed the essential problem—limited medical resources—more explicitly. However, while decisions about futility involve moral judgments about right or good care, decisions about rationing are about distributive justice: how to best use scarce and valuable resources.[20]

One study speaks of futility in the context of a medical condition in which the diagnosis of a fatal and incurable disease was ascertained, death was expected to occur within three months, and survival was not expected to be affected even by aggressive treatment.[21] The problem is that doctors quite often are not able to ascertain that these conditions are satisfied. Moreover, a treatment like cardiopulmonary resuscitation (CPR) is futile when it offers no benefit to the patient because maximal therapy has failed and no physiological improvement is possible. Under these circumstances, a unilateral decision by physicians to withhold therapy is argued to be in order. The question arises, then, whether we should consider a treatment futile if its likelihood of success is close to zero. Are treatments futile if they have a one percent chance of success, or two percent, or three percent?[22]

Schneiderman and his colleagues argue that a treatment should be considered futile when one hundred consecutive patients do not respond to it, or if the treatment fails to restore consciousness or alleviate total dependence on intensive care.[23] Robert D. Truog and his colleagues wonder how similar these hundred patients must be. They press the question of whether, in assessing the efficacy of mechanical ventilation to treat pneumonia, it is sufficient simply to recall the one hundred most recent patients who received artificial ventilation for pneumonia, or if this group must be stratified according to age, etiologic organism, or co-existing illness. Clearly, many of these factors will make an important difference.[24]

I wonder at which point one could determine that a given treatment had failed to restore consciousness. Relatively young PCU patients, who suffer from a trauma that brought about their unawareness, should have a grace period of two years to recover consciousness. It might be the case that short-term treatment will produce no positive results. The unqualified statement made by Schneiderman et al. opens the gate to stop treatment prematurely. Furthermore, what if the treatment alleviates significant dependence on intensive care, but not total dependence? Why such treatment would still be considered futile is unclear. After all, even according to Schneiderman and Jecker's general definition, it is possible to discern a benefit to a patient whose condition progressed from total dependence to some independence, and there is no reason to think that such treatment is necessarily likely to fail.

Futility is an elusive concept. As an evaluative instrument, it is used to justify the idea that a certain treatment would be ineffective because it would not yield any significant positive results or that the treatment would be inappropriate because its benefits are questionable. In public policy, the concept of futility can sanction restrictions in the allocation of health care resources. Patients cannot demand futile therapy, and society and doctors are under no obligation to provide such therapy. In ethics, policy, and law, the physician's opinion that a treatment is futile may lessen his or her obligation to the patient. The futility claims are supposed to rest on reasonable medical judgment. The problem is that physicians disagree about the type of clinical evidence necessary to justify a futility claim. Doctors often disagree not only about their evaluation of the likelihood of treatment success, but also about the value of outcomes. Some physicians would consider a treatment futile if it could provide a chance only for a couple of weeks of extended survival. Others would consider this a reasonable goal. Dying patients might consider this prolongation of life to be of supreme value.[25]

Recently, members of the AMA Council on Ethical and Judicial Affairs concluded that it is very difficult to assign an absolute definition to the term *futility*, as it is inherently a value-laden determination. Thus, they sensibly recommended a fair process approach for determining, and subsequently withholding or withdrawing, what is felt to be futile care. The fair-process approach insists on giving priority to patient or proxy assessments of worthwhile outcome, accommodating community and institutional standards, and the perspectives offered by the quantitative, functional, and interest approaches that involved parties may bring to the decision-making process.[26]

In her powerful critique of the concept of futility, Susan B. Rubin argues that futility is an insufficient ground for physicians' unilateral decision making. That is, physicians would not be justified in a unilateral refusal to provide treatment solely based on their opinion that the treatment would be futile. According to Rubin, the concept of futility distracted us from addressing ethical questions about the role of medicine and the framework of relationship between physicians and their patients. She is disturbed by the simplistic terms in which clinicians are encouraged to make judgments and is skeptical of attempts to divide judgments of futility into factual and evaluative statements. She rightly suggests that, at a minimum, patients must always be given an opportunity to participate in the decision-making process, insisting that the opportunity to participate must be genuine and meaningful.[27] That is, it must be genuine and meaningful for the patients, not for the health care system or for the caregivers.

Likewise, in a postscript written after he had published essays on futility, James F. Childress argues for restricting the term more narrowly than he intended at first, in part because appeals to futility have become ways to restore a kind of medical paternalism, to reinstate medical authority over patient and familial decision-making, to mask value-laden judgments as value-free and objective, to disguise rationing decisions, and so forth. Childress maintains that appeals to medical futility serve to stop conversation rather than to invite open discourse about values in treatment and nontreatment decisions, whether in caring for particular patients or in rationing care.[28]

Some maintain that the situation of PCU patients is futile. By resorting to the term *futility*, physicians promote a certain attitude to persons in need. The Santa Monica Hospital Medical Center's Futile Care Guidelines address situations in which the attending physician deems further treatment to be futile, but the patient or his/her loved ones insist on continuing treatment. These guidelines were formulated in response to the hospital's best interests, not patients' best interests. The policy defines futile care as "any clinical circumstance in which the doctor and his consultants, consistent with the available medical literature, conclude that further treatment (except comfort care) cannot, within a reasonable possibility, cure, ameliorate, improve or restore a quality of life that would be satisfactory to the patient." One such clinical condition is "persistent vegetative state."[29]

I contest this unqualified statement. Studies show that physicians are required to have some data about prolonged unawareness: the causes for this condition, the age of the patient, and the time factor since the onset of the unawareness, before concluding that treating PCU is futile (see chapter 2).

Double Effect

The ethical concept of double effect is used to justify medical treatment designed to relieve suffering where death is an unintended, though foreseeable, consequence. It comes from the double-effect doctrine developed by Roman Catholic moral theologians in the Middle Ages as a response to situations requiring actions in which it is impossible to avoid all harmful consequences. The doctrine makes intention in the mind of the doctor a crucial factor in judging the moral correctness of the doctor's action because of the Roman Catholic teaching that it is never permissible to "intend" the death of an "innocent person." An innocent person is one who has not forfeited the right to life by the way he or she behaves—for example, by threatening or taking the lives of others.[30]

The double-effect doctrine is based on two basic presuppositions: The doctor's intention is to alleviate suffering, and the treatment must be proportional to the illness.[31] The doctrine applies if the desired outcome is judged to be "good" (e.g., relief of suffering); the "bad" outcome (e.g., death of patient) is not intended; the "good" outcome is not achieved by means of the "bad"; and the "good" outcome outweighs the "bad." I am not in principle opposed to the double-effect doctrine, although my lack of opposition stems from practical, rather than ethical, considerations.[32] I think it is a different terminology and also a practical way—not altogether always sincere—to deal with a pressing problem. Religious authorities speak of double effect, and practical doctors use this idea in their practice. This doctrine serves both spiritual leaders and careful healers as a way to avoid dealing directly and sincerely with the question of mercy killings and physician-assisted suicide. Undoubtedly the doctrine provides a better solution than letting people die slowly in terrible agony. Doctors prescribe large doses of medication knowing that, as a result, suffering will be lessened and also that life will be shortened. They feel comfortable with what they are doing: They are not breaking the law; they are acting in accordance with their medical understanding and perceive themselves as providing solace to suffering patients.

Some patients do not want to play the doctors' game and speak of double effects that would allow a doctor to prescribe them a lethal dose of drugs, which, in turn, would shorten their lives while protecting the doctor's legal position. They seek a way out of a troubling existence. Why should their fate be worse than that of those who are able to commit suicide without assistance? Is it right that their inability to terminate their own lives forces them to continue to live in conditions they see as humiliating and pointless? (For further discussion of this issue, see conclusions.)

In their critique of the double-effect doctrine, Timothy E. Quill, Rebecca Dresser, and Dan W. Brock argue that the doctrine's complexities and ambiguities have limited its value as a guide to clinical practice and impaired care. They conclude that the rule is not a necessary means to adequate pain relief because informed consent, the degree of suffering, and the absence of less harmful alternatives suffice.[33]

Brain Death

More than thirty years ago, an ad hoc committee at Harvard Medical School promulgated criteria for the transplantation of vital organs from a donor.[34] Although the Harvard committee described the necessary condition of the donor as a state of irreversible coma, in the years that followed, this condition came to be known as brain death. The Harvard committee was explicit in noting that one of the important purposes of its document was to enable the nascent field of organ transplantation to develop.

Although the diagnosis of brain death is among the most straightforward in the practice of medicine, there is evidence that clinicians are frequently confused by the concept. One study of physicians and nurses who were frequently involved with questions of brain death and organ donation found that only 35 percent were able to correctly identify the legal and medical criteria for determining death. Most of the respondents used inconsistent concepts of death, and most did not believe that the brain-dead patients were really dead, but nevertheless felt comfortable with the process of organ procurement, on the basis that the patients were permanently unconscious and/or close to imminent death.[35] Rather than conclude that these clinicians were either unsophisticated or poorly trained, an editorial that accompanied this article expressed the view that this confusion about the concept was actually appropriate, given the inherent inconsistencies within the concept itself.[36]

Robert Truog explores the reasons that the concept of brain death was developed in the first place.[37] Truog returns to the work of the 1968 Harvard committee. In his review of the committee's paper, he indicates four questions that it was trying to address with this new notion:

1. When should life support be withdrawn for the benefit of the patient?

2. When should life support be withdrawn for the benefit of society?
3. When is a patient ready to be cremated or buried?
4. When is it permissible to remove organs from a patient for transplantation?

Truog argues that in 1968, the first question was very important, because removal of a ventilator from a living patient was legally viewed as a homicide. Now, however, the situation is entirely different. In most ICUs, more than half of the patients who die have had some form of life-sustaining therapy discontinued. The relevant question before removal of a ventilator in an intensive care unit is not "Is the patient dead?" but rather "Do the burdens of mechanical ventilation exceed the benefits?" The notion of using brain death to address the question of when to withdraw life support for the benefit of the patient, so central to the reasoning of the Harvard committee in 1968, has become virtually irrelevant over the last three decades.

In contrast, the second question about the allocation of scarce resources is perhaps even more important now than it was in 1968. Yet the problem is not that ICUs might be overrun by brain-dead patients on ventilators occupying ICU beds that are needed by others. Nowadays the question is whether we can continue to provide expensive treatments with marginal benefits to individuals at the extremes of their life span or with profoundly diminished capacities. Truog thinks that these difficult questions cannot be solved by holding on to the concept of brain death.

The third question differs from the first two in that it is essentially uncontroversial. We have always buried or cremated our loved ones after they have ceased to have pulse and respiration. Even when a person is diagnosed as dead by neurological criteria, the ventilator is removed and the clinicians wait until the patient is pulseless and without breath before removing the body to the morgue. Again, Truog contends that the concept of brain death is irrelevant to this question posed by the Harvard committee.

Finally, we are left with the question of when it is permissible to remove vital organs from one patient for transplantation into another. The sole reason for maintaining the concept of brain death is to identify a category of persons from whom this is possible. No wonder clinicians are confused by a category of death that is important, not for making the diagnosis of death per se, but solely to facilitate the procurement of organs for transplantation. At the very least, Truog maintains, this type of convoluted reasoning should prompt us to reevaluate whether the link between brain death and organ transplantation still makes sense, or whether there might be better ways to address the need for transplantable organs. Truog also notes that clinicians have observed that patients who were said to fulfill the tests for brain death frequently respond to surgical incision at the time of organ procurement with a significant rise in both heart rate and blood pressure. This suggests that integrated neurological function at a supraspinal level may be present in at least some of those patients. This means that there is a significant disparity between the standard tests used to make the diagnosis of brain death and the criterion these tests are purported to fulfill. Faced with these troublesome facts, we need to acknowledge that the criterion for whole-brain death is only an approximation.[38]

Conclusion

The current health care environment presents many dilemmas and challenges concerning possible conflict of interest between the medical staff, the patients, and other elements of the economic structure within which they operate. Ethics entail taking responsibility for our actions and speech, being sensitive to the people with whom we are dealing, and not offending them without justifiable grounds.

More consideration of ethics should be introduced into medical school curricula, and knowledge and understanding of ethical principles should be improved, while the medical staff should be equipped with communication skills. Research shows positive correlations among teaching higher-level moral reasoning, development of moral reasoning in medical students, and, in turn, good clinical performance.[39] The ethics education should be integrated into the curricula of each year of the medical school, where courses in progressive years build upon prior knowledge. Successful medical ethics teaching requires medical schools to invest in resources, time, and moral support for students.[40] The education can take the form of lectures that include pertinent films and video clips[41] as well as recent fictional and autobiographical literature about doctors and medicine.[42] Small group tutorials and clinical visits, discussing potential case vignettes as well as real situations and patients in wards, should be offered with the lectures.[43] The traditional model of ethics teaching, case based and issue oriented, emphasizing the knowledge and cognitive skills necessary for ethical decision-making, should be maintained.[44] In addition, the presentation of workshops and ethics rounds in hospitals in which a medical ethicist discusses ethical dilemmas with residents is a solid way to provide ethical education in a practical way.[45] Several studies evaluating the effect of medical ethics education have shown that both lectures and discussions of cases improved the moral reasoning scores of medical students and that small-group case study promotes the development of moral reasoning more than the lecture format.[46] In controlled trials, Daniel P. Sulmasy et al. found that lectures and discussions on ethics increased medical residents' knowledge and confidence in addressing ethical issues.[47] Similarly, Neil S. Wenger et al. argued that a medical ethics curriculum can increase residents' knowledge and awareness. Their study shows that residents who received educational intervention improved their knowledge of ethics, particularly in the areas of informed consent and physician-patient relationships.[48]

One of the main problems in patient-doctor relationships is that often doctors can be oblivious to the feelings of their patients, unaware that their own behavior and language cause patients anguish. That is not to say that the medical personnel are intentionally unethical. Instead, they are aethical, not appreciating the power of words and the consequences that words have on their patients. Because doctors lack time, they adopt short, concise terms that they themselves understand well and that serve their own interests. These terms do not necessarily serve the patients' best interests.

The lack of time is a crucial factor. As Stephen Wear notes, not only does it usually preclude the growth of an in-depth relationship between physician and patient, but it has other detrimental effects. All communication or counseling between the parties, including informed consent, must be sandwiched between many other diagnostic and therapeutic agendas. This dictates that communication will not occur in the unfolding process of mutual exploration, feedback, and understanding that we might hope for, the sort of intervention that might truly be expected to produce patient understanding.[49]

Studies consistently show that effective communication between clinicians and patients is a critical determinant of patient satisfaction.[50] Many health care organizations are aware of the need to promote communication skills and provide condensed training programs of a few hours each (e.g., "Thriving in a Busy Practice: Physician-Patient Communication") in which tens of thousands of clinicians take part.[51] However, this is not enough. Communication skills programs need to be longer and more intensive, teaching a broader range of skills and providing ongoing performance feedback.[52] More time should be invested in talking with patients and their loved ones. Honesty, the keeping of promises, confidentiality, caring, and empathy are essential for effective communication, which is the essential building block for an effective physician-patient relationship.[53]

Jay Katz writes in his landmark work of the silence that for many years surrounded patients and of the doctor-patient relationship, which has historically been based on one-way trust. Physicians have conversed with patients about all kinds of things, but they have not, except inadvertently, used language that invites patients to participate in making joint decisions.[54] Katz criticizes doctors for encouraging patients to relinquish their autonomy, and he demonstrates the detrimental effect their silence has on good patient care. He acknowledges the growing need in this age of medical technology for more sincere communication and a new, informed dialogue that respects the rights and needs of both physicians and patients.

The new ethos of patient autonomy and the emerging doctrine of informed consent have contributed in recent years to creating better communication between doctors and patients. In the United States, the Patient Self-Determination Act and managed care have heightened the awareness of communication. The act, which was passed by Congress on 5 November 1990, and went into effect on 1 December 1991, is based on the principles of informed consent. It lays the foundation for the exercise of the patient's decision-making authority, which will affect the course of treatment for all patients whether or not they possess decisional capacity.[55] In turn, managed care has heightened the awareness of communication because of the direct links among communication, outcomes, and malpractice liability.[56] As the silence at the bedside is replaced by mutual exploration and discussion, patients' concerns and fears should become more apparent to clinicians, and can be formally anticipated, rather than being allowed to fester unnoted and to cause trouble later.[57] A strong connection exists between the soul and the body, and doctors who are educated to fight for the life of their patients should not resort to terms that might weaken the will to live. Doctors should strive to use not only nontechnical terms to insure that patients understand the information they are given, but also terms that are not offensive to patients and/or to their loved ones.

Death with dignity is the subject of this book. Most patients hang on to life even in the most dreadful circumstances. At the same time, we should not ignore the small minority of patients who feel that their lives have no meaning and would opt for death rather than live a life that they regard as devoid of dignity. Patients who ask to die and plead for help in preserving what they perceive as their dignity are the focus of this discussion, not care providers. It is the patients who should evaluate the quality of their lives, not other people. The role of the doctor is ethically and analytically different and must be addressed after we agree that physician-assisted suicide is the right solution for the defined category of patients (competent, suffer from incurable disease, and reiterate their desire to die). All relevant circles of society should hold serious, open, and frank discussions on this painful topic. One preliminary discussion should be on terminology, making sure that everyone understands it the same way. Dehumanizing terms like PVS and *vegetable* should be excluded from the medical discussions for ethical reasons. Patients should not be labeled as "terminal," thereby delivering the message that there is no point investing work in preserving their lives. This is not to say that patients and their loved ones should not be provided with the relevant medical information. Instead, elaborate explanations would replace the concise and brutal word *terminal, which* falls like an axe on patients and their loved ones. Terms like *double effect* and *futility* should be explained in detail and with sincerity. The motivation for using these terms and others, like *brain death*, needs to be clarified. Doctors and patients, public leaders and religious figures, ethicists and intellectuals with a background in sociology and philosophy, psychologists, social workers, and others who care about patients should all take part in these discussions.

2 | Post-Coma Unawareness Patients

It has been argued that consciousness is the most critical moral, legal, and constitutional standard for human personhood, that consciousness is the most important characteristic that distinguishes humans from other forms of animal life, going beyond the vegetative functions of heartbeat and respiration, and that permanent loss of all consciousness is just as significant as the loss of all cardiopulmonary functions (the cardiopulmonary standard for death), and all brain functions (the neurological standard for death) in determining the moral and legal status of a human being.[1]

This chapter concerns unconscious, severely ill people who are in the twilight zone between life and death. These people constitute a moral problem for all those involved in deciding their destinies: families, their other loved ones, the medical staff, ethics committees, and sometimes the courts. There is an important distinction between patients in prolonged and/or persistent unawareness, as opposed to permanent unawareness. Physicians tend to confuse the two and conclude, sometimes prematurely, that for patients in prolonged unawareness there is no hope of regaining consciousness.

Indeed, in many countries it is normal clinical practice to withhold every form of care from patients in post-coma unawareness (PCU). In Norway, for example, once the diagnosis is established, the patients receive no further active treatment, not even artificial nutrition and hydration. The wide social acceptance of this practice leads health care professionals in Norway to consider it as the preferred choice of the reasonable person in that society.[2]

Research shows that PCU patients may improve their condition within two years of the event that caused the damage to their brains. The evidence I gathered in several countries shows that PCU patients may regain some of their faculties within this period of time and that afterward the chances for even minimal rehabilitation are very slim.

Cognitive recovery after six months is extremely rare in patients older than fifty, so there is no need to wait the suggested two-year grace period if the patient's condition is stable and if loved ones consent to stopping treatment.[3] Withdrawal of therapy from PCU patients younger than fifty could take place after two years with the consent of the patient's loved ones if the patient's situation did not improve during those two years. In the current state of medicine, the poor prognosis of some PCU patients is a self-fulfilling prophecy; they often fail to get adequate rehabilitative care early on. Improvement in their condition may require long months of continuous treatment, and this grace period is not always granted to them. Maybe in the future, when we know more about the brain, we will be able to make a firm judgment in a shorter period of time than is possible today.

A working group convened by the Royal College of Physicians in the United Kingdom held that in patients who are in a continuing "vegetative state" after head injury, the chances of recovery after six months are extremely low, and after twelve months "non-existent."[4] The medical ethics committee of the British Medical Association recommended in 1992 that decisions on withdrawing treatment should wait until the patient was thought to have been in PCU (the term they used was PVS) for at least a year. The committee thought it would be reasonable to remove invasive treatment, including artificial nutrition, if the doctor caring for the patient judged that there was no reasonable chance of improvement and two other doctors independently concurred.[5] However, this policy was criticized; opponents argued that the withdrawal of treatment after twelve months would be very dangerous. There are reported cases in which patients regained consciousness after a more prolonged length of time.[6]

A comprehensive study conducted by Andrew Grubb and his colleagues showed that only 17 percent of 1,027 responding doctors expressed confidence about predicting an ultimate outcome within the first three months of unawareness. The degree of confidence rose to 40 percent for patients in PCU for four to six months, and to 82 percent after one year. Eleven percent of respondents were uncertain about predicting an ultimate outcome when the patient was in PCU more than a year.[7]

In contrast, the American Academy of Neurology adopted the position that the vegetative state should be termed persistent at one month post-injury, and that it can be considered permanent after three months following nontraumatic injuries and after twelve months following traumatic injuries.[8]

Some specialists speak of a persistent or permanent vegetative state as if it were a defined condition, without looking at the variations of the condition, and without paying any attention to what caused the condition, whether it involved head injury, the length of the condition, and other factors that are pertinent for the evaluation of the state of unawareness.[9] Others hold: "Persistent vegetative state . . . should be considered a form of death."[10] This is not an illogical step to take after legitimizing the term PVS and describing human beings as vegetables. These scholars suggest redefining death, away from whole-brain death toward the recognition that patients who are in PCU are actually dead. They speak of a trend, through court decisions, of slowly moving toward a re-formulation of the definition of death. Financial costs play a crucial role in their considerations. This approach is reflected in the reports of the Hastings Center and the Society of Critical Care Medicine concluding that providing intensive care to patients in persistent vegetative state is generally a misuse of resources. Consequently, treatment of such patients could be withdrawn even without patients' advance directives and without the approval of surrogates.[11] Indeed, research indicates that resuscitative treatment was withheld from PCU patients without prior directives from the patients or without the consent of their families.[12]

I find these approaches alarming. The basic problem is that economy overshadows the differences between patients. *Post-coma unawareness* is a general term describing the condition of some patients, but various parameters must be taken into account in the evaluation of each individual patient's condition. We must be aware of the variations that led to this situation, the condition of each patient, the age of the patient, the length of time the patient has been in a state of unawareness, and other relevant criteria.[13] We must resist the temptation to resort to a single criterion simplified by a special term—PVS—that might lead to treating patients unjustly. This chapter calls upon physicians to think twice before withdrawing life-sustaining treatment from PCU patients. It questions the British one-year waiting policy and the position of the American Academy of Neurology. I suggest, as an alternative, that we should adopt a two-year waiting policy with patients who are younger than fifty and whose situation was caused by trauma.

If the patients left any form of advance directives declaring that they would find no benefit in hanging on to life on reaching such a stage, then their request should be honored. However, the majority of family members of PCU patients want life-saving therapies for their loved ones.[14] Therefore, whenever we are unsure about a patient's preferences, life should be maintained as long as some probability exists that the patient could regain at least some capacities.

When we deal with matters of life and death, we should be extra careful in our observations. The data and human stories gathered during my fieldwork in Israel, Canada, the United States, the Netherlands, and England illuminated the discussion and provided me with a better understanding of the issue. The cases presented here in no way exhaust all the cases I encountered during my fieldwork. Rather they illustrate a phenomenon not to be ignored. I hope this discussion will cause people like Ronald E. Cranford and David R. Smith to rethink their sweeping generalizations: "A patient in a persistent vegetative state has no health; health is an empty concept for a patient without consciousness."[15] Their conclusion is that preservation of life is an empty proposition for these patients. Although I agree with Cranford and Smith that cognition is the most valued human quality, I also think that we need to distinguish among three situations of lasting absence of cognitive ability: brain death, intractable coma,[16] and prolonged unawareness. Health is an empty concept for patients in the first two groups, but it might be meaningful for patients who belong to the third. It seems that Cranford and Smith confuse permanent unawareness and prolonged unawareness, treating these different situations as one and the same.[17]

Cranford and Smith present their arguments in explicit, conclusive language. I argue with no less conviction that current medicine is far from fully informed about problems concerning the brain. Therefore, the plea raised here is a plea for caution. In more than a few cases physicians are unable to safely conclude that PCU patients are irreversibly incapable of experiencing anything. Chris Borthwick argues that there are unquestionably hundreds of people in the United States who are being treated as if they were in PVS when they are not.[18] Electroencephalograms and scans cannot be diagnostic, although they may support a diagnosis. There is some hope that the new functional magnetic resonance scans will make an important contribution to diagnosis, but this has yet to be investigated formally.[19] It has been documented that some patients diagnosed as PCU patients do regain their consciousness. Thus we should be very careful when we decide to terminate life. In any event, families and other people close to patients in a state of unawareness should be informed of the existing likelihood, however meager, of the return of cognition. Many people are not at all aware of this possibility.

Post-Coma Unawareness

PCU patients have suffered brain injuries from various causes: trauma, cerebral anoxia from hypotension or cardiac arrest, cerebrovascular accidents, or dementia. These patients have periods of wakefulness and physiological sleep/wake cycles, but at no time are these patients aware of themselves or their environment. Neurologically, being awake but unaware is the result of a functioning brain stem and the total loss of cerebral cortical function. No voluntary action or behavior of any kind is present. Although PCU patients are generally able to breathe spontaneously because of the intact brain stem, some claim that the capacity to chew and swallow in a normal manner is lost because these functions are voluntary, requiring intact cerebral hemispheres.[20] In 1993 the American Neurological Association issued a report that contradicts part of this assertion, stating: "Primitive reflexes such as sucking, rooting, chewing and swallowing may be preserved."[21] Although I tend to think that the 1993 report is correct, the contrasting views show that we are still in the process of learning about PCU patients.

Once qualified clinicians have determined that a person is awake but unaware, the prognosis as to the permanence of the vegetative state depends on the age of the patient, the nature of the brain injury, and the length, so far, of the period of unawareness.[22] Irrespective of cause, in the United States the Council on Scientific Affairs and Council on Ethical and Judicial Affairs held that PCU patients younger than forty have a better chance than others of recovering self-aware consciousness after a delay of several months. Similarly, those who become vegetative following brain trauma or subarachnoid hemorrhage are more likely to show a long-delayed return of consciousness than are patients who have suffered severe asphyxial injury, such as the injury that follows cardiac arrest.[23] D. E. Levy and associates reported that patients with traumatic coma seem to do somewhat better than patients with nontraumatic coma.[24] Patients with intractable degenerative diseases of the central nervous system (Alzheimer's disease, Creutzfeld-Jacob disease, Ganglioside storage disease, etc.) will inevitably deteriorate. Therefore, patients in PCU resulting from these disorders have no possibility of recovery.[25]

PCU patients are not brain dead. PCU patients may show no behavioral response whatsoever over an extended period of time. They may continue to survive for a prolonged period as long as the artificial provision of nutrition and fluids is continued and proper nursing care is provided. On the other hand, brain death is a specific form of permanent coma in which coma is not only irreversible, but also the most severe—the absence of all brain stem functions. As was discussed in chapter 1, death of the brain is deemed equivalent to death of the patient. In contrast with brain stem death, PCU is associated with severe and irreversible damage to the cerebrum with or without the diencephalon, while many brain stem functions, such as spontaneous ventilation, chewing, coughing, swallowing, regulation of temperature and respiration, and cranial nerve reflexes, may be largely preserved.[26]

Research indicates concerns on the part of medical professionals over the possibility of inaccurate diagnosis of PCU, which might lead to the termination of life of patients who might improve and might have some opportunity for a meaningful life.[27] A study conducted among nurses at Toronto Hospital on the question of whether they support organ donation from patients in PCU revealed that a major cause of concern was the lack of certainty in diagnosis and the varying degrees of PCU.[28] There is no mention in this study of whether the time factor, for instance, played any role in the nurses' considerations. The lack of consideration in the study of this as well as other factors is quite alarming, because there is a difference between patients who have been in PCU for some years and patients who entered this condition only a few months ago. Patients in the latter group have a much better chance of regaining some of their faculties and of returning to some form of meaningful life. In addition, nothing was said in this study with regard to the cause of the patients' condition, whether it was traumatic or nontraumatic.

Research also indicates the confusion among professionals over the definitions of death and forms of prolonged unawareness. In their survey of 195 doctors and nurses likely to be involved in organ procurement and transplantation, S. J. Youngner and his colleagues asked respondents the factual question "What brain functions must be lost for a patient to be declared brain-dead?" They also measured the knowledge by presenting two cases and asking respondents whether each patient was legally dead. Patient A sustained irreversible loss of all brain function, including the brain stem and higher structures, such as the cortex. Patient B had sustained irreversible loss of all cortical brain function, and was unconscious and unresponsive, but breathing was spontaneous and internal regulation of blood pressure and temperature was intact. Youngner and his associates found that only 35 percent of respondents both knew the whole-brain criterion of death and were able to apply it correctly to identify the legal status of patients A and B. The others failed to correctly identify the legal and medical criteria for determining death. The majority of respondents (58 percent) used the two concepts inconsistently. A substantial minority (38 percent) said that patient B, who had irreversibly lost brain cortical function, was dead, and 36 percent held that it was morally permissible to retrieve organs from that patient.[29] These figures are disturbing. This and similar studies were conducted between 1989 and 1991, and it is to be hoped that the medical staff is more educated today with regard to PCU patients. Still, the data constitutes a cause for concern when the possible consequences of this confusion and lack of knowledge are considered.

One of the most crucial considerations prominent in physicians' minds when they are making health care decisions is the control of pain. If we could prove that PCU patients suffer, then we might think they are better off dead. We would not like to think that these patients would be sustained for months and years while suffering great pain. The problem, however, is that current medicine is unable to provide data in this regard. Disagreement exists regarding the question of whether PCU patients have the capacity to experience pain or suffering. The opinion of the American Academy of Neurology is that these patients do not. In their position paper, members of the executive board wrote: "Pain and suffering are attributes of consciousness requiring cerebral cortical functioning, and patients who are permanently and completely unconscious cannot experience these symptoms."[30] But then a question arises as to how it is possible to safely conclude that the patient is indeed in a state of permanent (to be distinguished from prolonged or persistent) unawareness. In a similar vein, Cranford and Smith also argue conclusively: "Persistent vegetative state patients do not have the capacity to experience pain or suffering."[31] My review of the literature and discussions with experts reveal that our knowledge is still very limited. Professor Martin Tweeddale, director of the critical care unit at the Vancouver Hospital, said in a private discussion that he simply does not know whether PCU patients suffer. In his opinion, we are in a position to say something in this regard when patients respond to certain stimuli, but when patients do not respond we are in no position to determine anything with regard to pain.[32] Tweeddale reiterates that because PCU patients (unlike coma patients) make some response to external stimuli, it is impossible to say they are unresponsive. On the other hand, because pain is totally subjective, we have no way of determining whether or not such sensations are present or whether there is any perception of them at all. Tweeddale concludes: "My own feeling is that these patients demonstrate complex, high level reflex activity only, but I am in no better position to defend that statement than are those who say there is no possibility of awareness, or those . . . who argue for some potential conscious activity, however rudimentary."[33]

Tweeddale admits he does not know the answer, but Joseph Alpert believes that PCU patients must be suffering at some level. He asks rhetorically: How could suffering not be present if any awareness exists of the extraordinary level of disability present?[34]

Kirk Payne and his associates surveyed physicians' attitudes about the care of patients in PCU. A substantial number of the medical doctors and neurologists who participated in the survey believed that these patients experience pain, thirst, and hunger, are aware of self and environment, and are made more comfortable by intravenous fluids and tube feedings.[35] Stephen Ashwal and his colleagues reported that 20 percent of pediatric neurologists in their survey believed that children in PCU experience pain and suffering, and 75 percent of the sample stated that they used medications to alleviate such symptoms.[36] There is a spectrum of views on this most crucial issue, which again shows that we are still in the learning process and hence need to be extra careful in making decisions with regard to the patients in PCU. PCU patients do not give any perceptible indication that they experience the cognitive and emotional concomitants of pain and suffering. But we cannot safely say that their inability to give any indication, or alternatively our inability to find any indication, may serve as sufficient grounds to conclude that these patients do not feel pain. I am not aware of any study in which patients who emerged from PCU were asked whether or not they felt pain while they were in this condition.

Scholars refer to the PCU state as vegetative because the body retains the functions necessary to sustain vegetative and homeostatic functions.[37] However, the term *vegetative* suggests some form of subhuman life. The connotation is that these people are no longer human beings.

Discussions with physicians reveal that some of them disagree with my position. Some physicians see nothing wrong with the term *vegetative*, which, to their mind, provides a medical account of a patient's situation. I am not sure to what extent they are aware of the offense caused to patients' loved ones who are told that the patient is in "a state of vegetable" or in "vegetative state." Some physicians also think this term is proper because it compels families to be realistic and does not raise their expectations. The families now understand that their loved one has little or no hope of recovery. From the physicians' point of view, the term *vegetative* is instrumental: It provides a medical account of the patient's condition, and at the same time delivers a message to the families and to other people concerned with the well-being of the patient.

My disagreement with this line of reasoning is deep and unequivocal. On the premise that physicians use the term *vegetative* to draw a medical distinction between higher and lower functions of the body, they may use this term in team conversations (although a proviso needs to be added: The very use of the term might imply that less effort should be invested in maintaining such patients). The terms *vegetative* and *vegetable* should not be included in the vocabulary of physicians and nurses who provide care and comfort. As for the "not raising expectations" rationale, physicians can resort to other terms and/or longer explanations to describe a patient's condition. They do not need to draw an analogy with vegetables. The inoffensive, conciliatory, tangible, and coherent terminology has to be acknowledged as mandatory for physicians and other medical personnel. One of the duties of the medical profession is to maintain the dignity of those who require medical care, either for themselves or for their loved ones.

The Israeli Experience

In Israel, an attempt is made to place all patients with prolonged unawareness in one critical care unit, at the Loewenstein Rehabilitation Hospital (LRH), where they stay for periods of up to one year. LRH was established in the mid-1960s and provides almost all the existing rehabilitation functions: a vocational rehabilitation center; an orthopedic center for the manufacture of artificial limbs; a biomechanics library; research functions; and all therapeutic functions: speech, vocational, psychological, psychiatric, and social work. LRH does not provide rehabilitation for blind persons or for patients who suffer from heart failure. The hospital has departments for patients with spinal cord injuries (SCI); rehabilitation of patients after strokes; fifteen beds for children, either disabled or suffering from brain injuries; a department of orthopedic rehabilitation; a department of traumatic brain injuries (TBI), and a critical care unit (CCU) to which patients in prolonged unawareness are transferred.

The CCU was established in 1973. First it was decided to treat patients for one year and then, if no progress had been recorded, to transfer them to institutions for patients with chronic illnesses. According to Dr. Leon Sazbon, director of the CCU at Loewenstein, experience showed that one year was too long. Brain-damaged patients may remain unconscious for years. If a patient does not show any progress within the period of six months from the day of the accident (or the stroke, or any other cause), the chance of functioning cognitively in the future is very slim. Thus, the tendency is to provide medical assistance for six months and then transfer those who have not returned to consciousness to hospitals for chronic patients. Dr. Sazbon explains that the six-month period is sufficient to identify 95 percent of the patients who have a chance to regain some of their faculties. He admits that there is a likelihood that 5 percent of the patients will regain consciousness at a later date, but maintaining them at LRH for two years would mean blocking the way for other patients who have a chance for rehabilitation.

Dr. Sazbon reiterates that none of the patients is in any way deserted, and that all patients receive the same treatment they get at LRH in the hospitals for chronic patients.[38]

The decision to relocate patients after six months is very difficult for the patients' loved ones, who understand this to mean that the physicians at Loewenstein have given up hope that the patient will recover. This, however, is believed to be necessary by the directors of Loewenstein because of the pressing demand for beds. The hospital asks the consent of the patient's family to transfer him or her to another hospital. The law demands the family's consent before relocation of patients can be made.

The CCU has fifteen beds. Patients who are in a coma owing to anoxia (shortage of oxygen) and patients who need artificial respiration are not admitted, because preference is given to patients with a reasonable chance of returning to social life. Patients who are not able to breathe without artificial respiration usually stay in general hospitals. The small number of available beds forces the medical staff to make the decision to invest efforts where the chances for success are relatively high. These beds are usually fully occupied, and there is a short waiting list (one to three patients in neurosurgery departments in general hospitals, i.e., hospitals that do not specialize in rehabilitation).

There are two types of causes of prolonged unawareness: traumatic and nontraumatic. Traumatic causes are commonly road accidents and IDF (Israel Defense Forces) training accidents or battle injuries. Nontraumatic causes include strokes, encephalitis, cardiac arrest, respiratory failure, complications of anesthesia and/or neurosurgery, poisoning, severe infections, and the like. On average, two of the fifteen patients are soldiers. In wartime, this number increases.

The CCU staff helps the families as well as the patients. Social workers accompany the families, explain the situation to them, and urge them to return to their own social life as much as they can. The directors at Loewenstein seek to establish close relationships with the families. Physicians and social workers explain to the families and other concerned people that their loved ones are receiving the best available medical treatment, and there is no need for them to remain near their beds around the clock. Families are allowed to visit their relatives only during specific visiting hours (three to seven P.M.). The directors at Loewenstein do not believe that talking to the patients and showering them with endless love can have any positive impact on them. They believe that if the patients wake up, they will require the close attention of their families; thus the families should preserve their own sanity by continuing to live as normal a life as possible. They should also take into consideration the possibility that their loved ones will never wake up.

The relationships between physicians and social workers, on the one hand, and the families, on the other, are extremely delicate. Trust and mutual understanding are extremely significant in maintaining a workable environment. When a person has died, a formal mourning procedure denotes the sad event, and afterward people continue to live their lives. A person in a state of prolonged unawareness hovers between life and death, and no defined custom exists to help people cope with such a tragedy.

Statistics and Human Stories

The Multi-Society Task Force, comprised of representatives of the American Academy of Neurology, the Child Neurology Society, the American Neurological Association, the American Association of Neurological Surgeons, and the American Academy of Pediatrics, considered data on 434 head injury patients and noted: "Three months after injury, 33 percent of the patients had recovered consciousness; 67 percent had died or remained in a vegetative state. Recovery had occurred in 46 percent of patients at 6 months, and in 52 percent at 12 months. Recovery after 12 months was reported in only 7 of the 434 patients." One patient recovered consciousness after thirty months.[39]

The recovery of only seven patients after twelve months, or 1.6 percent of the total number, does not sound like a lot. However, as Chris Borthwick notes, the relevant figure is not the number who recover in any period as a percentage of the whole but that figure as a percentage of the ones available to recover—that is, those who had not died or recovered already. Accordingly, at the end of the first year 52 percent of the patients had recovered consciousness, 33 percent had died, 15 percent were still in PVS, and 10.6 percent (seven out of 65) recovered after twelve months.[40]

U. T. Heindl and M. C. Laub studied two groups of children: eighty-two patients with traumatic brain injury (TBI), and forty-five patients with hypoxic brain injury (HBI). They found significant differences between the two groups. The TBI patients progressed better than the HBI patients. 34 percent of the patients in the TBI group (compared with 13 percent of the HBI group) regained consciousness after three months. One year after trauma, 80 percent of the patients in this group had left PCU. Even after being in PCU for a period up to nine months, eight children of the TBI group achieved independence in everyday life. Heindl and Laub conclude that after nine months in PCU it is possible to make a prognosis with a relatively high reliability (in both groups the number of patients who left PCU after nine months was less than 5 percent), but not with certainty. They contend that some patients can make clinical improvement after this time.[41]

Stephen Ashwal and his colleagues did a survey of members of the Child Neurology Society regarding aspects of the diagnosis and management of PCU. The minimum observation period recommended for infants and children younger than two was five to six months. Eighty-six percent of the neurologists in the sample believed that the age of the patient would affect the duration of time needed to make the diagnosis of PCU.[42]

G. A. Rosenberg et al. describe the case of a forty-three-year-old man who was in prolonged unawareness for seventeen months following anoxic brain damage before showing the first signs of awareness. He progressed to being able to tell stories and jokes, though he was unable to recognize complex collections of objects in pictures and was unable to read.[43] In another case, a forty-four-year-old man in prolonged unawareness showed signs of recovery one year following a subarachnoid hemorrhage to regain nearly normal physical and mental capabilities.[44] Nancy L. Childs and Walt N. Mercer reported the case of an eighteen-year-old woman who suffered a traumatic brain injury in a motor vehicle accident. After fifteen months, the medical staff reported some responses on her part. Seventeen months after the injury, she was able to follow simple commands and could complete simple arithmetic problems and multiple-choice sentences using eye blinks. She communicated: "Mom, I love you."[45]

Information from the Traumatic Data Bank Study of eighty-four PVS patients who were followed up long term found that 41 percent became conscious by six months, a further 11 percent between six months and a year, and an additional 6 percent between one and two and a half years.[46] In a five-year follow-up of thirty patients in PVS, five recovered between one and five years, though only two recovered enough to communicate. One was a sixty-one-year-old woman who was in prolonged unawareness for three years following a subarachnoid hemorrhage. The other was a twenty-six-year-old man who was in prolonged unawareness for eight months due to anoxia before he began to respond. Both eventually were able to read, watch television, write, perform simple addition and subtraction, tell the time, and feed themselves; were wheelchair independent; and could speak well.[47] In another study of 110 PCU patients, K. Higashi and associates found that eight patients were assessed as no longer vegetative at the end of the three-year follow-up study.[48] S.

Sato and colleagues reported that fourteen of 216 patients (6.5 percent) recovered from PCU within a year. Among them, seven patients achieved good recovery.[49]

Estimates about the number of patients in PCU in the United States range from ten thousand to twenty-five thousand.[50] Most of these patients are cared for in chronic care institutions, but the proportion of these patients cared for by families at home is unknown.[51] Data gathered in Israel show that every year some three hundred persons are in a state of PCU. This number is more or less fixed, because some patients regain consciousness or die and others enter this state.

Dr. Leon Sazbon has served at the Loewenstein hospital since the day the CCU opened. More than five hundred patients were treated in the unit between 1974 and 1993. According to his evidence, the introduction of mobile intensive care, modern technology, and advancement of knowledge brought about great improvement and increased the likelihood of saving people whose brains were damaged owing to both traumatic and nontraumatic causes. The prognosis of nontraumatic PCU is much worse than that of the same duration of unconsciousness following trauma. On average, patients who show immediate progress wake up after eleven weeks.[52] Others can remain in a state of PCU for many years, the longest on record being over forty years.[53] This is why Dr. Keith Andrews, director of the Royal Hospital for Neurodisability in Putney, London, argues that life expectancy of PCU patients depends very much on the attitude of the family and clinicians—that is, on how long the patient is allowed to live rather than how long he or she can live.[54]

A study conducted at LRH describes the functional outcome of 72 patients comprising 53.7 percent of a group of 134 patients in a state of post-traumatic unconsciousness. They were treated between 1974 and 1983 and recovered consciousness after spending more than one month in a state of prolonged unawareness. Most of the patients (68.7 percent) were victims of motor vehicle accidents. Penetrating war injuries were present in the second largest group (11.9 percent), and 5.2 percent of the patients had work-related accidents. The rest of the patients (14.2 percent) had suffered brain trauma from other causes. Almost half the patients were independent in activities of daily living, and another 20 percent were only partially dependent. Eight patients (11.1 percent) were able to resume paid work, and 35 (48.6 percent) were engaged in sheltered workshops. Most of the patients (72 percent), including those working for pay, lived with their families. Although the mean rehabilitation period was about fifteen months, over 70 percent of these severely injured patients were considered to be socially integrated, and thus were able to enjoy a reasonable quality of life.[55]

The fate of patients who entered a state of unawareness due to nontraumatic causes is much more gloomy. Leon Sazbon and associates conducted a study that included one hundred patients who were admitted to the critical care unit of Loewenstein Rehabilitation Hospital in a state of PCU lasting at least thirty days following anoxia. They were admitted to the hospital between 1974 and 1987. The etiology of PCU was cardiac arrest or respiratory failure in thirty-four cases, complications of anesthesia and/or neurosurgery in thirty-four, stroke in fifteen, encephalitis in eight, and various other causes in nine cases.[56]

Twenty of the patients recovered consciousness within five months of injury. Seven of them were over the age of forty-five. The younger patients achieved more independence in ambulation than the older ones. The younger patients also attained a greater degree of independence in daily living activities. Thirty-one of the remaining patients died within six months following injury, whereas forty-nine remained unconscious until death. The mean life expectancy of these forty-nine was twenty-six to thirty-four months from the time of the injury. All twenty patients who recovered awareness continued to suffer from major disability. Among those who recovered consciousness, the younger patients showed somewhat better results in three parameters of function: locomotion, ADL (activities of daily living), and day placement (sheltered employment or school setting), but not in cognition, behavior, or speech accuracy and fluency. Six of the seven patients over the age of forty-five remained bedridden, while the seventh was restricted to a wheelchair; six of the eleven patients aged seventeen to forty-five were bedridden, four were wheelchair-bound, and one achieved assisted walking. By contrast, both of the children attained at least partially independent walking. All of the seven older patients remained in nursing care, compared with none of the patients under sixteen.[57]

According to Dr. Sazbon and his associates, if a patient wakes up within six months, we can expect rehabilitation: integration into the family, the job market, and general society. Those who recover between the sixth and the twelfth month suffer grave deficiencies to the extent that they are not able to return to their families, to work, or to integrate into the society at large. In the following discussion, however, I will present cases of patients who regained consciousness and returned to a substantial way of life after the twelfth month. There are not many cases of this kind, but those to be presented still illustrate my thesis that we should not cease treatment of PCU patients prior to the two-year period in cases involving patients younger than fifty who have left no directives that they would rather die upon entering such a state, and whose loved ones wish to keep them alive. I reiterate that this policy should be fostered especially with regard to post-traumatic patients. If a crude line for policy purposes needs to be drawn, it is safer to draw it at the two-year period than at one year, better serving the best interests of the patients concerned.

The data gathered in Israel was substantiated by research conducted in Canada, implying that this rationale is valid. Professor Frederick Lowy, former director of the Center for Bioethics at the University of Toronto, and currently rector and vice chancellor of Concordia University, agreed with me in a private conversation that it is a wise policy to provide a two-year period for PCU patients to recover. Policies that endorse a six-month or even one-year period might cause the loss of lives that could be saved if patients were given a period of two years to recover. With patients who show no progress in their condition after two years in prolonged unawareness, we may conclude that the possibility of some recovery is so small that we are unable to justify a longer maintenance policy.

One of the Israeli hospitals for chronic patients is Lichtenstaedter Hospital in Tel-Aviv, which serves as a nursing home as well as a rehabilitation center.[58] Lichtenstaedter has room for 220 patients and is usually fully occupied. Seven physicians and some eighty nurses and auxiliary helpers care for the patients. Most of the patients are chronic, bedridden, unable to function by themselves, and cannot do the simplest tasks (in the terminology of the hospital director, Dr. Nachman Wilensky, they are unable to "scare off a fly"). The department that cares for brain-damaged patients, including PCU patients, comprises twenty-five beds, with one doctor, seven nurses, and several assistants on each shift. Most of the patients in this facility do not show signs of improvement, although some do, and the records show a few cases of patients who succeeded in regaining consciousness and returning to life.

One patient, L.S. (the full name is on record), a member of a religious family, suffered from postpartum depression after her eighth delivery, when she was thirty-eight years old. She went to a hotel in Jerusalem, where she tried to commit suicide by hanging herself. She was rescued, and on 6 October 1986, she was admitted to a hospital, suffering respiratory arrest. On 4 November 1986, L.S. was moved to Loewenstein, and on 21 November, she had a CT (computerized tomography) examination and other medical examinations that showed significant brain atrophy, caused by symmetric, central, and cortical injury in the brain stem and the cerebral hemisphere. This CT result convinced the physicians at Loewenstein that the patient's condition was irreversible and that she was not a candidate for rehabilitation. Accordingly, on 9 December 1986, she was transferred to Lichtenstaedter, suffering from prolonged anoxic unawareness. She was in a state of prolonged unawareness for eighteen months, during which, as time elapsed, she slowly regained consciousness. In 1994, she was still at Lichtenstaedter, blind, bedridden, able to speak and to communicate, able to remember things that happened to her in the past, and clear-minded to the point of refusing to have a sexual relationship with her husband.

Another incident involves Z.B., a fifteen-year-old boy who in March 1985 was brought to a hospital with a severe head injury. In the hospital he lost consciousness, suffering from bleeding into the brain. He underwent two operations and in May 1985 was transferred to Loewenstein Hospital in a state of PCU, accompanied by epileptic seizures, and with a tracheotomy. The patient was diagnosed as having no prospect for rehabilitation, and consequently, in November 1985, was moved to Lichtenstaedter. In August 1986, seventeen months after the trauma that caused the dramatic deterioration of Z.B.'s health, his condition began slowly to improve. He regained consciousness and resumed talking, and was able to relate for the first time what brought about his tragic fate. He told the physicians that he had been attacked by two teenagers who wanted to take his watch. When he resisted, one of them struck him on the head with a large stick. The young patient stayed one year at Lichtenstaedter and was then relocated to Loewenstein for rehabilitation. By 1994, he was half paralyzed but able to talk and to communicate, was clear-minded, and lived with his parents. Dr. Wilensky thought he would be able to attend a mainstream school.

A third story concerns M.B., a thirty-seven-year-old patient who, in November 1988, delivered a healthy baby by Cesarean section. During the operation she went into cardiac arrest. M.B. was resuscitated but remained in a state of PCU. In June 1989, she was moved to Lichtenstaedter, still in PCU. After fourteen months in a state of PCU, M.B. slowly recovered. She began to respond; she was able to see, to communicate, to move her limbs, and to walk a few steps with a walking aid. She was clear minded and enjoyed the company of her family. She needed constant support and treatment, and her father resigned from work and was with her almost constantly. When he was not present, her mother stayed with her.

These three stories illustrate the thesis presented here for medical and social debate. The three patients were younger than fifty years old. They were in a state of prolonged unawareness for a period longer than one year but shorter than two years, and they regained consciousness. All of them were grateful to the physicians who kept them alive. Critics would say that it is hard to build an argument on the basis of three cases. There are not dozens of such cases, but there are enough to justify the policy recommend here. These cases are illustrative; they do not exhaust all cases I encountered during my research in Israel, the United States, the Netherlands, England, and Canada. Patients in prolonged unawareness deserve a fair chance to regain their faculties. According to the current state of knowledge a two-year maintenance period constitutes such a fair chance.[59]

Conclusion

Many believe that because of the costs involved we should not waste our resources to keep PCU patients alive. Other patients, who have a stronger chance of enjoying a better quality of life, should get treatment at the expense of PCU patients. We must decide on priorities. We must allocate scarce resources in a logical way. We cannot keep all people alive, no matter what costs are involved. In the survey conducted by Payne and associates, about 94 percent of the physicians thought that PCU patients would be better off dead; almost half of all respondents thought that they should be considered dead; and almost all of them would agree to the explicit rationing of most treatments for PCU patients.[60]

The story of L.S. is arguably the most difficult of those discussed so far, because of her very limited quality of life. Nevertheless, L.S.'s family and physicians felt that hers was a worthwhile quality of life. Should we cut L.S.'s thread of life? I think not, for two reasons: L.S. found pleasure and meaning in her life, and obviously, we cannot disregard the family. How could we face them and say at any given point during the eighteen months of unawareness that L.S.'s life was not worth living, considering the endless attention they invested in her care, and at the same time being ourselves unsure of the prognosis that presumes that the patient would never regain consciousness?[61] Every human life counts, and we should do our utmost to safeguard them when patients have not voiced their desire to cease living. When they wish to die, then we should respect their request, acknowledging that by doing so we respect them as human beings, respect their autonomy, and respect their dignity. But when we have no reason to believe these patients would opt for dying, we should keep them alive. Respecting their lives and their dignity is a compelling obligation. And in any event, the patients' loved ones should be aware of all relevant data in deciding the patients' fate.

Dr. Keith Andrews gives an account of patients (seventeen of forty, 43 percent) who have been misdiagnosed as being in PCU. He describes the results as "frightening," saying that some were missed cases of locked-in syndrome,[62] in which the patient is profoundly paralyzed, unable to speak or to move any muscle, but the brain may be functioning normally.[63] D. D. Tresch and associates examined sixty-two patients identified as having PCU by their nursing home medical personnel and found that eleven of these patients were misdiagnosed.[64] N. J. Childs and associates reviewed the experience of the diagnosis of PCU in patients referred to the Healthcare Rehabilitation Center in Austin, Texas. Eighteen (37 percent) of the forty-nine patients referred to the center were misdiagnosed.[65] Adrian Treloar of Bexley Hospital, in the United Kingdom, said that patients who could not express their wishes were being killed without their consent and without evidence of any benefit to them.[66] These testimonies are, indeed, frightening. I can understand the pressures not to sustain unconscious patients, pressures resulting from financial considerations, among other things. But with all due respect to financial considerations, human life is more important.[67] With the current state of knowledge, caution is a basic requirement not to be ignored.

A caveat regarding living wills is pertinent. Many people are signing living wills stating that upon reaching a stage when they are unable to communicate with their surroundings, and/or unable to recognize their loved ones, and/or unable to control their body's functions, they prefer to cease all treatment and be allowed to die. People who sign such living wills will probably not receive the recommended grace period of two years if they enter a state of prolonged unawareness. Living wills resort to simplistic formulations that could be suitable for all diseases and conditions. The problem is that life, with all its complexities and challenging illnesses, is not simple. Here I address only the state of PCU, but each deadly disease has its own characteristics that decide the fate of the patient. The formulations need to be far more complex and detailed. Most laypeople, however, lack the required knowledge to draft detailed living wills.

One of the arguments frequently mentioned with regard to PCU patients is that their quality of life does not justify maintaining them. The next chapter probes the quality-of-life argument, contrasting it with the sanctity-of-life model, and offering a middle ground for analysis.

3 | Sanctity and Quality of Life in Medical Ethics

Modern medicine can extend the lives of patients whose illnesses would have been incurable and would have resulted in death in the past.[1] Today it is possible to sustain and resuscitate patients using machines. Should doctors always use the knowledge and technology to add a few weeks, days, or hours to a patient's life, especially when that life has lost its quality, and involves continuous suffering?

In recent years, there has been an increase in the number of requests by patients and their relatives for what they call mercy killing, often involving the termination of life-prolonging treatment. Their assumption is that death is preferable to life when life becomes devoid of quality. In contrast to this quality-of-life argument, those promulgating the sanctity-of-life argument claim that life has intrinsic value and must be preserved in any form, regardless of its quality. The dispute between the two approaches is still very lively. How is it possible to evaluate quality of life, and what criteria can be used to distinguish between a life of quality and a life that is devoid of quality? Can euthanasia, physician-assisted suicide, or the withholding of treatment be justified based on the quality of a person's life, or must life be preserved without question? Does the same argument apply to all three methods of ending life? How can the tension between the sanctity-of-life principle and the quality-of-life argument be resolved? This chapter presents both religious and secular views, and then suggests an interpretation of the sanctity-of-life principle that does not necessarily lead to a blanket prohibition of physician-assisted suicide. It proposes a golden path between the sanctity of life and the quality of life that reflects the balance struck between the two extreme positions. Doctors and nonprofessionals are already devoting considerable thought to the quality-of-life issue and have come to distinguish between lives with quality and those without it. We argue that life is important, but it is not sacred. Life can be evaluated, but quality of life is not the sole criterion.

It is difficult to draw the line between a life of quality and a life devoid of quality because the concept of quality life is necessarily subjective. The most basic components for determining the quality of life are consciousness, lack of pain and suffering, and human dignity. Does the absence of any of these components mean that life has lost its quality, therefore justifying physician-assisted suicide when the patient finds death the more desirable alternative?

Most people find some meaning in their lives even when they are severely impaired, bedridden, limited in movement, and in constant need of help. Only a small percentage of the patient population asks to die under circumstances of severe illness. These patients are competent adults who have expressed a will to die or who had expressed such a will while they were conscious, before reaching a stage when the quality of their life was diminished, and with a full understanding of the meaning of their request. These patients face a narrow array of alternatives: lives of suffering or unconsciousness, or death. Can death in these cases be preferable to life? The quality-of-life argument is one of several interconnected considerations in decisions regarding physician-assisted suicide. In one such consideration, when patients feel that they are a burden on their loved ones, on the medical staff, or on society at large, this feeling could lower the quality of their lives (see chapter 6).[2]

Is Quality of Life Measurable?

The idea of comparing a specific life with the so-called good life is not at all new. Socrates, Plato, Aristotle, and many others have dealt with it.[3] The issue has become prominent as medical technology has created new options. A request to terminate a life-sustaining treatment assumes that in the given situation, death is preferable to life. These patients differentiate between a good life and a life that is not so good; and in the absence of the good life, some of them prefer to die. The phrase *good life* in this context does not imply a life of luxury but rather a conscious life (or, in the case of PCU patients, potential for a conscious life) that has some meaning for the patient, and that includes more than physical pain or numbness.

In contrast to the quality-of-life argument, the sanctity-of-life principle conceives of human life as sacred and holy and therefore as something not to be harmed. As discussed earlier in the introduction, life in itself is conceived as valuable, regardless of its content. Human value is not determined by subjective or utilitarian criteria. The advocates of this view think that the recognition of the sanctity of life is essential, lest distinctions be made between superior and inferior life, putting some lives in jeopardy.[4]

Those who hold life sacred do not argue for this principle without qualifications. Instead their assertion is that human life must not be harmed without proper justification, meaning that there are cases in which this might be permissible. The clear example is the death penalty, issued to murderers in some liberal societies. The rationale for the death penalty is accepted by many who endorse the sanctity-of-life principle in medicine. Judaism promotes the view that life is sacred while still permitting killing under certain circumstances (i.e., for self-defense). The question, then, is: What is the underlying difference between the two approaches? The advocates of the quality-of-life approach also agree that human life must not be harmed without proper justification.

The difference between the two approaches lies in their justifications for harming human life. According to the sanctity-of-life principle, these justifications are based on defending life itself. A murderer is sentenced to death because he or she took life, and capital punishment is designed to punish the murderer as well as to deter others from committing a similar offense. Under this rationale, capital punishment helps to promote and secure the value of human life. Similarly, killing in self-defense and at times of war is permissible because the purpose is to protect human lives. There is no justification for taking human lives outside the context of protecting life.[5]

On the other hand, the advocates of the quality-of-life argument base their justifications on considerations regarding the content of life, and not on the very fact of living. For instance, preserving the patient's dignity as a human being would be considered a relevant justification for shortening human life by the quality-of-life advocates, but it would not be taken into consideration by the advocates of the sanctity-of-life principle.[6] Life as such is not important. What is important is what we do with our lives. Having a life is a precondition for self-realization, for fulfilling our ambitions, for developing ourselves, advancing our character and personality. Similarly, the body as such is not important. It is merely a capsule, and what is important is the enterprise of body and mind: what we do with our bodies to develop our faculties and enrich ourselves and, inevitably, others.

The Sanctity-of-Life View: Life Cannot
Be Evaluated

Monotheistic religions uphold the sanctity-of-life principle. God created life and death, and we must not take His place.[7] The Christian church, particularly after St. Augustine, advocated absolute respect for the sanctity of human life and condemned suicide under all circumstances.[8] Theologians have seldom challenged the Christian tradition condemning medical assistance or action that is intended to end life. Earlier this century a few church leaders in Britain, such as Dean Inge and W. R. Matthews, did challenge it, as did Joseph Fletcher in the United States. They were exceptions, however. For most church leaders and theologians the tradition was intact, and voices challenging it inside and outside church institutions were unusual. It was widely argued that it was not a proper or appropriate role for medical staff to end human life that had been given and sanctified by God. The proper role for medical staff was to save life and not to destroy it.[9]

The Christian tradition emphasizes these guidelines:

1. Life is a God-given gift. It is given to people "in trust." Hence people do not own their lives. Life is a gift over which we are to exercise stewardship, not dominion. That stewardship demands that we be responsible for life—its protection and enhancement. We will in turn be held accountable before the Creator not only for how we protected and developed our individual lives, but for all life. We cannot do with our lives as we will.[10] As the Sacred Congregation for the Doctrine of the Faith wrote in the Vatican Declaration on Euthanasia: "Most people regard life as something sacred and hold that no one may dispose of it at will, but believers see in life something greater, namely a gift of God's love, which they are called upon to preserve and make fruitful."[11]

2. All human life is equal, because every human creature is a creation of God.[12]

3. Because God created human life, even the most miserable of lives is worth living.[13]

4. Life itself is holy. God granted the respect, value, and sanctity of the human being to people, and they are not subject to human measurement. Life is not sacred because of something it includes, because of its content; rather, life is sacred because God created it: God is holy, and He has sanctified life. Human life has worth because Christ died to redeem it, and it has meaning because God has eternal purpose for it.[14]

5. The life that God gives human beings is quite different from the life

of all other living creatures, inasmuch as we, although formed from the dust of the earth, are a manifestation of God in the world, a sign of His presence, a trace of His glory. We have been given a sublime dignity based on the intimate bond that unites us with our Creator: In us there shines forth a reflection of God Himself. Life is the Lord's image and imprint, a sharing in His breath of life.[15]

6. Life is indelibly marked by the truth of its own. By accepting God's gift, we are obliged to maintain life in this truth, which is essential to it. To detach ourselves from this truth is to condemn ourselves to meaninglessness and unhappiness, and possibly to become a threat to the existence of others, as the barriers guaranteeing respect for life and the defense of life, in every circumstance, have been broken down.[16]

7. People must not "play God" by determining when someone should die.

From a secular point of view, it is difficult to argue with religious approaches, because matters of belief do not necessarily involve logical reasoning. Belief in the existence of God leads people to accept God as part of reality. As Nathan Rotenstreich observed: "Holiness is a matter of belief. Belief does not demand explanations. It anchors people and the world, and the unknown is another separate aspect. Using holiness to describe life is not an explanation but a fortification."[17] In the face of the glorified term *sanctity*, it is difficult to juxtapose the competing secular concepts: autonomy, human dignity, and quality of life. Despite this difficulty, there are possible answers to the religious arguments, especially regarding those holding that we must not play God, and that people are God's possessions and therefore have no control over their deaths.

There are many similarities between the Christian and the Jewish points of view. Both Judaism and Christianity affirm creation as the necessary background for their respective revelations. Both share beliefs about the sanctity of human life, the integrity of the family, and the right to a variety of individual and cooperative achievements. One of the basic theological affirmations that is shared by the Jewish and Christian ethical traditions is that persons are created by God for the primary purpose of being related to God.[18] The notion of a person includes not only the soul, spirit, and cognitive and intellectual capacities, but also a living body. Human life is intrinsically good and valuable, and society is obliged to respect a living body irrespective of the person's cognitive capacities.[19] These intrinsic values do not imply interests. Life is intrinsically valuable, without regard to a person's interests. In this view, taking one's life, alone or with the help of others, is considered to be wrong in itself. Even if people have deliberately chosen to die, it is nevertheless bad for them to do so. Euthanasia is conceived as an insult to the sanctity of human life. It is also an insult to God, usurping His authority.

There is a code of Jewish law dealing with this issue. It is important to note that although I have great respect for the integrity of the Orthodox tradition, I nevertheless join the views of the Conservative and the Reform movements in Judaism that Jewish law (*halacha*) would benefit from some accommodations and qualifications, as a response required by modern life.

In Judaism, the basis for the value of the life of every individual is that human beings were created in God's image.[20] Therefore people must not be differentiated from one another according to any perceived value of their lives. We must not harm the godly image of our fellows, and we must not harm our own godly image. The value of human life is immeasurable, and the sanctity of life overshadows all other considerations.[21] Life is not relative to something else; nor can it be equated to another life. Consequently, the value of seventy years is equal to the value of one second, and the value of a sick person's life is equal to that of a healthy one. As soon as we agree on any relative criterion upon which we may evaluate life, a dangerous distinction may be drawn between inferior and superior people. If we accept the presumption that we must not take lives, then this presumption applies to seconds and minutes as well. By this principle, it is impossible to agree on criteria for the taking of lives.[22]

A Talmudic passage regarding the creation of Adam appears in the Sanhedrin religious tractate: "Therefore only a single human being was created in the world, to teach that if any person has caused a single soul to perish, Scripture regards him as if he had caused an entire world to perish; and if any human being saves a single soul, Scripture regards him as if he had saved an entire world."[23] Human life is not a good thing to be preserved as a condition of other values but must be preserved as an absolute. The obligation to preserve life is commensurately all-encompassing.[24]

According to the Jewish tradition, the very existence of a person, his or her essence as a human being, is a natural fact that does not depend on any human evaluation or social institution. This principle is valid and should not be questioned. Once we start to question it, we undermine its validity. Hence, halacha holds that we should conceive of the dying person exactly in the same way as we conceive of any other person.

Jewish law distinguishes between two kinds of patients who are doomed to die shortly (*morituri* in Latin): the moribund, or *gossess*, who

are already dying; and the incurable, or *tereifa*, who suffer from lacera-
tion of a vital organ or any other lethal injury, but in whom the process
of death has not yet set in. Elaborate rules have been enumerated to prohibit active intervention in the process of death of the gossess. We must
not take any actions that might hasten someone's death even if we are
certain that death is near, even if the person has only minutes left to
live, and even if our intention is in the person's best interest.[25] We may
not wash or anoint the person, or pry open the jaws or plug any ori-
fices, or remove pillows from underneath the person, or lay the person
on the ground or on sand or salt, or put anything on the abdomen—all
actions supposedly calculated to hasten death.[26] Nor may we close the
person's eyes: Closing the eyes of a dying person is like putting one's
finger in a flickering flame—the touch of the finger will extinguish it.
Rabbi Meir said: "It is like a dripping candle, if a man touches it—the
candle is snuffed. So is the case when you are making an effort to close
the eyes of a dying patient; it is as if you take his soul."[27] According to
the halachic view, even the dripping candle burns; even the dripping
candle is capable of shedding light.[28]

No such rules were enunciated with respect to the tereifa, but we
can infer from the discussion on the gossess that if it is prohibited to
do any act that may shorten life even only by a few minutes, it must
surely be prohibited to do any act by which life may be shortened by a
longer period. Even in regard to the gossess, however, the prohibition
applies only to active intervention; it is not forbidden to cause the hastening of death by abstaining from any intervention. The reason is that
the soul of the dying person must be presumed to be desirous of leaving the body, and one must not impede its departure. In other words, as
one ought not to do anything to hasten death, one need not and may
not do anything to delay the due completion of the death process.[29]

In halacha, several other principles teach us not to take life:

1. People do not own their bodies, so they are not permitted to harm
   themselves. The body was given to a person "in trust" in order to
   fulfill certain tasks and missions defined by the commandments of
   the Bible. This trust should not be harmed in any way.[30] The human soul is a godly possession.
2. There is merit in the very existence of a human life in any form and
   under any circumstances. There is always a possibility for further
   spiritual elevation. The patient has a moral obligation not to give
   up, but to continue hoping. The continuation of life might make it
   possible to gain complete redemption.[31]
3. We must recognize that there are things beyond our understanding:

The assumption is that a person's suffering is the will of God, and the taking of his or her life constitutes a rebellion against His will. "This is His wish, Blessed be He": God gives each of us what we deserve on the basis of our actions. A person who died an "easy" death without suffering might suffer greatly in the next world, whereas another person who suffered severely from a prolonged disease might be rewarded in Heaven. Alternatively, maybe someone who experienced a pleasant death has more "rights" in this world. Rabbi Halevi further explained: "If we conceive of the soul as a being that existed before entering this body, and a being that will exist after departing from this body, and if we bear in mind that we do not know why the soul came into the world at all, what it supplements in this body, what awaits it in that world, what value has every hour and minute spent in this body (these are the mysteries of the soul and its puzzles), then it is easier for us to understand why it is forbidden to bring closer, even one minute closer, the parting of the soul from this world."[32]

As Maimonides declared categorically: "The killing of any person, whether healthy, mortally sick, or even in the final throes of death is an act punishable by death."[33]

A contemporary prominent philosopher and Orthodox thinker, Yeshayahu Leibowitz, argues that life as such is sacred. It is sacred not because of its history, or its biography, or because it constitutes an enterprise of body and spirit. Human life is sacred because it is produced by God. Leibowitz contends that human existence is a natural fact. This is the meaning of the contention in Pirkei Avot (Sayings of the Fathers): "Against your will you have been created; against your will you are born; against your will you are alive." Because the existence of a person is a natural fact, not an institutional product, conceptions of right, duty, or prohibition are meaningless and invalid, irrelevant regarding natural things. The sky, the earth, and all that exists in them are part of reality, beyond these legal conceptions. They exist because they exist, not because we grant them some value. Human beings are part of this natural reality, and one should not question their existence. Certain principles are of immense importance and validity as long as we do not question them. When we start to doubt their meaning, we nullify them. Leibowitz maintains that the right of persons to live is not a rational principle. Because human life is something that cannot be rationalized, we cannot determine boundaries to life. The postulate "Do not take human life" is an absolute that cannot be rationalized. We should never question its validity and try to qualify it.[34]

Several criticisms of Leibowitz's claim may be advanced: First, the fact that life is a constitutive element within a given reality does not imply that it is impossible to interfere with this reality or to change it. Second, Leibowitz claims that objects, plant life, and animals also are part of this reality, and they could be harmed unless the judicial system prevents it. The question then arises: Why can we not end human life if, as Leibowitz holds, life as such does not have a rational base but rather is protected by a moral postulate that we took upon ourselves?[35] If the prohibition on the taking of lives is accepted as part of some sort of social pact that includes human moral rules, it is not clear why we cannot change the moral postulate. After all, a moral postulate is not a natural reality, but rather an institutional reality. Moreover, the postulate is not absolute, because it is violated at certain times (war) and toward certain groups (criminals in certain countries) as a policy.

A principle in Judaism that prima facie contradicts all that has been stated until now is that of consideration of sorrow and human suffering. The term *pleasant death* is Talmudic, referring not to euthanasia but to the mercy shown at the time of death.[36] There is a conflict in halacha between its principles regarding the sanctity of life, their importance and endless value, the great merit embodied in life itself, and the duty of doctors and other people to preserve and nurture the life entrusted to them by God, and the principle of striving to ease pain and diminish all suffering.

Several answers are presented to answer this conflict. While active euthanasia is strictly prohibited, withholding and withdrawing treatment (passive euthanasia) is allowed under certain circumstances (for a fuller account of these concepts in the medical ethics discourse, see chapter 4). Although we should abstain from taking measures that impede the departure of the soul from the body, it is permitted, for example, to take a grain of salt from the tongue of a dying person, so as not to prolong the suffering; it is prohibited to cut trees near the house of a dying person, so that the noise will not disturb the departure of the soul.[37] The conclusion is that the balance in halacha is between the sanctity of life and the suffering and pain of the patient. A balance must be struck even if the patient's mind or body is impaired, such as when he or she suffers from paralysis or unawareness.[38]

Several comments regarding the halachic stance are pertinent. First, the assumption that the value of life is immeasurable is debatable. There are cases, even according to halacha, in which other values exceed the value of life, not only when the justification is the preservation of human life. For instance, the value of minimizing suffering and pain might outweigh the value of life, or the biblical commandment to "wipe out the memory of Amalek."[39] So the prohibition on taking lives is not absolute, and the value of life can be measured against other considerations.

Second, regarding the dripping-candle argument, there are cases in which its assumption is incorrect. A "shining life" is a life consisting of more than biological functioning. The halachic scholars did not refer to, nor did they pretend to represent, the subjective viewpoint of the patient with regard to his or her life. In doing so, halacha ignored the will of the patient. The *Cruzan* case is a pertinent example.[40] As a result of a traffic accident, Nancy Cruzan suffered from irreversible, permanent, and progressive cerebral cortical atrophy of the brain. Prior to the accident, Cruzan expressed the opinion that "she would not wish to continue living if she couldn't be at least halfway normal." It was maintained that her lifestyle and other statements to family and friends suggested that "she would not wish to continue her present existence without hope as it is."[41] Cruzan's family and friends asserted that her prior statements and everything they knew of her convinced them that she would not want continued life support, including nutrition and hydration. Thus, it is difficult to understand how it is possible to speak of Cruzan in terms of "a shining candle." The doctors and Cruzan's relatives did not think of the body sustained by mechanical means as a shining candle, and we can assume that Nancy Cruzan herself would not have described her situation in such terms. These are subjective conceptions and, indeed, the criticism of the halachic perspective is that it ignores the subjective opinions of the patients and their families when they feel that the candle has ceased to burn and shine (the *Cruzan* case is further discussed in chapter 5).

Third, concerning the idea that human life has been entrusted to us by God: When a patient's life is prolonged artificially, when the patient's existence depends on machinery, we meddle with the will of God, we "play God," and interfere with the "gift." Without such machines, the patients would have returned their souls to the creator. The words of Rabbi Haim David Halevi support this opinion. According to him, when the patient is connected to a ventilator and no longer feels a thing, he must be disconnected from the machine for his soul, which belongs to God, has already been taken back by God; as soon as the machine is removed he will die: "And by continuing to resuscitate artificially we keep the soul in him and cause it (the soul, not the patient) grief since it cannot part and return to its peace."[42]

This opinion is somewhat problematic because it assumes that the taking of the soul has already taken place. The acceptance of this opinion would have ramifications on many other actions of modern medicine. For example, someone in need of dialysis, or someone who has a pacemaker implanted, theoretically should not be kept alive artificially, because as soon as the machines are removed, the patient will die. Therefore we must not go as far as Rabbi Halevi, who claims that the soul has already been taken. Plainly stated, the proscription against playing God loses its validity, because in many instances doctors most certainly do interfere with natural processes. In this context we can distinguish between giving (or granting) the soul, and preserving the soul. It could be argued that God is the giver and the taker of the soul. But the role of preservation of the soul was given to people, to doctors. Disconnection from a life-support system is therefore forbidden by religious authorities because it is conceived as a preliminary step to the exit of the soul; but installing a pacemaker in someone's body is an example of an act of preservation that does not take God's place.

Concerning the belief that people are the possessions of God, a belief prevalent in other religions as well, Noam Zohar claims that people are considered "the possession of God" only in the context of mercy killings, because this statement has nothing to do with other meanings of ownership. For instance, there are no similar claims over the control and possession of human assets.[43] Zohar further explains that it is possible to understand possession and ownership in terms of sovereignty and authority. It is possible to claim that a person is the possession of God in the sense that he or she is within His authority, meaning subordinate to Him and required to obey Him. A person's aspiration to determine his or her own time of death could accordingly be understood as a private case of mutiny against God's authority. Just as people must obey God throughout their lifetime, so must they accept godly control over their time of death. The problem, argues Zohar, is that this unqualified claim is valid only if we assume that subordination to godly authority requires total human passivity. In other words, people must do nothing regarding their own lives, and among other things they must not take their lives. But this assumption is absurd. Subordination to godly sovereignty means not abstaining from any action but accommodating the actions to the will of God, who wants us to perform certain actions and forbids others. If so, is it clear that the termination of life-prolonging treatment when the patient wishes to be redeemed from suffering is contradictory to the will of God? Zohar claims that in the traditional Talmudic framework, it is possible to accept the sovereignty of God without concluding that actions that prevent or shorten the suffering of a dying person are necessarily contradictory to His will.[44]

This discussion concerns not only physical torment, but also spiritual torment, including psychological suffering caused by loss of autonomy and self-control, loss of human dignity, and the degradation and humiliation that cause patients to feel their lives are continuing against their will. Often it seems that religious deliberations are not sufficiently mindful of mental distress.

Even if the religious doctrines are not accepted today as they were in the past, the ethical questions they raise still affect secular thought. Many secular people believe in the sanctity of life. Although secular approaches consider principles such as respect and sanctity as intrinsic to people, neither depending on God nor created by Him, there are many similarities between the religious and secular approaches. The sense of great respect for life is emphasized in both approaches. They share the belief that life is a great thing: amazing, majestic, respectable, mysterious, and, therefore, worthy of being protected. The religious and secular approaches also share the assumption that the sanctity-of-life principle, at least in general, is the basis and the starting point for every medical decision.[45] Many secular individuals accept the idea that people should not "play God." The sanctity-of-life principle's deep roots are evident in the rationale for forbidding legislation allowing euthanasia.[46] Courts speak of the interest of the state in preserving life. The majority opinion in the *Cruzan* case asserted that the state may properly decline to make judgments about the quality of life that a particular individual may enjoy, and simply assert "an unqualified interest in the preservation of human life" to be weighed against the constitutionally protected interests of the individual.[47]

The vitalist approaches interpret the sanctity-of-life principle in the most meticulous and ostensible manner. According to the vitalist interpretation, the principle means that from the moment human life is created, it is our duty to preserve it. When we are confronted with deciding the fate of a patient who asks to terminate treatment, the sanctity-of-life principle is not merely one of several considerations; it is the only and final consideration. Therefore, quality-of-life considerations are of no significance.[48] Jewish theologians are not vitalists, although they believe that life has absolute value, because one is not obligated to undertake heroic measures to prolong the life of a patient. Vitalism becomes medically problematic when it insists on aggressive treatment to prolong the life of a dying patient and on continuing physical life without respect for the patient's biological, psychological, spiritual, or social prognosis. This approach is also called biologism, a concern only for the bodily life of the patient.[49]

Many people in the religious and secular communities believe that life is not subject to rationalization. Secular approaches that believe in the sanctity-of-life principle base their reasoning on the belief that life has intrinsic value, that harming life may cause anarchy and undermine world order, that life could be harmed only if weighty justifications are found. As a general rule, we must keep and preserve human life. This belief does not necessarily have a rational basis. Rather it is a natural feeling about the order of things as they should be.

The quality-of-life approach holds that life can be evaluated. Consequently, it is possible to determine that, under certain circumstances, some lives are not worth prolonging.

The Quality-of-Life View: Life Can Be Evaluated

The adoption of the intrinsic-value view leads to a single stance: We should do our utmost to safeguard and to save life. We are obliged to think of life in terms of intrinsic value, not in terms of the magnitude of the loss. Thus some people object to the idea of abortion, under all circumstances, and no matter in what stage of pregnancy it is contemplated. The claim that life has an intrinsic value implies that killing is wrong in itself. The argument here bears some similarity to the argument used to promote art: Art is a good thing; therefore, we want to bring it into existence. Life is a good thing; therefore, we want to bring it into existence. And we should not destroy either (for further discussion, see chapter 5).

However, people do refer to the magnitude of the loss when someone dies, and when a piece of art is destroyed. With regard to human life, the general feeling is that, on the whole, it is a sad thing when a fetus is miscarried or aborted. It is worse to have a late abortion than an early one. It is worse to die in infancy than to have an abortion. Many also feel it is worse to die in adolescence than to die in infancy or in old age.[50] Here we speak only in terms of comparison. The general feeling is that for a person to die when she begins her course of life, starts to make plans, establishes contacts with family and friends, begins to see the results of her deeds, is a worse thing than dying as an infant, or as an old person who achieved something in her life.

Thus people are constantly evaluating life, even if they do it subconsciously or by intuition. People do it in present terms, in past terms, and in future terms. For instance, when a person dies, people ponder various considerations in evaluating his or her life. They see importance not only in whether he or she was old or young, an adult or a child; they also ponder whether the person lived alone or with a family, whether death came swiftly or salvaged the person from misery; whether the person "died proud," with dignity; what that person accomplished in life; to what extent the person actualized his or her potential, and many similar questions. Why are these questions important, and why do they affect the way we conceive of death? Perhaps because we ask ourselves what that person lost with death.

Roy Perrett pushes the issue further by arguing that it is morally permissible to put a price on a person's life, and that there is a theoretically adequate way of determining such a price.[51] He maintains that the value of a person's life has two components: its personal value, its value for the person whose life it is, and its social value, its value for others: "Thus the total value of a person's life is the sum of its personal and social values."[52] Perrett explains that the personal value of life is concerned with the happiness of the life, and the pursuit or accomplishment of the person's objectives, whereas the social value of life involves the emotional and psychological value that a person's life has for others, the economic value of a person's life to others, and the recognition that the lives of some special individuals have a personal service value.

Ranking lives in accordance with their social value is a dangerous policy that could increase existing inequalities in society, could serve the best interests of the elite, and could discriminate against so-called common people. We may speak of the subjective value of a given life in accordance with how the person who leads that life appraises it. All considerations of the social value of life and of supposedly objective utilitarian rankings of life should be excluded from medical decision-making processes.

Helga Kuhse and Peter Singer are among those who assert that life can be evaluated and that we can compare lives.[53] They rightly argue that a conscious life is preferable to an unconscious life,[54] and that people do make moral judgments when they refer to a specific life and sometimes compare it with other lives. In their opinion, those who speak of the sanctity of life do not really mean that all kinds of life are sacred and are of the same value; rather, they mean that human life, as opposed to that of a sheep or a head of lettuce, is sacred.[55] In other words, different types of life are judged differently. By explaining the basis for the different judgment between human life and other kinds of life, Kuhse and Singer reach the conclusion that a moral judgment regarding the quality of human life is possible. Thus, for instance, most people would agree that the life of a mature, autonomous, and healthy person is of higher quality than the life of an infant who is born anencephalic, without most of a brain. Kuhse maintains that it is morally proper for parents, in consultation with their doctor, to decide that their disabled infant should not live. It is unacceptable that societies continue to pay lip service to the sanctity-of-life view while practicing a quality-of-life approach.[56] Kuhse and Singer offer two possible answers in response to the question of what gives value to human life:

1. A human life is sacred because it is a life of a creature that belongs to *Homo sapiens*. It is clear that this definition includes all humans. But in Kuhse and Singer's opinion, the fact that a creature belongs to *Homo sapiens* and not to another species does not say a thing about the value of that creature's life. The value of human life should not be based on the view that human life has a special value simply because it is a human life. Giving preference to the life of a being simply because that being is a member of our species would put us in the same position as racists who give preference to those who are members of their own group.[57] Belonging to a particular species is not important in itself; what is important is the quality and nature of the creature's life. The same principle applies in medical decisions: What is important is the quality of the patient's life (a life of pleasure as opposed to a life of suffering) and the kind of life (a life of an adult as opposed to that of a baby or a fetus).[58]
2. Human life has special value because people are rational creatures, self-conscious, autonomous, moral beings, who have ideals, goals, ambitions, and many other qualities that make them persons.[59] Each one of these qualities (or a combination thereof) could serve as a basis for a moral distinction between persons and other creatures. For if the value of life were based on mere biological life, the life of a head of lettuce would be equal to that of a person.

In *Practical Ethics*, Peter Singer addresses the question of whether we can accept the idea of ordering the value of different lives.[60] Singer assumes a hypothetical neutral ground in which a person could choose between being a horse and being a human, when it is known to that person what being a horse is composed of (as far as the horse is concerned, with the consciousness of a horse, etc.), and what being a human is all about (from a human perspective). This choice is actually an evaluation of the life of a horse against the life of a person. Singer concedes that there are comparisons that are difficult to draw, such as whether it would be better to be a fish or a snake. But in general it seems that the more highly developed the conscious life of the being, the greater the self-awareness and rationality, and the more one would prefer that kind of life. He maintains that if it is true that we are capable of understanding a choice between two forms of life, then we can understand the idea of one form of life having greater value than another form of life. So, in effect, Singer admits that it would not necessarily be "speciesist" to rank the value of different lives in some hierarchical order.[61]

Kuhse and Singer hold that it is reasonable to say that the life of a rational conscious creature is of greater value than the life of a creature lacking those characteristics. If we accept this view, we are saying not that human life is sanctified, but that we must examine whether human life has been blessed with rationalism, consciousness, and desires.[62] They also emphasize the sanctity of a spiritual life, as opposed to a physical life, and in doing so they are giving another interpretation to the sanctity-of-life principle.

Some scholars have tried to establish that there are different levels of concern for humans and nonhumans. For instance, R. S. Downie and Elizabeth Telfer acknowledge three such levels. On the lowest level are the animals that are regarded as having a presumptive right not to suffer.[63] Next we have, in Downie and Telfer's terminology, "sub-normal" humans who are not accorded full respect but are not treated as animals either. Downie and Telfer have made a shift from concern to respect, as if both terms have the same meaning, which is false (see the introduction of this book). They say that we can distinguish three levels of concern but then continue speaking of respect. Downie and Telfer maintain that it is not meaningful to attribute to infants, the severely mentally ill, the senile, and those in terminal coma a capacity for self-determination. Finally, there are the normal humans who are accorded full respect, and they are called persons.[64]

Downie and Telfer assert that what makes people worthy of respect is their capacity for self-determination and for the adoption of ideals.[65] When certain capacities are lacking or cease to exist, people are no longer worthy of full respect. On this issue, Downie and Telfer's view comes close to that of Joseph Fletcher, Helga Kuhse, and Peter Singer.

Fletcher has listed fifteen "indicators of humanhood." His list includes such attributes as self-awareness, self-control, a sense of the future, a sense of the past, the capacity to relate to others, communication, curiosity, and minimal intelligence.[66] According to his view, it is questionable whether anyone with an IQ below forty is a person, and he does not consider anyone with an IQ below twenty a person. But even if an infant does qualify as a person according to this checklist, taking the infant's life may still be justified in some situations, taking into account not only the good of the child in question, but also the family's economic resources and the welfare of other children involved, as well as the parents' physical and emotional capacity to cope. Therefore, physicians should have only a qualified respect for human life.[67]

Kuhse and Singer accept Fletcher's reasoning and further maintain that it is "entirely reasonable to suggest that it is much more serious to take the life of a being possessing all or most of these characteristics than it would be to take the life of a being possessing none of them."[68] This is a questionable position. What makes people worthy of respect is their humanness, the fact that people are people, whether or not they have a capacity for self-determination, adoption of ideals, curiosity, or a sense of the future. When human life begins, it is important that it will continue with dignity and with respect. We give people respect because we value life as such, in itself.[69] Is killing a retarded person less serious than killing a person of greater intelligence? Certainly not. It constitutes a more serious offense, because the killer is taking advantage of the deficiencies of a person who is unable to defend herself/himself. Defenseless individuals need more concern, not less. This is not to endorse the sanctity-of-life approach, or to leave no place for physician-assisted suicide in a liberal society. We may start to question the quality of human life when, for instance, our lives are saturated with incurable suffering and pain. In such circumstances the underlying assumption that existence is better than nonexistence is questionable. We may think that it is in our best interest to opt for death because life is no longer an attractive option. When life becomes a burden for the patient, some patients are no longer sure it possesses any meaning or value (see conclusions).

Downie and Telfer connect capacity for self-determination to the notion of respect. A direct connection of the kind that they suggest exists between self-determination and self-rule, but the criterion of capacity for self-determination should not decide how much respect a person should be accorded. Those who lack self-determination may need the advice, support, and assistance of others, but they should not be accorded less respect. These persons may be accorded different kinds of respect and concern, involving more compassionate elements, but not less respect, as Downie and Telfer argue. Gross paternalism is inappropriate when rational persons are considered, but more acceptable when our concern lies with mentally retarded persons or with children.[70] People deserve the same respect—to be seen as ends, rather than means, whatever their capacity for rational decision-making may be. They deserve more concern when this capacity is lacking.

The notions of respect and concern are in the foci of Paragraph 9 of the regulations issued in 1974 by the U.S. Department of Health, Education, and Welfare for skilled nursing facilities. It holds that each patient is to be treated "with consideration, respect, and full recognition of his dignity and individuality, including privacy in treatment and in care for his personal needs."[71] This document regards human beings as ends rather than means and does not speak of different kinds of respect to be accorded to different patients depending on their existing capacities. Liberal democracies have a duty to protect weak third parties, especially minors.[72]

In light of this document and of the generally accepted duty to protect the weak, Kuhse and Singer's views on infants are most disturbing.
They argue that "nothing in the views we express in this book in any
way implies a lack of concern for disabled people in our community.
On the contrary, it is our view that affluent nations should be spending
far more than they presently allocate to assist disabled people to live
fulfilling, worthwhile lives, and to enable people with disabilities to develop their potential to the utmost."[73] How should this statement be
reconciled with Kuhse and Singer's statement regarding human characteristics? ("It is entirely reasonable to suggest that it is much more serious to take the life of a being possessing all or most of these characteristics
than it would be to take the life of a being possessing none of them.")

Furthermore, immediately after making the humane statement that
it is appropriate to care for disabled people, they qualify their statement
by saying that their discussion refers only to disabled infants. They seem
to try to dehumanize such infants, and they do it by arguing more generally that infants have no right to life.[74] But surely, if certain disabled
infants were killed, there would be fewer disabled adults in society, so,
in a way, their prescription is designed to decrease the number of disabled individuals and thus enable society to allocate the same (or more)
resources to less afflicted people. Only those who became disabled at a
later stage in life would get better treatment.[75]

Kuhse and Singer employ an interesting method to convince their
readers of the merits of their disturbing suggestions. They submit even
more radical and shocking propositions, and in comparison, their thesis sounds almost bearable. Alternatively, they offer outrageous positions,
then say they do not endorse them (so why bring them up at all?), only
later to qualify them, or further say that these positions are as senseless
as the one endorsing sanctity of human life. This methodology is especially evident in their discussion of infanticide.[76] Kuhse and Singer explain that they decided to dedicate a chapter to infanticide in order to
see "how other cultures would handle the problems" that they discuss;
to obtain "a broader, less culturally-bound perspective on these problems"; and to gain "a better grasp of the historical framework within
which these issues continue to be discussed."[77] They find that most cross-
cultural studies of non-Western societies show that "the majority accepted
infanticide in at least some circumstances."[78] This survey also shows
that "infanticide is compatible with a stable, well-organized human society,"[79] as if this is the prime aim of Western societies, to maintain sta-
bility and organization. There are few, if any, feelings of compassion and
mercy in this utilitarian, cold, detached, and most troubling discussion.[80]

Kuhse and Singer quote the geneticist J. V. Neel, who argued that because infanticide is much easier to carry out and requires a considerably less sophisticated understanding of human reproduction than abstinence, contraception, or abortion, we first became "truly human" when we began deliberately killing our children. In response, Kuhse and Singer write, "We do not endorse Neel's suggestion, but it is no more far-fetched than the idea that belief in the sanctity of all innocent human life is a prerequisite for any civilized society."[81]

The discussion offers the reader food for thought on the issue of infanticide, if not its legitimacy. Kuhse and Singer do not question the argument in favor of infanticide; they fail to discuss the hypothesis that infanticide might become an almost too easy solution that would contribute to irresponsibility on the part of parents to bring babies to this world. In a world where infanticide would be legal, what would prevent parents who are told there is a 90 percent chance their newborn will have a serious genetic disease from bringing children into the world, knowing they could just throw away the damaged babies? Should we allow this gambling? Should we allow them to destroy one, two, three, or more babies, and continue to gamble until they achieve the right result? Moreover, women who become ill with diseases that might put their fetus at risk will opt for continuation of the pregnancy, knowing that infanticide is an option if something goes wrong. Is this a moral option? Parents could relieve themselves from taking responsibility for and caring about the consequences of their decisions.

Unlike Kuhse and Singer, we have no qualms about describing ourselves as "speciesists," as people who think first of all of our own species, the human race. The very birth of human life is morally significant, something of great importance.[82] Contrary to their view, we think that newborn infants do have a right to life merely because they are human and have emerged from the womb.[83] This humane natural affinity is shared by many people who adhere to the Kantian notion of perceiving human beings as ends in themselves. It is only a humane and preferable inclination to think first about our fellow humans. It is also natural for an elephant to think first and foremost about its fellow elephants. This view is very different from that of Kuhse and Singer, who differentiate between babies and persons and hence do not recognize the babies' natural right to life simply because they are human. The very title of their book, *Should the Baby Live?*, is highly provocative, problematic, and offensive, although they apparently have no qualms about it. From their point of view, babies are more similar to fetuses than to people and, therefore, it is not directly wrong to end the lives of babies with birth defects.[84]

According to Kuhse and Singer, the life of a brain-damaged baby, or indeed, of normal healthy babies,[85] or the lives of PCU patients are not comparable to the life of an autonomous, conscious person. In Singer's eyes, killing a chimpanzee, an animal with "human" qualities, is a more serious act than killing a person who, for reasons of intellectual defects, lacks these characteristics.[86]

We reject these claims completely. We do not accept the notion that any person whose mind stopped functioning is equivalent to a head of lettuce. Saying such a thing is a terrible blow to human dignity. A woman born with a mental defect could undergo certain experiences, and as a person she is an entity with meaning to her loved ones. It is possible that her life has meaning, taste, and quality, even if a bystander does not recognize it. Treating her as a person rather than a vegetable could possibly improve her condition. Furthermore, although a life consisting of physical function alone is devoid of quality, it is not logical to conclude, as Singer does, that killing a person in this condition is comparable to "killing" a head of lettuce. A person could have a family and friends who care greatly for her, regardless of her condition. Most of the population, unlike Singer, accords enormous value to human life, much greater value than is accorded to heads of lettuce or sheep. The fact that most people appreciate human life more than plant life or animal life does not necessarily stem from the two possibilities listed by Kuhse and Singer—belonging to *Homo sapiens* or possessing mental capacities. Religious people see human beings as created in God's image, unlike animals and plants, and for them this is the source for the special value of human life.

Kuhse and Singer represent the most radical view within the quality-of-life approach. It is possible to be much more cautious: Quality of life is an important consideration, but it is not all there is. On the other hand, life as such does not have absolute value. We were not asked whether or not we want to be born, but from the moment when we are able to make decisions regarding our health care, we should be free to do as we wish with our lives, including forgoing life when we feel that it is a life we no longer wish to lead. With this proviso in mind, the starting point in pertinent medical discussions should be the sanctity of life: Life has great value; it should be respected and preserved, but there are cases in which another value might exceed it in importance. When, for instance, it is asked that a ventilator be withdrawn, the claim is that the ventilator is burdensome. We agree with the words of Judge Uri Goren in the *Eyal* case: "This important 'sanctity-of-life' principle is limited to cases in which it is in the power of medical care to save a life or to better the medical condition of a patient. When doctors' actions cannot help to heal the patient and cannot improve or even stabilize his (or her) condition—the 'sanctity-of-life' principle is no longer so holy."[87] (For further discussion on the *Eyal* case, see conclusions.)

The state's interest in preserving life is meaningful, but it is not absolute. In certain cases it is possible to evaluate life and to determine that a certain characteristic could make it better or worse in comparison with other lives. The Kantian view that conceives of people as ends rather than means leads to the conclusion that life is not sanctified when the continuation of life harms human dignity and contradicts the patient's best interests.

Scales for Measuring Qualitative Life

Which components of human life, when they are lacking, take the quality out of life? Critics might argue that in the absence of information about existence after death, it is never possible to claim that death is preferable to life, even if it is an extremely difficult life. Despite the difficulty of evaluating life without being able to evaluate "non-life," it is possible to examine the meanings attached to life and the elements that make people think that the unknown afterlife is a better alternative than the existing life.

A "good life" is conceptually distinct from mere biological life. Many think that a life of biological existence alone does not encompass the full meaning of life. Ronald Dworkin claims that there is no point in continuing to live when only a body remains, without autonomy and spirit.[88] Although it is easy to sympathize with such an opinion, making an objective determination of when life loses its quality altogether is problematic. There are those who think—like John Finnis—that the body itself is valuable, even if it is devoid of mental capacities. No consideration should serve as a trump card to override the intrinsic right to life (see chapter 5).

Disagreements on this issue are not confined to philosophers. Physicians, jurists, judges, and laypeople hold various views. However, courts are often asked to decide on matters of life and death. In this context, Justice Antonin Scalia expressed the opinion in the *Cruzan* case that nine Supreme Court judges are no more competent to determine at what point life becomes "worthless" than any nine people, randomly chosen out of a phone book, would be.[89] It may not be possible to speak of a general and objective criterion for quality of life. The question of whether there is a point to life or a point to a certain kind of life does not have a single answer that would satisfy all people. Most patients opt to fight for every further moment of life. At times it is more than a will; it is a living instinct.

Given that *quality of life* is a subjective term, there is no point in asking what the boundaries of quality are. And here is where the importance of the will of the patient comes in: Did that subject of life express his or her will, explicit or implicit, that under certain circumstances he or she would rather die? Patients who have expressed a will to die at a point when they were mentally competent to do so are the subjects of this discussion.

There are three fundamental elements in determining quality of life: consciousness, lack of suffering, and dignity. To what extent could lack of these cause lives to be devoid of quality? There is no sharp distinction among these elements, and at times the differences between them are blurred. For example, if we include emotional suffering in the element of suffering, it could connect to dignity as well: A feeling of lack of human dignity leads to emotional suffering. Experiencing great suffering that takes over the patient's being is almost like losing consciousness. It is important to remember that there could be different extents and degrees of suffering, dependence, and so on, and each patient has a different chance of recovery.

These three components—consciousness, lack of suffering, and dignity—are interconnected, and together compose the quality of life. The relative part of each and the importance of each element in the whole quality of life could differ from one person to another. Although some may claim that it is necessary for all three components to exist in order for it to be a life of quality, others would claim that partial existence or certain degrees suffice. Those who oppose euthanasia and physician-assisted suicide may claim that when patients ask to die, the very fact that they can express themselves, communicate, and formulate a request implies that they are aware of their state and understand its meaning for them; therefore, their wish must not be granted because the element of consciousness exists in these patients' lives, and their lives contain some quality. This claim does not respect the will of the patient and ignores the fact that consciousness is only one of the components of quality life. If a person is aware of his or her condition and is able to communicate, yet life is saturated with continuous suffering and the patient regards this situation as harmful, as contradictory to his or her dignity, then from this patient's perspective consciousness might not be enough to justify continuing to live.

Consciousness

Consciousness includes the following mental qualities: awareness, the ability to communicate, autonomy, rationality, the ability to choose, to decide and to act according to the decision, and the ability to grasp past and future. Those who suffer brain damage may lose these qualities, completely or partially.

When people are aware of what goes on around them and can understand and communicate, they are often able to cope with difficult, even humiliating, physical conditions. For example, during the Holocaust some people found meaning and purpose in their lives despite their suffering even in the hellish concentration camps. They managed to explore spiritual experiences that gave meaning to their lives.[90] Consciousness is therefore a necessary element in shaping a will to live. Nonetheless, many people wish to continue living even when they are not conscious. The primary motivation in many cases is the hope for a medical miracle, the discovery of a new cure, and so on. There are known cases of PCU patients who remained alive for many years; still, their relatives insisted on sustaining them, hoping they would return to a state of awareness.[91]

Lack of Suffering

In the *Cruzan* and *Scheffer* cases, the tendency of the American and Israeli Supreme Courts was not to terminate treatment, although the patients appeared not to suffer. In the *Saikewicz* case, the court referred to the quality-of-life argument and interpreted a reduced quality of life to be defined as a continuous state of pain and disorientation caused by the patient's chemotherapy. Only upon such interpretation was the court willing to accept the quality-of-life argument.[92] The following questions arise:

1. Is a life of suffering equivalent to a life devoid of quality? Not necessarily. Many people are willing to suffer continuous and severe pain in order to see one more smile, to read another book, to enjoy another meeting with relatives, to enjoy the blue sky, and so on.[93]
2. What about PCU patients who did not leave instructions that they would rather die upon reaching this situation? At this stage we cannot conclusively determine whether or not they experience pain (see chapter 2). It is clear that their quality of life is diminished; some might say that their lives are devoid of any quality. In these cases, the components of awareness, consciousness, and human dignity must be taken into consideration. In other words, the existence of suffering diminishes the quality of a given life, but lack of suffering and pain does not in itself guarantee a life of quality.

Doctors often say that pain and suffering are complex matters, because different people have different abilities to cope with pain. It is difficult to point to a specific level of pain after which there is no more quality. But there are states of staggering pain caused, for instance, by cancer, in which the pain overshadows patients' existence and fills their lives to the extent that they are unable to do anything else or to think about other matters. In such a situation, we could claim that life is devoid of quality because it is similar to unconsciousness, but worse. The patients are constantly busy fighting against the enormous pain that overpowers their physical and mental existence without being aware of what goes on around them. In many cases medicine can ease physical pain, but at times the struggle against the physical pain arouses unbearable emotional suffering. This kind of suffering is not always curable by medicine.

Those advocating the sanctity-of-life approach might respond that suffering is a constitutive part of life. Life is not a rose garden. From the moment of birth we confront pain and suffering. But surely these clichés do not suffice. We should recognize the difference between living and suffering. Once they become one and the same, we speak of a very different meaning of life. We all aspire to reduce suffering, and when we are unable to cope with it, a question then arises as to whether this life is worth living. The answer to this question should be left to the sufferer.

Some religious authorities find meaning and value in suffering. Suffering is viewed as symbolizing the triumph of the spirit over the body, a recognition that God's actions must not be questioned, a matter of reward and punishment: Although the body might suffer, the soul is being rewarded. According to the Christian belief, suffering can bring redemption; it is a source of spiritual elevation, providing a chance for penance for past sins.[94] Killing a suffering person is wrong, therefore, because it deprives the person of the divine rewards for suffering and also deprives the souls in purgatory of potential favors.[95] Edmund Pellegrino quotes Miguel de Unamuno: "Suffering is the substance of life and the root of personality. Only suffering makes us persons,"[96] maintaining that this is not an argument for letting patients suffer, but it does suggest that inevitable suffering may serve some purposes that are not immediately apparent. Pellegrino argues that the lives of many of the handicapped, the retarded, and the aged teach us much about courage and personal growth and give some substance to Unamuno's observation.[97]

We see suffering differently. Most handicapped, retarded, and aged people do not see death as an appealing option, so they courageously fight for life. For them it is simply the lesser evil. Generally speaking, suffering is an ugly matter, humiliating and degrading. It is difficult to find anything beautiful, pure, or holy in it, and we have no duty to search for meaning in it. Those who believe that an incurable patient who wishes to die must continue to suffer, because life must never be shortened, do not dignify life. On the contrary, these people not only harm life and its meaning, they harm the will of individuals and human dignity as well.

Dignity

The right to die with dignity is, in essence, a right not to live in indignity. In the *Scheffer* verdict concerning whether to terminate the treatment of a Tay-Sachs baby, it was asserted that Yael Scheffer's dignity was not disgraced by the continuous treatment. A doctor was quoted as saying: "From a nursing point of view, she is a patient in better than fair state. She is not degraded or humiliated; her dignity is preserved carefully."[98] What are the components of human dignity? For instance, are the facts that the room is aired and clean, that the patient is carefully washed, that her clothes are changed, and that she receives intravenous nourishment sufficient to determine that her dignity is preserved?

The concept of human dignity encompasses a range of human sentiments with regard to people's place in this world, their relatives, the environment in which they live, and their conception of the past, the present, and the likely future. People are sensitive not only to pain and physical discomfort. Most of us care how others see us, what they think of us, and how they will remember us.[99] For sick people, the concept of human dignity includes the desire not to become a burden and the desire that their own suffering will not cause their loved ones to suffer. They also fear developing dependency on others or on machines; they want their death to somewhat reflect the way they lived; they want to control the process of death as much as possible; they fear dying without control over their bodies, and they fear continual suffering.

The Implications of Evaluating Life

As it has been established that life can be evaluated, and that there is a place to respect patients' requests not to prolong their lives when they find them not worth living, it is important to examine the ramifications of this view and the hazards it entails. There are several grounds for warnings: the financial aspects; the doctor-patient relationship; patients' relationship with their surroundings, and the effects of this outlook on the patients themselves.

Financial Considerations

The assumption that it is possible to evaluate the worth of a life could lead to a situation in which the value of life would be measured in financial terms, setting a price on human life. Only patients whose lives were deemed to be worthy would be cared for. People who were perceived as weak, such as the elderly, the poor, patients in locked-in syndrome and PCU patients, would be most likely to be neglected (for further discussion, see appendix).

Doctor-Patient Relationship

The assumption that certain lives are worthless might affect, even subconsciously, doctors' attitudes toward their patients. Once they concluded that the patients' lives were of little or no quality, they might cease to provide caring treatment, and from that very moment the patients might be conceived of as a burden. Doctors might distance themselves from their patients, physically and emotionally. An implicit signal to patients that they constituted a burden and were unwanted might shorten their lives, whereas a friendly environment could improve a patient's condition. We need to ensure that the physician healer sees interpersonal sensitivity as an important means to the therapeutic end.[100]

Patients' Relationships with Their Loved Ones

Loved ones are those who are close to the patient; these are mainly, but not exclusively, relatives. Using this term rather than the term *relatives* is especially important in reference to AIDS patients.

Having accepted the assumption that certain lives are not worth living, the patients' loved ones might give up on them too soon. Relationships between patients and the people close to them could affect the treatment given by doctors. Research shows that in the decision to terminate the treatment of a certain patient, doctors are affected by the family stance: If family members treat their loved one as a person and are hopeful, doctors tend to continue treatment. If the family treats the patient as a "vegetable," doctors tend to terminate treatment.[101]

In the past there have been cases in which families used quality-of-life reasoning to shorten the life of their disabled children. The case of *In re Phillip* is pertinent. It concerned a twelve-year-old with Down's syndrome who also suffered from a congenital heart defect that could lead to early death if it were not corrected by surgery. The parents chose not to authorize the surgery. Implicitly, their reasoning was that the quality of their son's life did not warrant its extension. Another significant factor that influenced the court's ruling was the testimony of an expert witness saying that Phillip's case was more risky than the average for two reasons: He had pulmonary vascular changes and thus the operation was prone to have more complications, and children with Down's syndrome have more problems than other children in the postoperative period. The court held that denial by the parents of approval for surgery was not failure to provide the required necessities of life, and it upheld the parents' choice against surgery.[102] Here the family ordered the death of a close relative who probably constituted a great burden, and the state chose not to object. The court obviously respected what the parents conceived to be their own best interest. Can we speak of the "best interest" of the patient in such a case? Can we say that it was in Phillip's best interest to die? The court should have at least contemplated removing the child from the parents' custody and finding a new home for him.[103] (For further deliberation, see chapter 6.)

Patients' Self-Perception

Assuming that a life could be worthless, patients themselves might give up too soon. A strong connection exists between body and soul; loss of hope might lead to loss of physical strength.

These concerns rightfully arise in almost every context of the right to die with dignity, and more powerfully so in the context of the quality-of-life argument. Therefore, it is important to be meticulous with these matters. At the same time, an outright rejection of physician-assisted suicide is not the solution. Rather, we must establish clear rules and guidelines and observe them carefully. The condition of each patient must be examined: the extent of his or her suffering, the doctors' projections concerning the possibility of recovery, the patient's will to live or die as expressed now or previously when the patient was competent to decide.[104] (For further discussion, see conclusions.)

There is certainly room for caution, and it is important to listen to the various concerns involved. Human life is too important to allow a callous outlook. Nonetheless, we should recognize the need of certain people to part from life in a way that they find respectful, when they feel that their lives are forced upon them and contradict their existence as autonomous beings. We must not ignore existing problems of some patients because of speculative fears that the situation might get worse once we address their wish. We must insist on clear guidelines that will not enable overly permissive decisions, while not resorting to excessive prohibition. Ignoring patients who wish to forgo treatment and end their lives might lead to the moral deterioration of a society that closes its eyes to the suffering of those patients. All decisions should be made on a case-by-case basis, in accordance with each one's special circumstances, mainly because most patients prefer to continue living and only a few ask to die.

Conclusion

Life can be evaluated. A life of quality is a life of consciousness, as free as possible from suffering and pain, and one in which human dignity is preserved. Through the philosophical and theological arguments as well as references to several Israeli and American court cases, the relevant considerations that should be kept in mind when evaluating life have emerged. Both the quality-of-life argument and the sanctity-of-life principle should be qualified, and policies should adequately respect the best interests of the patients. Undoubtedly, the courts will need to address repeatedly the challenging question of death with dignity and its relationship with quality of life. Their decisions would benefit from discussions among other circles of society.

It is important to maintain an open and sincere discussion of the issue of physician-assisted suicide for competent, adult patients who suffer from an incurable disease, are unable to commit suicide without help, and repeatedly voice a desire to die. These patients do not want to ask their doctors or loved ones to commit a criminal act. They pose a need that society must address. Human life is too precious to allow a sweeping permissive attitude toward ending it; yet we must recognize the need of certain people to part from life in what they consider to be a dignified manner. For these people, physician-assisted suicide is more dignified than maintaining a condition of mere existence in circumstances that contradict their perception of life. Their present and real voices must not be ignored because of hypothetical future fears. Closing our eyes to their suffering might lead to the moral deterioration of our society.

4 | Passive and Active Euthanasia

This chapter addresses the way various democracies view active and passive euthanasia and the right to die with dignity. Attention is given to the familiar distinction between active and passive euthanasia, and then the current legal positions in the Netherlands, the United States, Australia, Switzerland, England, and Canada are analyzed.

Some patients may feel that they are about to die, or wish to hasten their death while maintaining their dignity. Faced with the deterioration of their bodily functions, patients may find it hard to maintain their dignity. Some feel exhausted and no longer wish to continue their struggle, especially when they are required (so they feel) to use their energies not only to fight against their diminishing strength but also to fight against relatives and nursing personnel, who sometimes tend to treat them as either infantile or senile, subjects worthy or unworthy of their mercy. Patients' motivations and inclinations help us recognize their right to die with dignity. A distinction should be drawn between the right to die with dignity and the process of dignified dying.

Active and Passive Euthanasia

Liberals consider first and foremost the rights and interests of the individual. It has been argued that respect for human life permits, and in some cases argues for, mercy killing (merciful treatment that results in death). In this context, a distinction has been made be-

tween active and passive euthanasia. *Euthanasia* is a Greek term meaning "easy death" (*eu*, good, easy; *thanatos*, death). Active euthanasia involves prescribing medication or treatment aimed at shortening life and
suffering. It may be done by the attending physician through, for example,
a poisonous injection or through prescribing large doses of drugs with
the intention of cutting the patient's life short. Some describe this action as killing.[1] Passive euthanasia (also termed forgoing life-sustaining
treatment) may take two forms: One is abstention from performing acts
that prolong the patient's life. An example may be refraining from connecting a patient to a ventilator or to a resuscitation machine. The other
form involves discontinuation of actions designed to sustain life, which
involves withdrawing machines to which the patient has already been
connected.[2]

A dispute exists as to whether the distinction between killing and
letting someone die is valid. Daniel Callahan claims that this distinction is valid, in that there is a fundamental difference between what nature does to us and what we do to one another.[3] James Rachels, on the
other hand, thinks that no moral difference exists between killing and
abstaining from action, thereby enabling a patient to die. He gives an
example of Smith, who drowns his six-year-old cousin in order to gain
a large inheritance, and of Jones, who, like Smith, plans to kill his cousin
for a similar reason by a similar method, but in the second scenario the
child slips, hits his head, and drowns by himself while the delighted
Jones stands by, ready to push the child's head back under the water if
necessary. Rachels rightly argues that for Jones to plead the moral defense that he, unlike Smith, did not drown the child but merely watched
him drown is a grotesque perversion of moral reasoning. The relevant
action could not be in itself worse than the relevant omission. By implication, Rachels persuasively writes that when a doctor lets a patient
die for humane reasons, he places himself in the same moral position
as if he had given the patient a lethal injection for humane reasons. The
motive is what is morally significant, not the action itself (or lack
thereof).[4] I will elaborate on the strength of this claim later in reference
to the *Benjamin Eyal* case (see conclusions).

Supporters of Callahan's stance will add that by performing active
euthanasia, we interfere with the process of nature. On the other hand,
Rachels's supporters will rightly claim that technology generally challenges nature. Attachment to life-support systems clearly constitutes interference with nature. Most of us do not live by the laws of nature most
of the time, and we allow ourselves to interfere with its course. Therefore such a statement contains a certain degree of self-righteousness.[5]

In arguing against active euthanasia, Callahan holds that the result of killing and the result of an act that lets the patient die may be the same, but this does not imply that the causal distinction between the two is irrelevant in moral terms. Callahan argues that Rachels is mistaken in claiming that identical intentions are at work when we let a person die and when we kill him. Rachels errs in assuming that the manner by which the doctor causes the patient to die "is not important in itself." For Callahan the manner is certainly important, because when we let a patient die, the illness is the agent that causes the death. Thus, the doctor's traditional oath and role that forbids killing patients remains unbroken. In cases of active euthanasia, however, the doctor's action causes the death.[6] In Callahan's opinion, all assumptions about the role of medicine in modern life must be reconsidered if we ignore this important distinction. Therefore, we must vigorously reject active euthanasia and assisted suicide. These acts are wrong and harmful reactions to a nasty death marked by pain and suffering.[7]

Another consideration that leads Callahan to categorically reject active euthanasia and assisted suicide is the fear of exploitation. He is concerned that once the authority to terminate life is granted, it might be used against the patient's wishes.[8] Many ethicists and doctors agree with this point of view.[9] From conversations I have had with dozens of doctors in Israel, the United States, Canada, the Netherlands, and England I have learned that many are indeed willing to refrain from attaching patients to machines or to remove them from ventilators, but most of them (with the exception of Dutch doctors)[10] refrain from declaring openly that they would be willing, under certain circumstances, to inject poison to shorten the life of a suffering patient.[11] Some clearly postulate that their calling is to preserve life, not to terminate it, and therefore active euthanasia is immoral, signifying betrayal of the education they received and the morals to which they adhere. Some doctors and ethicists mention in this context the section of the Hippocratic Oath that forbids euthanasia. The oath states: "I will neither give a deadly drug to anybody if asked for it, nor will I make a suggestion to this effect."[12] It is interesting that many doctors are in favor of abortion, even though the same clause of the oath also forbids abortions ("Similarly I will not give to a woman an abortive remedy").[13]

In certain cases, in contradiction to this view, the necessity for voluntary physician-assisted suicide (PAS) should be recognized. On such occasions, which should be clearly defined, PAS is morally permissible, and killing and letting die are morally on a par. (For further discussion, see conclusions.)

Using this logic, it might be argued that if PAS is sometimes morally permissible, then active euthanasia is also sometimes morally permissible. A few years ago I endorsed this view in some of my publications. The study in the Netherlands caused me to change my views, not on the ethics of euthanasia but rather on the practicality of its implementation. To secure patients against fears of abuse, we should grant them control over their lives until the very last moment. Hence the argument is circumscribed to PAS only. Undoubtedly the role that the consenting doctors would be expected to play is great and onerous. Doctors who agree with the rationale presented here would argue that while it is true that the doctor's job is to prolong life, it is also the doctor's job to prevent suffering and ensure the preservation of human dignity. Sometimes, however, prolonging life and preserving human dignity are mutually exclusive.

Consider James, who suffers from a malignant disease that spreads through his body and slowly destroys it.[14] The doctors must amputate his leg, but they cannot stop the endemic process that paralyzes his limbs and destroys his body. The physicians are able only to relieve his pain. They explain to James that the disease is without remedy. James obviously suffers but, acknowledging his fate, refuses to accept treatment. He wants to die. James shares his feelings with the doctors, telling them that his suffering is both physical and emotional because it is difficult for him to witness the anguish of his loved ones, who surround his bed day and night. This patient specifically states: "I have lived my life; I have said what I had to say; I feel I lived a full and meaningful life to the best of my abilities. In my current position, I no longer find life an appealing option. I suffer, and my condition causes my loved ones to suffer as well. In essence, all I do is wait for death to redeem me from my misery. There is no point in prolonging this situation. Allow me to die with dignity. Dying will dignify me more than the continuation of a pointless life that damages my bones, my body, my soul, and my mind. If I were able, I would commit suicide, but I cannot. Please help me die now."

The doctors suggest the option of a hospice, but James declines the offer.[15] He wants to die now, not in several months. James explains that the medicine meant to help him cope with pain is not a useful solution for him, because the suffering is not only physical. He is appalled at his own feebleness, wretchedness, and dependency upon others. The suffering is psychological, too, deeply touching his soul, causing him to feel that one of the things dearest to him—human dignity—is disappearing, while no one can stop the process of his physical deterioration.

The suffering that James causes to others does not constitute the final reason for his will to die. In this hypothetical case, as in many real cases, the patient's loved ones are clearly dear to the patient, and their suffering is inseparable from his. A significant part of patients' dignity is their continued ability to do good for those around them. Most of us find positive elements in life when we are able to share—to give and receive. In this case, James, in his ongoing condition, becomes increasingly convinced that he has lost his humanness, because even his ability to give to his loved ones, in a way he considers meaningful, has been taken from him. On the contrary, his growing feeling is that he causes them only pain and sorrow.[16] This increases his distress and strengthens his opinion that it is time to bid them farewell. This does not mean that a patient's life should be terminated because of the suffering endured by his loved ones. Rather, the suffering caused to the family plays at least some part in the patient's considerations when he requests termination of treatment, and this consideration must not be ignored.

In such a case, the correct policy respects the patient's wish and includes measures to hasten the end. The doctors should be allowed to provide assisted suicide. The important thing is to ease the patient into a final, peaceful rest, and to show respect by fulfilling his request.

Doctors who would be willing to entertain this reasoning would also recognize their duty to help the patient when he could not help himself. Although this example is hypothetical, it nevertheless characterizes a group of patients who suffer from incurable diseases and express a similar desire (see, for instance, the Canadian Sue Rodriguez case, discussed later in this chapter).[17] For a small minority of patients, the continuation of living at all costs is not an appealing option. These patients should not be ignored. Medicine and ethics should address their needs. Although this is not an easy task, the solution must not be beyond our reach, either medically or ethically. That solution might change the nature of medicine, but the nature of medicine is not a static concept. It is in constant flux, and through the ages it has developed through the use of various standards and norms (e.g., for instance, the agenda and terminology of the Hippocratic Oath). The history of the last thirty years shows that medicine has changed dramatically due to rapid technological developments, which make it possible to prolong life in difficult situations. An acrobatic argument that acknowledges technological advances but dismisses the evolving ethical issues that pose uncomfortable and disturbing questions is unfair to the patient community.

Comparative Law

Active euthanasia is considered a criminal offense in most countries of the world. The Netherlands exhibits the most permissive attitude in this sphere. Euthanasia and assisted suicide have been practiced and tolerated in the Netherlands over the past twenty years, even though, until November 2000, it remained an illegal act, under Articles 293 and 294 of the Penal Code. Several lower court decisions, supported by a Supreme Court decision and reflected in the policies of the regional attorneys general and further promulgated by the Royal Dutch Medical Association, have held that when euthanasia meets a certain set of guidelines, it may be defended under a plea of *force majeure* and so is reasonably sure of being subjected to prosecution.[18] The euthanasia law, which was approved by the Dutch Parliament on 28 November 2000, places euthanasia outside the Dutch Penal Code when doctors follow a specified administrative procedure. Euthanasia would be supervised, not as in the past by the public prosecutor, but by a public committee consisting of a doctor, a lawyer, and an ethics expert. Doctors must be "convinced" that the patient's request is voluntary and well considered and that the patient is facing "unremitting and unbearable" suffering; must have advised the patient of his or her situation and prospects; and must have reached a firm conclusion with the patient that there is "no reasonable alternative." At least one other independent physician must have examined the patient. It also ensures that parental consent will now be required before incurably sick minors aged twelve to sixteen can request euthanasia[19] (see chapter 7).

In the United States, attempts made in 1988–1992 in the states of Washington and California to pass laws recognizing the possibility of active euthanasia were unsuccessful.[20] In November 1994, voters in Oregon approved the first American law allowing doctors to hasten death for the terminally ill. The Oregon Death with Dignity Act (Measure No. 16) was designed to protect these patient interests: avoiding unnecessary pain and suffering; preserving and enhancing the right of competent adults to make their own critical health care decisions; avoiding tragic cases of attempted or successful suicides in a less humane and dignified manner; protecting "the terminally ill and their loved ones" from financial hardships they wish to avoid, and protecting "the terminally ill and their loved ones from unwanted intrusions into their personal affairs" by law enforcement officers and others.[21]

In 1994, the Oregon law was approved by a 51 percent to 49 percent vote of the state residents, but it was promptly put on hold amid great legal wrangling.[22] Two days before the Death with Dignity Act was to take effect, a lawsuit was filed by a group of physicians, residential care facilities, and terminally ill Oregon residents challenging the act on constitutional grounds.[23] The federal district court granted a temporary injunction and eight months later struck down the act on equal protection grounds.[24]

This decision was subsequently vacated for procedural reasons, remanding the judgment of the district court for lack of jurisdiction.[25] Then, in 1997, the state's voters backed the law again, this time by a decisive margin of 60 percent to 40 percent (see chapter 8).

Following the passing of the Oregon Death with Dignity Act, attempts to legalize assisted suicide were made by many other states, among them Alaska, Arizona, California, Colorado, Connecticut, Illinois, Massachusetts, Michigan, Mississippi, Nebraska, Washington, and Wisconsin. All attempts were rejected.[26] A bigger setback for assisted suicide advocates came in the summer of 1997, when the U.S. Supreme Court upheld laws in Washington State and New York banning physician-assisted suicides. The Court reversed decisions of the lower courts that held those laws unconstitutional.

In 1994, the U.S. District Court was asked to rule on the constitutionality of the state of Washington's criminal prohibition against physician-assisted suicide. Specifically, the plaintiffs asserted that the Fourteenth Amendment to the Constitution guarantees mentally competent, terminally ill adults who act under no undue influence the right voluntarily to hasten their death by taking a lethal dose of physician-prescribed drugs. Chief Judge Rothstein held that such a right for these patients was liberty interest protected under the Fourteenth Amendment, and that the 140–year-old anti-assisted-suicide Washington statute violated equal protection by prohibiting these patients from seeking physician-assisted suicide but allowing withdrawal of life-support systems.[27] Later, this judgment was reversed by the U.S. Court of Appeals, Ninth Circuit, under Judge Noonan, saying that the Washington statute did not deprive patients of constitutionally protected liberty interest. The panel majority found that the statute prohibiting suicide promotion furthered, among other things, the interest of denying to physicians "the role of killers of their patients."[28]

Under the argument posited by Rachels, physicians do not fulfill the role of killers by prescribing drugs to hasten the death of patients who voluntarily choose this option any more than they do so by withdrawing life-support machines. The court clouded an important issue by resorting to this radical language instead of probing the complexities involved and establishing procedures to ensure patients against possible abuse.

The Ninth Circuit Court reheard the case, reversed the panel decision, and affirmed the district court ruling.[29] Circuit Judge Reinhardt opened his judgment with these thoughtful words:

> This case raises an extraordinarily important and difficult issue. It compels us to address questions to which there are no

easy or simple answers, at law or otherwise. It requires us to confront the most basic of human concerns—the mortality of self and loved ones—and to balance the interest in preserving human life against the desire to die peacefully and with dignity. People of good will can and do passionately disagree about the proper result, perhaps even more intensely than they part ways over the constitutionality of restricting a woman's right to have an abortion. Heated though the debate may be, we must determine whether and how the United States Constitution applies to the controversy before us, a controversy that may touch more people more profoundly than any other issue the courts will face in the foreseeable future.[30]

The court held that there was a constitutionally protected liberty interest in determining the time and manner of one's own death, an interest that must be weighed against the state's legitimate and countervailing interests, especially those related to the preservation of human life. After balancing the competing interests, the court concluded that insofar as the Washington statute prohibited physicians from prescribing life-ending medication for use by terminally ill, competent adults who wish to hasten their deaths, it violated the Due Process clause of the Fourteenth Amendment.[31]

Finally, the Supreme Court, per Chief Justice William Rehnquist, reversed the judgment yet again, holding that the asserted right to assistance in committing suicide was not fundamental liberty interest protected by the Due Process clause, and that Washington's ban on assisted suicide was rationally related to legitimate government interests, among them the preservation of human life; the protection of the integrity and ethics of the medical profession; the protection of vulnerable groups from abuse, neglect, and mistakes; and furthermore, the protection of disabled and terminally ill people from prejudice, negative and inaccurate stereotypes, and societal indifference.[32]

Interestingly, Chief Justice Rehnquist chose to conclude his opinion by calling on the public to continue the debate in earnest: "Throughout the Nation, Americans are engaged in an earnest and profound debate about the morality, legality, and practicality of physician-assisted suicide. Our holding permits this debate to continue, as it should in a democratic society."[33]

In 1996, Dr. Timothy Quill and his colleagues appealed to the courts to declare two New York statutes penalizing assistance in suicide unconstitutional in part. The physicians argued that the statutes under examination were invalid to the extent that they prohibited them from acceding to the requests of terminally ill, mentally competent patients for help in hastening death. The court struck down the statutes, finding that they violated the Equal Protection clause of the Fourteenth Amendment because they were not "rationally related to a legitimate state interest." Quoting a series of precedents from 1914 onward, the court said that the right to refuse medical treatment has long been recognized in New York,[34] holding that physicians who are willing to do so may prescribe drugs to be self-administered by mentally competent patients who seek to end their lives during the final stages of a terminal illness.[35]

New York public officials appealed to the Supreme Court, which reversed the decision. The Court, per Chief Justice Rehnquist, held that New York's prohibition on assisted suicide did not violate the Equal Protection clause of the Fourteenth Amendment. The Court maintained that the distinction between letting a patient die and making that patient die was important, logical, rational, and well established.[36]

As a result of the two Supreme Court decisions, *Washington v. Glucksberg* and *Vacco v. Quill*, both given on 26 June 1997, by a 9 to 0 vote, the states have responsibility for insuring that the interests of all patients near the end of their lives are not imperiled. In American pluralistic society there are widely differing values and sharply clashing views on mercy killings, physician-assisted suicide, and the right to die with dignity. Oregon Measure 16 represents one aspect of this conflict. In Michigan, a special statute was passed in 1993 to stop Dr. Jack Kevorkian from helping patients to die.[37] However, Dr. Kevorkian subsequently stood trial several times, and in all instances the juries refused to convict him of violating that statute, although Kevorkian admitted he had indeed assisted people in committing suicide. Kevorkian was acquitted on the grounds that his main intent was to relieve pain, not to cause death.[38] In November 1998, he actively euthanized Thomas Youk, stood trial, and was convicted of second-degree murder and for delivering a controlled substance for the purpose of injecting Youk with lethal drugs. Kevorkian was given a jail sentence of ten to twenty-five years on the second-degree murder conviction, and three to seven years on the controlled-substance conviction (for further discussion of Kevorkian's campaign, see conclusions).

In Australia, the Legislative Assembly of the Northern Territory passed on 25 May 1995 the Northern Territory Rights of the Terminally Ill Bill 1995, the world's only law allowing terminally ill patients to commit suicide with a doctor's help. The legislation, applied only in the Northern Territory, allowed a terminally ill Australian adult, experiencing "unacceptable" pain, to be examined by a qualified physician to determine whether the patient could be cured.[39] The act required confirming examinations by two other independent physicians, one specializing in treating terminal illness and the other a qualified psychiatrist, to confirm that the patient was terminally ill and not clinically depressed.[40] After considering the advice of the consultants, medically assisted suicide could not take place if there were palliative care options "reasonably available to the patient to alleviate the patient's pain and suffering to levels acceptable to the patient."[41]

The act also included provisions intended to ensure that the patient was making an informed choice. The doctor had to have informed the patient of the nature of the illness, its likely course, and the medical procedures available. Upon having the pertinent information, the patient could indicate a wish to end his or her life. The doctor had to be satisfied that the patient had considered the possible implications of the decision for the family, and that the decision had been made freely, voluntarily, and after due consideration.[42]

The act provided for a nine-day cooling-off period comprised of two stages. Seven days had to elapse between the initial request and the signing of the certificate of request, and a further forty-eight hours had to pass before the patient was provided with assistance to terminate life.[43] The signing of the certificate had to be witnessed by two doctors. If the patient was physically unable to sign the certificate, a person other than the doctors and psychiatrist referred to, who was at least eighteen years old, could sign it on behalf of the patient.[44] The person could not be likely to receive any financial benefit from the patient's death, and forfeited any benefit if he or she would in fact have received it.[45] The statute provided that the patient could rescind the request to die at any time and in any manner, and that the physician was under no obligation to assist suicide.[46] If the physician chose to comply with the patient's request, death could be hastened by prescribing or preparing a lethal substance, giving the substance to the patient for self-administration, or administering the lethal substance to the patient. The doctor had to remain present until the death of the patient.[47]

The legislation became operative in July 1996, and in the following nine months, four patients who requested to die received help under the provisions of the act by Dr. Philip Nitschke.[48] The act was subsequently annulled in March 1997, when federal parliamentarians, by thirty-eight votes to thirty-four, with one abstention, passed the Commonwealth Euthanasia Laws Bill 1996.[49] That act effectively prohibits Australian territories from enacting legislation that permits "the form of intentional killing of another called euthanasia . . . or the assisting of a person to terminate his or her life," but allows the making of laws regarding the withdrawal or withholding of life-sustaining treatment and the provision of palliative care to the dying, provided these do not sanction the intentional killing of the patient.[50] After the Northern Territory's euthanasia law was overturned by Federal Parliament, Dr. Nitschke revealed that he had helped fifteen patients, including some from Victoria, to end their lives.[51]

While the United States struggles with controversy regarding the legality of assisted suicide, the Swiss legal system has condoned the practice for more than sixty years. In contrast to practices in the Netherlands, Australia, and the various U.S. proposals under which assisted suicide is limited to physician-assisted suicide, Swiss law permits laypersons to aid the dying in this way. Since 1937, assistance to suicide has been governed by Articles 114 and 115 of the Penal Code. Although under Article 114 anyone taking another person's life, even if for honorable motives of pity and at the request of the sufferer, is liable to imprisonment,[52] still the judge will consider whether the patient is a mentally competent adult who suffers from intolerable health problems and voluntarily asks to shorten his or her life. This is under Article 63 of the Penal Code of 1937, which instructs the judge to mete out punishment in accordance with the guilt of the actor, considering the motives, the prior life, and the personal circumstances of the guilty person. The Swiss Penal Code says that "assisted suicide is not punishable, provided it is not done for enrichment purposes and that the person [who wishes to commit suicide] carries out the final death act."[53] Swiss law permits both passive euthanasia—deliberate renunciation or interruption of measures to preserve life, and active indirect euthanasia—the administering of substances to reduce suffering whose secondary effects may reduce the period of the patient's survival.[54]

Although Swiss law permits physicians and nonmedical persons to assist suicides, the Swiss Academy of Medical Sciences, like many other medical organizations, including the American Medical Association, opposes doctors helping patients to die.[55] Swiss laws stipulate that persons who assist a suicide do so for humane reasons with no chance of personal gain.[56] The Swiss Society for Human Dying, EXIT, requires that the applicant wishing to die with EXIT's help be at least eighteen years old, a Swiss resident, mentally competent, and suffering from intolerable health problems. He or she must personally apply for the service and convince the administrators of EXIT that there is no coercion or third-party influence involved in the decision. An EXIT physician considers the application and decides whether or not assistance can be offered. In doubtful cases, a team composed of a lawyer, a psychiatrist, and another physician will jointly make the decision.[57] Between 100 and 120 people are openly helped in this way each year, and so far no member of an EXIT team has had to appear before the court for helping a person to commit suicide.[58]

Belgium has no formal registration and authorization procedure for end-of-life decisions in medical practice. Although euthanasia is illegal and is treated as intentionally causing death under criminal law, prosecutions are exceptional. Legalization of euthanasia is intensely discussed, both by the official Advisory Committee on Bioethics and by the Belgian Parliament.[59]

English criminal law does not recognize active euthanasia as a defense in a murder charge. Lord Devlin directed the jury in *R. v. Adams* that no doctor, nor any man, no more in the case of the dying than of the healthy, has the right to deliberately cut the thread of life.[60] This argument was restated in *R. v. Cox*.[61] At the same time, it is established that passive euthanasia may be allowed in certain circumstances. Precedents prescribe withholding medical care if such a course of action represents good medical practice,[62] and if it is done "in the best interests of the patient.[63] This reasoning, which emphasizes the best interests of the patient, has been reiterated in several court decisions and has become a cornerstone in English law. In determining these interests, the court balances the benefit of continued treatment against the pain and suffering of the patient concerned. In *In re J.*, Lord Donaldson of the Court of Appeal delivered an opinion against resuscitating a severely brain-damaged child because the pain and suffering likely to be experienced exceeded any benefit accruing from prolonging his life. Lord Donaldson argued that there are cases "in which the answer must be that it is not in the interests of the child to subject it to treatment which will cause increased suffering and produce no commensurate benefit, giving the fullest possible weight to the child's, and mankind's desire to survive."[64]

In England, all requests for withdrawal of tube feeding must go through the courts. In the *Airedale NHS Trust v. Bland* case involving a football fan who was severely injured in the Hillsborough stadium disaster of April 1989, both the Court of Appeal and the House of Lords upheld a declaratory judgment by the Family Division of the High Court that withdrawing artificial nutrition and hydration from a patient in a severe, persistent vegetative state (PVS) did not constitute an unlawful act. The court held that artificial feeding and the administration of antibiotic drugs could lawfully be withheld from an insensate patient who had no hope of recovery when it was believed that the result would be that the patient would die shortly thereafter. It was also emphasized that by virtue of his condition, a PVS patient would not suffer as a result of being deprived of food and hydration, and that the major consideration in determining the best interests of the patient are medical: The opinion of the physicians decides the course of the treatment.[65] The court explained that relevant considerations for deciding the best interests of PVS patients include the avoidance of invasive and undignified procedures, which would have an adverse effect upon the way such patients would be remembered by their loved ones. Lord Goff saw no reason to maintain medical treatment simply to prolong a patient's life when such treatment had no therapeutic purpose of any kind, "as where it is futile because the patient is unconscious and there is no prospect of any improvement in his condition."[66] Lord Mustill argued that Anthony Bland had no best interests because the loss of all cognitive functions meant that he had "no best interests of any kind." Because the patient had no interest in staying alive, no legal justification existed for any invasive life-supporting treatment.[67]

In Canada, Parliament debated a private member's bill (C-261) to legalize active euthanasia. The bill was not adopted, but legislators became aware that physician-assisted suicide had widespread support in Canada. By 1999, about three quarters of Canadians (77 percent) believed that doctors should be allowed to end the life of a patient whose life is immediately threatened by a disease that causes the patient great suffering. Canadians are less likely to support physician-assisted suicide if the patient is suffering from a disease that is not immediately life threatening, such as a chronically debilitating illness. Still, 57 percent of Canadians believed that doctors should be allowed, by law, to end the life of a patient who suffers from a disease that does not immediately threaten his or her life. This figure had not changed since 1995.[68]

One Canadian court case concerned Nancy B., a twenty-five-year-old woman who had had generalized polyneuropathy for two and a half years as a result of Guillain-Barré syndrome. She initiated a legal action for an injunction permitting her physicians to withdraw her respirator. The Quebec Superior Court granted the injunction, her respirator was withdrawn, and Nancy B. died.[69] In Justice Dufour's opinion, Nancy B.'s refusal of treatment was not an attempt to commit suicide but rather an attempt merely to allow a disease to take its natural course.

The most known death-with-dignity case in Canada concerns Sue Rodriguez, who was dying from amyotrophic lateral sclerosis (ALS), a disease that causes progressive muscle paralysis in the face, the tongue, the throat, the respiratory system, the shoulders, hands, and legs. In its final stages the patient cannot swallow, speak, cough, or breathe unassisted.[70] One specialist described this situation as "a living hell."[71] As her condition deteriorated, Rodriguez publicly expressed a wish to have a physician assist her in ending her life at a time of her choosing, when she herself would be unable to do so, rather than waiting helplessly to die by suffocation or choking. Rodriguez sought to challenge the Criminal Code of Canada prohibition on assisted suicide, on the grounds that it violated the Charter of Rights and Freedoms. The specific section of the Criminal Code is 241(b): "Everyone who aids or abets a person to commit suicide, whether suicide ensues or not, is guilty of an indictable offence and liable to imprisonment for a term not exceeding fourteen years."[72]

The appeal was rejected in a five-to-four landmark decision. The Court did not want to intervene in this delicate public matter, on the grounds that it should be up to the legislature to change the law if such a change was deemed necessary.[73] I discussed her case with three of the justices in the Canadian Supreme Court. One of them told me that this was the toughest decision this judge had ever made, and that the Court might overturn the decision if the legislature failed to address the issue adequately and another case came up.[74]

The media took much interest in Rodriguez's tragedy and discussed at length the ethical dilemma involved in her appeal to be assisted to die. Her case exemplifies the kind of story that the media seek: It involved a human drama of a person who became a public figure whose story had ethical and societal implications.[75] Rodriguez was well aware of the media interest in her story and cooperated with them fully until her very last days. On 5 February 1994, one week prior to her death through assisted suicide, she advised a member of the media that a physician had agreed to assist her in her death, but she would not divulge the physician's name or the details of the suicide plan.[76]

Margaret Somerville, who regularly appears in Canadian media voicing her adamant views against euthanasia, attests that it was difficult to argue against Rodriguez when they were face-to-face in a television debate.[77] Rodriguez implicitly asked: "Why would you deny this to me when I want it so much and it is the only way that I can see to relieve my suffering?"[78] Somerville later wrote that it was hard to say no, but because she believed that legalizing euthanasia would do great harm to society and to our respect for human life, and because she thought it would change one of the most fundamental norms on which society is based, namely, that we must not kill one another, she remained firmly in her position against active euthanasia.

Because it is important that the patient have control over his or her life until the very end, and due to a fear of the abuse of this process, this book does not advocate active euthanasia but rather physician-assisted suicide. Nevertheless, it is striking to see how liberals like Somerville, who ordinarily conceive the individual as the prime subject, are willing to overlook Rodriguez's misery because of hypothetical societal concerns. Fearing harmful consequences to the society at large brings Somerville and others to ignore the real and agonizing voice of people who suffer from incurable diseases and who seek death as refuge from their undignified situation. The present individual is lost, sacrificed, in favor of possible future harmful consequences to the public. In addition, Somerville overlooks the fact that democracies do acknowledge that there are circumstances under which it is permissible for one human being to kill another. Accepting voluntary physician-assisted suicide would not constitute the dramatic revolution that she is describing. All democracies accept the right to self-defense. Some democracies accept capital punishment. Some democracies go to wars and kill their enemies. These, of course, are regarded as exceptional cases in which the taking of human life under special and justified provisions is permitted. Physician-assisted suicide should be regarded in the same light.

Patients in a devastating situation who wish to cease living, if they are helped by a physician, are helped to relieve their suffering. The physician's motivation in this case is to assist a fellow human being by providing relief from prolonged suffering. The decision to perform physician-assisted suicide is first and foremost a moral decision. The physician who provides the assistance is convinced that this act is justified not only medically but also morally; otherwise he or she would not have agreed to assist the patient in the first place.

Conclusion

This chapter surveys the attempts that have been made around the globe to facilitate death with dignity. Oregon's Measure 16, which allows assisted suicide, is facing a challenge. In Australia, the Northern Territory Bill, which allowed terminally ill patients to commit suicide with a doctor's help, was declared void. The legislatures of Canada and England have consistently resisted attempts to legalize assisted suicide and euthanasia. The Netherlands remains the only country in the liberal world that generally accepts the policy and practice of both euthanasia and physician-assisted suicide, without seeing much difference between the two, and whose legislatures have advanced more bills that would further legitimize euthanasia, while broadening the scope of the practice.

The next chapter analyzes and criticizes Ronald Dworkin's distinction between experiential and critical interests.[79] The discussion raises doubts as to the importance of the role that should be assigned to living wills. It is argued that present wishes should have precedence over past wishes, and that living wills should be honored only when we can assume that the patient did not change her or his mind after signing the will.

5 | What Interests Do We Have?

This chapter discusses Ronald Dworkin's distinction between experiential and critical interests, further contemplating the analogy he draws between the destruction of life and the destruction of masterpieces of art. Specific attention is given to what Dworkin terms "critical interests" and to the notion of dignity. The intention is to refute Dworkin's contentions that a life that comprises only thin pleasures is not worth living, and that the priorities held by a competent person in the past should be held decisive when it is decided whether to treat this person when he or she becomes incompetent. Dworkin's assertion is refuted by the argument that even meager pleasures are worth living for, and that whenever we are unsure of whether the patient concerned wishes to die, we should err on the side of life. In any event, the patient's present order of priorities should override past considerations. In this connection, a caveat is made regarding advance directives (ADs), Do Not Resuscitate orders (DNRs),[1] and living wills.

Experiential and Critical Interests

According to Dworkin, most of us think it is important to achieve something in our lives. We all want a decent life upon which we can look with pride and satisfaction. We have two kinds of interests: We want to derive pleasure and enjoyment from the fulfillment of our desires and ambitions, and we also want to live worthwhile lives.

That is, we look at our lives as a kind of assignment, a mission. The first kind of interests are experiential; the second, critical.[2]

Thus, playing basketball and sailing are experiential interests. Sheila enjoys both, but she does not think her life would be less worthwhile if she did not play basketball or sail. She does not think the lives of others who do not enjoy these experiences are defective because of that. But she may think that her sense of living a good life would be diminished if it did not include enjoying the company of her children. We have a critical interest in having children and in spending time with them. We have a critical interest in having a family, in giving and sharing. This critical interest is connected to our convictions about the intrinsic value of our own lives.

Intuitively, Dworkin seems to be right. We all have interests that we believe will make our lives genuinely better. This does not mean that we have to find our place only by bringing children into the world. But it seems right to say that most of us have a critical interest in having a family, in being part of a social framework to which we can contribute, both giving and taking. We all want to succeed in our relationships with people who are dear to us. Familial attachments as well as frequent encounters with people in our social activities make us feel more comfortable with some people than with others. Social encounters may take place at work and outside work, and personal acquaintance makes some people more important to us than others. In some things the sense of enjoyment is dominant and central. In others, the sense of obligation—to ourselves and to others—is central and dominant. We strive to find joy in things we want to achieve in life. With experiential interests, the sense of obligation is not necessarily present.

Another relevant differentiation is Bernard Williams's distinction between ambitions and values that are contingent on the prospect of being alive, and categorical desires.[3] The first group includes, for example, the ambition to have a Chinese meal or to go abroad, whereas categorical desires have values that are not dependent on the fact of living, but give us an incentive and reason to continue living. Saving the world from an atomic or ecological disaster comprises a categorical desire.

There is much similarity between Dworkin's and Williams's distinctions. Dworkin's experiential interests bear a resemblance to Williams's ambitions and values that are contingent on the prospect of being alive. Likewise, Dworkin's critical interests are not significantly different from Williams's categorical desires. The interests that Dworkin defines as critical give us an incentive and reason to continue living.

This point of view brings Dworkin to think that human life as such is not sacred. Life that includes only animal-like experiences without any critical interests is not sacred. He implies that the view that human life is intrinsically good and that taking one's own life (or ending one's life with the help of others) is a wrong deed in itself, may be analogous to the common view regarding the destruction of masterpieces of art: The owner of a painting should not exercise the liberty to destroy it, because the painting possesses an intrinsic value that is universal, that belongs to our culture, and is beyond the possession of a single human being. Destroying a masterpiece robs, in a sense, the human race. Such an action diminishes a certain value that belongs not to the owner of the painting, but to art as such: art for art's sake. We are not able to say how much better the world is because of this painting or how great the loss would have been if it had not been painted. We value the painting in itself, intrinsically, in the sense that it does not serve any ulterior purpose. Dworkin does not suggest that a human life is literally a work of art. He regards such an idea as dangerous, because it suggests that we should value a person in the same way as we value a painting or a poem, for beauty, style, or originality, rather than for personal, moral, or intellectual qualities. But we do treat life as a creative activity that we respect as we respect artistic creation. Dworkin holds that both art and living species are inviolable to us not by association, but by virtue of their history, of how they came to exist. We see the evolutionary process through which endangered species developed as itself contributing, in some way, to the shamefulness of what we do when we cause their extinction. Dworkin maintains that people who are concerned about protecting threatened species (especially their own) often stress the connection between art and nature by describing the evolution of species as a process of creation.[4] Like art and life, the notions of knowledge, love, friendship, and the prosperity of our country also seem to possess an intrinsic value.

Past Wishes, Present Concerns

In *Life's Dominion*, Dworkin emphasizes the notion of dignity. Dignity is the central aspect of the intrinsic importance of human life.[5] A person's right to be treated with dignity is based on others' acknowledging the person's critical interests: They recognize that he or she has a moral standing, and that it is intrinsically, objectively important how his or her life goes. Bearing this view in mind, I ask you to consider the following issue: Most of us have a critical interest in having a family. This critical interest is connected to our convictions about the intrinsic value of our own lives. We are concerned with how people look at us. We all have an interest in the way we will be remembered after death. We do not want to be remembered as people who were dependent on others, unable to perform the simplest actions. Patients prefer to have the memories of their loved ones filled predominantly with thoughts about their past vitality, rather than their present condition. Thus, many are inclined to minimize the burden their illness imposes on others. Dworkin writes that many people do not want to be remembered as living in circumstances they perceive as degrading. At least part of what people fear about dependence is its impact not on those responsible for their care, but on their own dignity. Dworkin contends that some people are horrified that their death might express an idea that they detest as a perversion: that mere biological life—just hanging on—has an independent intrinsic value.[6]

Dworkin maintains that when we think of dignity, it is not just life in any form that is important. Anyone who believes in the sanctity of human life believes that once a human life has started, it is intrinsically important that that life goes well, that the investment it represents is realized rather than frustrated.[7] Dworkin's contention comes close to that of a British court ruling that the avoidance of invasive and undignified procedures that would have an adverse effect upon the way the patients concerned would be remembered by their loved ones, counted among the relevant considerations in deciding about the best interests of post-coma unawareness (PCU) patients.[8]

Dworkin has no qualms about referring to some patients as vegetables.[9] He assumes that harm is being done when a patient is living as a vegetable.[10] In his criticism of the *Cruzan* ruling, Dworkin contemplates a case in which a woman named Margo had executed a formal document directing that if she should develop Alzheimer's disease or any other life-impairing disease, she wanted to be killed as soon and as painlessly as possible.[11] Dworkin asks whether autonomy requires that her wishes be respected now when she is ill, even though she seems perfectly happy with her dog-eared mysteries, the single painting she repaints, and her peanut-butter-and-jelly sandwiches. In such a case an apparent contradiction seems to exist between past and present wishes, between past and present autonomy. Dworkin endorses respecting Margo's past wishes, arguing that a competent person making a living will to provide for her treatment if she becomes demented is making the kind of judgment that autonomy, in the integrity view, most respects: a judgment about the overall shape of the kind of life she wants to have led.[12] In other words, Dworkin implies that a life lacking critical interests is a poor life in terms of its quality. What we seek is not just any form of life, but rather life in earnest. This reasoning brings him to conclude that a life that includes peanut-butter-and-jelly sandwiches and similar trivial things is not worth living. Eating these sandwiches cannot bring a person to consider his or her life as a kind of assignment, as a mission.[13]

Contrary to Dworkin's arguments, my contention is that even the small pleasure of peanut butter and jelly is indeed worthwhile. Evidence shows that many people who reach the stage of permanent dementia and live nonautonomous lives nevertheless hang on to life and find pleasure in things that had no importance for them in the past. Their present priorities should win over past considerations. Dworkin seems to think that our directives are predetermined and unchangeable, but this is not necessarily the case. We are not able to know how our lives will look when we are about to die. We cannot say that values and priorities that are important to us now will be equally important to us until the very last day. The notion of an unchangeable, unified personality is questionable. People do change, and these changes may become meaningful to us in circumstances that we cannot envisage. Indeed, the very idea of autonomy reflects our ability and desire to construct and reshape realities, to reevaluate values and ideas, to renounce old beliefs, and to accommodate ourselves to new situations.

Dworkin assumes that people, as rational agents, may have certain attitudes regarding dementia and may decide beforehand that some kinds of lives are repugnant, meaningless, and not worth living. People try to assess how their situation might look in the future and decide on their destiny according to the data they currently have on the demented state. However, people are not only thinking creatures. Not all factors can be grasped by our rational faculties. Not all data can be digested by the application of reason and judgment. Sometimes people do things they could not have imagined doing. Sometimes people act in accordance with their sentiments, rather than their brains. Sometimes people are pushed to do something by their instincts, their impulses, factors that they find difficult to explain in rational terms. On some occasions people are overpowered, overwhelmed by the reality they confront. They accommodate themselves to situations imposed on them.

We should acknowledge that a person's priorities are not always fixed, and, therefore, we should not renounce the possibility of changing them. People are not prophets. We can appraise possibilities based upon evidence, data, and experience, but we cannot know with absolute certainty that these assessments will prove to be true for us.[14] Most people are willing to make a commitment that they think and hope will last a lifetime when they marry, but often they have negative experiences and, at a later point in their lives, revise their commitment. We may try to imagine how we would feel in the future upon reaching a certain condition, but on many issues our imagination does not suffice to fully comprehend the future new reality. A parallel example may be the thought of becoming a parent and then actually being a parent. We may think that we understand what becoming a parent entails, what it involves. We may try to exercise our cognitive capacities to imagine ourselves as parents. But we can really grasp the sense of obligation, of love and affection involved in becoming a parent, only when we become parents. This is because we are not merely thinking creators, but also passionate, emotional beings. We love and like to be loved, to give and to share, and these positive feelings can be appreciated only when we actually experience them. Applying cognitive faculties would be a good start for fathoming what is involved in being a parent, but having the actual experience is a different matter. The same reasoning holds when we lose a father or mother. We can fully grasp the notion of being an orphan only upon experiencing such a grave loss. The same reasoning holds for the thought of becoming demented, as opposed to the actual suffering of dementia.

In coming to decide the fate of incompetent patients such as those who are suffering from dementia, consideration should be given to whether the patient's condition is irreversible, whether a chance exists for rehabilitation of some constitutive, vital elements of human life, whether the patient previously expressed a desire to die upon reaching a certain state of living, and also whether we feel the patient's current interests are similar to the interests expressed in the past. These preconditions affirm values that liberals so much appreciate—for example, autonomy and respect for others. Other relevant considerations include the opinions of physicians and of the patient's loved ones.

A caveat has to be made regarding living wills (or advance directives)[15] and DNR orders. The strengths of these directives are the compelling moral force they possess on the way caregivers participate in medical decisions concerning their patients; and their ability to provide help to the clinician in the end-of-life treatment decisions. A difficult question is whether advance directives are invalid and should not be enforceable when the patient in question is incompetent.[16] In the case of patients with chronic disabilities, such as PCU patients, we are not dealing with patients who are about to die, so the concerns revolve around quality-of-life questions—a much less objective field of clinical evaluation. Furthermore, ADs are often formulated without the opportunities for informed consent required for competent patients. On what basis did the patient make the decision against treatment? The decision not to receive treatment should be based on a clear understanding of the situation. It is essential that the patient really understands the disorder, the available alternatives, the chances of survival, and the risks involved in a given treatment. This can be rather complicated in situations in which the physicians themselves do not have a clear picture about the condition and cannot provide a reliable prognosis. Keith Andrews, director of medical and research services, Royal Hospital for Neurodisabilities in Westhill, Putney, in London, contends that with PCU, oftentimes the clinician giving the advice has very little experience, if any, of the condition and is not knowledgeable enough to give informed guidance.[17]

Andrews also voices concerns about the patient's opportunity to change his or her mind, the potential for scientific developments, and the clarity of the advance directive. In the case of a patient who is mentally alert and who makes a decision not to receive treatment, there is always the opportunity for the clinician to consider with the patient the reason for the decision in light of the patient's particular clinical features. The clinician also has the opportunity to discuss with the patient why he or she does not want treatment. Is it due to fear of pain, concern about the loss of dignity, concern for others, or some other reason? In these circumstances, the clinician is in a better position to ensure that the patient has carefully thought out the decision. This possibility is removed in the case of an incompetent patient with a previously formulated AD.[18]

As for potential for scientific progress, competent patients have the advantage of making their decision on the basis of up-to-date knowledge. Advance directives may be made many years prior to the time for their implementation, a period during which new treatment or changes in quality-of life opportunities may have occurred. In addition, ADs do not always make clear the patient's intentions. Andrews testifies that he saw an advance directive stating that, if the person developed severe brain damage, she would not want to continue living. There was no statement as to whether this decision was to be made on the first day or after a period of several days/weeks/months in which the patient would be given the opportunity to recover. The general statement about severe brain damage gives wide latitude for widely differing views, even among clinicians experienced in the management of brain damage.[19]

Advance directives, DNR orders, and living wills reflect competent values and interests in circumstances in which they may no longer be applicable.[20] Because the patient is incompetent at the time these procedures become effective, the withdrawal or withholding of life-sustaining therapies under DNR orders or living wills constitutes a form of imputed consent. The situation of the incompetent patient is viewed as it was by the prior competent self rather than in the light of the patient's current state. It is usually assumed that the justification for giving the competent person power over decisions to be made in the future, when he or she is incompetent, is that the competent person is best situated to identify what those future interests will be. The problem, however, is that the incompetent patient's interests are no longer informed by the interests and values he or she had when competent. The values and interests of the competent person are no longer relevant to someone who has lost the rational structure on which those values and interests rested. Although the patient is still the same person, the patient's interests change radically when he or she becomes incompetent. Thus there is a possible conflict between past competent and current incompetent interests.[21]

To resolve the conflict between past competent and current incompetent interests, I suggest, along with John A. Robertson, James F. Childress, and Sanford H. Kadish,[22] that instead of simply enforcing all prior directives, doctors, family, and others involved in the care of incompetent patients should be able to examine whether patient interests would best be served by actions contrary to the living will, in situations in which the incompetent patient appears to have an interest in further life.[23] On this issue my view differs significantly from that of Dworkin, who endorses precedent autonomy as genuine. In his view, the decision made earlier while the patient was competent remains in force because no new decision by a person capable of autonomy has annulled it. A competent person's right to autonomy requires that his past decisions about how he is to be treated if he becomes demented be respected, even if they contradict the desires he appears to have at that later point. If we decide to honor the patient's current decision, then we violate his autonomy. While criticizing the Supreme Court ruling in *Cruzan*, Dworkin argues that "just as Justice Rehnquist was wrong to assume there is no harm in a patient's living on as a vegetable, so it would be wrong to assume that there is no harm in living on demented." Demented people have no sense of their own critical interests, but before that, when they were competent, they did have such a sense, and we cannot disregard this or think it no longer matters.[24]

Dworkin backs his reasoning by the findings of a poll he conducted among people he knows. Roughly half were repelled by the idea of living demented, totally dependent lives, speaking gibberish, incapable of understanding that there was a world beyond them, let alone following its course. Dworkin says these persons think a life ending like that is seriously marred, that the critical harm is even greater than "living on as a quiescent vegetable." They do not think the possible childish pleasures of dementia would redeem its course.[25]

In response, I first demur with regard to the use of the term *vegetable* to describe a life, poor in quality as it might be (see chapter 1).

Second, it seems that Dworkin's personal poll is highly selective. No conclusion should be drawn from it because it does not represent the population as a whole. From my own research conducted at Loewenstein Rehabilitation Hospital and at Israeli, English, American, and Canadian hospitals for chronic patients as well as in intensive care units, I learned that most patients hang on to life. In most cases, it is possible to alleviate emotional, psychological, and spiritual suffering. Once these parameters are controlled, the vast majority of patients will continue to have the urge to live. Patients find pleasure in things they never appreciated before. As Pellegrino argues, requests for euthanasia are often the result of desperation that the medical staff and the patients' loved ones can forestall by providing the understanding, support, and sharing that will assure the patients that they are still members of the human community.[26]

Zev Susak, general director of the Loewenstein Rehabilitation Hospital, asserted that in his more than twenty years of experience very few patients had expressed a desire to die. When I pressed him for numbers, his answer was that, on occasion, when patients were in deep depression (when, for example, they were told they would always be lame), they asserted they would rather die. But many of these patients did not persist with their wish for long. After some period of reconciliation, they learned to cope with their new situation and wanted to continue living.[27] Similarly, Nachman Wilensky, director of the Lichtenstaedter Hospital for chronic patients, told me that in twenty-one years of experience, only a handful of his patients had insisted that they wanted to die. Lichtenstaedter Hospital does not keep records of such requests, but in any event, the number is no more than ten patients among thousands.[28] Charles Sprung, professor of medicine at Hebrew University and director of the intensive care unit, Hadassah Hebrew University Medical Center, told me that although most of his patients are unconscious, he holds many discussions with families and has never had a request for euthanasia or assisted suicide.[29]

Keith Andrews testified that in thirty years of practice in geriatric medicine and chronic disability of young disabled people, he could only remember having come across four patients who made a definite request to die—and three of these were elderly. All of the three elderly people changed their minds after a period of discussion. One asked to die because, at the age of eighty-five, she felt that her symptoms of incontinence, unsteadiness, dizziness, and a tendency to fall were too much for her. However, Andrews said, "once we treated the bio-chemical abnormalities her symptoms ceased, she wished to continue living." One of the other elderly patients was more frightened about what would happen in the future and was frightened of developing severe pain. Andrews explained that "once we reassured her that we would treat all pain she withdrew her request to die." The third patient felt she was being a burden on her family, but once her family reassured her that they loved her and wanted her to remain alive, she also withdrew her request. The fourth patient was an eighty-five-year-old professor of medicine who developed severe brain damage, despite which he had insight into his condition. He felt that life was not worthwhile living if he was not able to continue his medical academic work. While this patient continued to hold this view, he made no adamant request to have his life ended. Andrews stated that in his 280–bed hospital for profoundly neurologically disabled people, studies by the in-house psychology department have demonstrated that nearly all the patients who are mentally alert but profoundly disabled consider that they have good quality of life. The factor that seems to differentiate between those who regard themselves as having a good quality of life and those who do not is the level of control they have over decisions affecting their lives.[30]

Canadian findings are not significantly different. Larry Librach, director of the division of palliative medicine at Mount Sinai Hospital, Toronto, told me that out of hundreds of patients treated annually, an average of two patients requested to die. Pat Porterfield, clinical nurse specialist in the palliative care unit, Vancouver Hospital, estimated that 99.9 percent of the patients want to continue living. David Kuhl of the palliative care unit at St. Paul's Hospital in Vancouver estimated that 98 percent of the patients cling to life. R. N. MacDonald, palliative care specialist at the Centre for Bioethics in Montreal, said he had never had a patient who insisted that he or she wanted assistance to die, and that in a period of thirty years, fewer than five of his patients actually committed suicide.[31]

Zail S. Berry, an American internist who had been involved in hospice work for ten years, caring for well over two thousand terminally ill patients during that time, said that scores of people had asked him to kill them. All but three completely withdrew the requests once their physical pain was under control.[32]

While these testimonials constitute anecdotal evidence and cannot be assigned the same weight as scientific statistical surveys, the pattern described by senior doctors and other health care professionals in various parts of the world about the wishes of patients whom they have encountered during their rich careers is strikingly similar.

In the Netherlands, the only country in the world where euthanasia and physician-assisted suicide have been practiced with increased openness during the past two decades, there are a relatively large number of requests for both procedures. The Netherlands is also the only country in the world where in-depth studies of a large scale have been conducted, trying to estimate the scale of the phenomenon, and learning from the experience of these practices. Paul Van der Maas and his colleagues testify in their 1995–1996 report that there were 34,500 requests for euthanasia at a later time in the course of disease and 9,700 explicit requests for euthanasia or physician-assisted suicide at a particular time. However, a relatively smaller number of the requests were granted: 3,200 cases of euthanasia and 400 cases of physician-assisted suicide, accounting for 2.4 percent and 0.3 percent of all deaths respectively. It is estimated that a third of Dutch physicians have never had a request or participated in actively ending life, and the total percentage of deaths shows that euthanasia and physician-assisted suicide remain relatively rare events.[33]

In this context, it is pertinent to make a distinction between a temporary and a consistent desire to die. Physician-assisted suicide can be contemplated on some occasions when patients freely and genuinely express their wish to die, and when they persist in expressing that desire. We all need time to digest major developments in our lives. That is why all cultures develop meaningful customs that enable us to come to grips with crucial experiences. All cultures have symbols and rituals that help people grow accustomed to new realities, such as birth, adulthood, love, disappointment, and death. Nature gives us nine months to anticipate the introduction of a new life into our families. In some cultures weddings last days, even weeks. Other cultures adopt the honeymoon concept to celebrate the occasion.

As we need time to grasp happy occasions, so we need time to comprehend somber ones. We mourn our dead to acknowledge their departure from our lives. Similarly we need time to digest the fact that some faculties we had are no longer present. Every person has weak moments. We should not immediately respond to impulses arising from shock, frustration, or dismay, for at such moments people may not be considered fully autonomous. The distinguishing feature of autonomy is the forming of insights in a way that is supported by reason, even though the person's rationality might be impaired.[34] Patients who express a desire to die out of emotional shock, depression, frustration, or dismay cannot be said to be using rational judgment. They do not form an opinion, but rather surrender themselves to circumstances. Caught in their feelings, some of these patients are too frail to resist. They are overwhelmed by the news conveyed to them. As has been shown here, however, almost all patients eventually become more accepting and become accustomed to the new reality. They prefer to live.

The insistence on a consistent desire to die is designed to overcome the influence of depression, allowing time for treatment to change this state of mind and to give patients the opportunity to regain a positive trust in the possibility of a good life. Robert G. Twycross argues that if patients are provided with good pain and symptom relief, the desire "to end it all" is generally associated with a transient mood disorder, a depressive illness, or delirium.[35] This argument coincides with the findings of Ezekiel Emanuel and his colleagues. They show that patients who had previously considered and prepared for euthanasia or physician-assisted suicide were significantly more likely to be clinically depressed. Depressed patients were more likely than nondepressed patients to find that discussions of euthanasia or physician-assisted suicide increased trust in their physicians. Conversely, patients experiencing pain were not inclined to opt for these measures. This suggests that having pain does not predispose patients to desire or take action to end their life. Pain does not seem to propel patients to perceive euthanasia or physician-assisted suicide as the appropriate response. Emanuel and colleagues added that cancer patients in pain might be suspicious that if euthanasia or physician-assisted suicide were legalized, the medical care system might not focus sufficient resources on provision of pain relief and palliative care.[36] This concern should be carefully addressed. Medicine today has the ability to cope with most pain symptoms, and this ability should be exhausted before the relatively few requests for euthanasia and physician-assisted suicide are considered. Obviously, these measures should not serve as a substitute for elaborate schemes of pain management.

Cruzan

In the *Cruzan* case, Chief Justice William Rehnquist ruled it was better to keep alive even the person who had expressed the wish to die should he or she reach this situation, because it is better to err reversibly on the side of life than to err irreversibly on the side of death.[37] The underlying assumption is that keeping someone alive in a state of PCU, even if that person had asked to die upon reaching such a state, causes no serious damage. In his criticism of the decision of the U.S. Supreme Court, Dworkin rightly attacks this assumption. In his opinion, mere biological existence, without intelligence or feelings, is neither valuable nor worthy of existence. Thus, Justice Rehnquist's assumption that people lose nothing when permission to terminate their lives is refused is mistaken. A great many people believe that a decision to keep them alive would cheat them forever of a chance to die with both dignity and consideration for others.[38]

Dworkin compares death with the final act of a play. He says that it is important to people that their lives end in a way that is compatible with the way they lived. The last stage of their lives affects their view of their lives as a whole.[39] These issues are related to the issue of human dignity: Some people find the end of their lives contradictory to their previous experiences to the extent that it constitutes an offense to their dignity.

The play metaphor is appealing, and it is obviously preferable that the final stage of life would suit the previous stages. In reality, however, the final stage of life is usually less appealing than the others. We may characterize life as comprising a continuum from beginning to end, which involves the deterioration of the body. The final scene could be tragic and painful, and it is our duty to treat patients with respect even at this last stage, regardless of the difficulties and the inconvenience encountered. It is at this stage of life that people, more than ever before, are in need of help in order to preserve their dignity.

Although the Supreme Court was wrong in not honoring Cruzan's right to die with dignity, I wish to raise unequivocal warning against simplistic and sweeping generalizations voiced by both parties in the controversy. Chief Justice Rehnquist did not grant Cruzan's motion because he thought the Missouri rule that favors keeping comatose people alive was in the best interests of the thousands of people who live in a permanent vegetative state and did not sign living wills when they could have done so.[40] Rehnquist's judgment ignored the data evinced by Cruzan's friends and family that she probably would not have wanted to remain in such a condition for many years and would opt for death if she were able to speak her desire. Preservation of life and body for its own sake was not an object for Cruzan. Chief Justice Rehnquist emphasized the public will of thousands of other people in Cruzan's condition and, at the same time, ignored the specific person named Nancy Cruzan. Research does not provide grounds to suspect that her family and friends were biased in presenting her best interest. Her condition remained stagnant for years without any significant signs of progress (the accident took place in 1983, and she died in December 1990, after nutrition and hydration were stopped). The Missouri trial court found that permanent brain damage generally results after six minutes in an anoxic state; the best estimate for Cruzan's anoxia was twelve to fourteen minutes. Over a substantial period of time, valiant efforts to rehabilitate her took place without success. She received all her nutrition and hydration through a gastrostomy tube.[41]

Cruzan's parents hoped she would get better and waited for four years before reluctantly accepting that she would not recover. Then, because of their love and respect for their daughter, they petitioned the courts

to allow removal of the feeding tube. The extensive documentation testified that her condition was hopeless, and that all the doctors could do
was preserve her existence.[42]

I would also like to warn against sweeping generalizations on the
other side of the spectrum of views. Dworkin argued that Rehnquist's
argument was implausible: "Many people who are now in that position
talked and acted in ways that make it very likely that they would have
signed a living will had they anticipated their own accidents," as Cruzan
did in conversations with her loved ones.[43] Dworkin maintained: "The
Missouri rule flouts rather than honors their autonomy. Many others . . .
almost certainly would have decided that way if they had ever considered the matter."[44] The problem, however, is that the public at large is
unaware of the relevant medical data for PCU patients and the chances
for some form of recovery, and, I suspect, so is Dworkin. PCU patients
have some chance, meager as it might be, to regain their consciousness
and possibly some of their faculties. The common practice in the United
States, however, often does not allow these patients the option of some
recovery, and the public is unaware of the complicated details (see chapter 2). Dworkin's research on the medical aspects of his theory is quite
deficient. Someone who deals with issues of life and death could be expected to be much clearer, and more careful and concise, in his definitions and categories.

Dworkin argues that it is not right, in the case of people in a situation like that of Cruzan, that public expenditure be used to keep them
alive. The state cannot afford to keep comatose people alive for months
and years.[45] On this issue, Dworkin's view is akin to that of Callahan,
who argues that modern medicine should be an option for severely deteriorated patients only if it promises clear benefit; it should not be an
imposed burden. Callahan contends that the costs of high-technology
terminal care are not a trivial consideration. Thus, with advanced dementia, the presumption should be against treatment unless there are
some compelling reasons to continue the treatment. Callahan concludes
that such costs can be justified only if some clear benefit is likely to
result, and there seems to be none where PCU patients are concerned[46]
(for further discussion, see appendix).

John Finnis disagrees, stating that affluent societies like the United
States can afford to care for comatose people. To abandon such people
is to deny them communal obligation, dignity, and respect. Only the explicit consent to be disconnected from the machine, previously communicated by the persons concerned, can justify the taking of life.[47] Finnis
finds value in mere physical existence. Being human includes being a
body. Human life is the actuality of one's body. The body is perceived

as a properly personal reality, a sign and place of relations with others, with God, and with the world. Human life is intrinsically good, and we have an obligation to respect a body, irrespective of whether a person has cognitive capacities, and without using the economic argument as a justification for terminating a life.[48] To use Dworkin's terminology, the economic burden of keeping people alive should not serve as a trump card to overrule other considerations, such as the dignity of persons as human beings.

Accordingly, we may discern two different arguments for keeping comatose people alive: First, we should keep people alive as long as there is a chance they could return to social life; and second, the imperative to keep people alive arises from a gut feeling, deriving from a strong sense of self-preservation of humanity, of our species.

Finnis conveys both ideas, while Dworkin does not see any value in self-preservation per se. The crux of the disagreement between Dworkin and Finnis lies with the issue of whether the body itself has a certain intrinsic value. Finnis thinks it does. Dworkin contends that what we value is the system—that is, a body and consciousness. We value the body because we see it as part of an enterprise, part of a system that is comprised of physical, biological components and cognitive faculties. The body as such does not have an intrinsic value. However, Dworkin's assertion that "life that is permanently vegetative is not valuable to anyone" is clearly mistaken.[49] It is valuable at least to John Finnis and to many other people who share his views.

Conclusion

Dworkin is right in asserting that patients suffering from severe dementia lack autonomy. But should this serve as the sole criterion for deciding their destiny when the patients concerned clearly want now (i.e., in their new situation) to continue living, no matter what? I think not. Many demented people are fundamentally happy. Some of them exhibit their happiness by singing and dancing. A competent person might say, "I don't want this singing and dancing body of mine to continue living when I no longer inhabit this body." However, most doctors will not terminate life simply because an advance directive was given when the patient who wrote the directive seems content with her present situation, and is not obviously suffering. It is not the role of doctor to abide by such a request. Doctors cannot be sure that the AD or living will is really what the patient now wants, and because of lack of communication, they would prefer to err on the side of life.

Experiential interests voiced in the present are more important than critical interests that were voiced in the past. We are in no position to disregard our future interests simply because we think they will be merely experiential. Something that has a limited value in the present may gain enormous meaning in the future, to the point of even becoming critical. What may seem experiential in one stage of life might in a marred, limited life become critical to our being. For some demented patients the taste of vanilla ice cream and the smell of lilies might be essential to the definition and conception of life. Life might seem significantly and genuinely worse without the ice cream and the lilies. The interest of having them becomes the most important one. Life is conceived as good when the interest of having certain things is satisfied, when life without ice cream and lilies would be much worse. We are not prophets, so we cannot put ourselves in a position we are unable to grasp before we actually experience it. We cannot say in advance that only a certain level of autonomy is worth living because life is in flux, circumstances are in flux, and personality is in flux. People do change. They change not only as a result of facing physical deterioration, but also as a result of social changes, of learning and of experiencing new things in life. Moreover, autonomy is important, but it is not the only consideration. As Joseph Raz, a prominent philosopher at Oxford University, once contended in a private discussion, many competent healthy persons find autonomy a burden and prefer to leave decision making in the hands of others. So autonomy is significant, but it is not more important than life when we have reason to assume that the patient concerned prefers to live. There can be life without autonomy, but there cannot be autonomy without life.

If a patient expressed in an advance directive in the form of a living will, a DNR order, a letter, and so on, that he or she would wish to continue living, no matter what, and we have no reason to believe that the patient ever changed his or her mind, then we should respect that wish.[50] If the patient prepared an advance directive saying that he or she would prefer that all treatment be terminated when the last stage of an incurable disease was reached, and we are uncertain about the patient's present wishes because, for instance, the patient is in PCU and the attending physicians think that the situation is irreversible, then we should respect the advance directives and let the patient die. For persons who prepared advance directives asking to die upon reaching a certain condition, death is not the worst possible outcome compared to being on the verge of death and then being stabilized without hope of ever really getting better. Patients who suffer from incurable diseases such as cancer may feel that their lives have become transient and that the thought of death brings them more comfort than alarm. They may feel that their dignity, their autonomy, their humanity will be better served if they are allowed to die. These patients' wishes must be respected. This is especially true if they have emphasized beforehand that their dignity cannot be separated from consideration of the suffering of their loved ones. For some patients, knowledge of the anguish their condition imposes on their families is such a heavy burden that they prefer to die and not be remembered in their diminished condition. Of course, this is not the sole consideration, but it is a significant additional consideration that needs to be taken into account.

If no advance directives are available, we should ask the advice of the patient's loved ones, who should know the patient better than anyone else. If they believe the patient would want to be kept alive, then we should respect their decision, even if the attending physicians disagree. In the event that the patient's loved ones wish to withhold treatment but the attending physicians think there is still a hope of recovery, then we have to respect the physicians' decision. The patient's best interests require erring on the side of life.

If the patient's loved ones and the attending physicians believe the patient's condition will only deteriorate, and that this condition negates the patient's dignity, the best interests of the patient require allowing the patient to die. It is the best interests of the patient, not those of the family or other loved ones, the physician, or the hospital or the society at large that are paramount.

6

The Role of
the Patients'
Loved Ones

This chapter explores the intricate issue of the right to die with dignity by focusing on the role of the patient's loved ones in three illustrative American court cases. In the first case, *Saikewicz*, the patient had neither family nor other loved ones, and this had a significant bearing on the court's ruling not to provide him treatment. The second case, *Spring*, involved a patient whose family wanted to withhold treatment from him. It demonstrates the importance of caution in incidents when the best interests of the patient's loved ones contradict the best interests of the patient. The third case, *Gray*, serves as an example in which the patient's best interests coincide with the best interests of her loved ones. Sometimes families need to consent to forgoing life support for their relative who wishes to die.[1] By granting their consent, they honor the patient's dignity, enabling the patient to maintain control over life as he or she desired. Consideration has to be given to the question of whether the patient's loved ones demonstrate a unified position in regard to the destiny of the patient.

The term the patient's *loved ones* refers to persons who are closely related to the patient emotionally. This does not necessarily mean that only those who have close biological and marital attachments should give their consent and advice. The opinion of a person who has lived with the patient for the past five years without formal ties will be much more germane than the opinion of the patient's sister who has lived abroad and has seen the patient only once in a while. The opinion of a very close friend in whom the patient has confided and whose advice she has sought is much more important than the opinion of a father who broke relations with the patient.

Patients' Wishes and the Commitments of Family and Friends

Grace is gravely ill. She suffers from a progressive dementia, and the attending physician is not able to provide her with treatment that may halt the progress of the disease. Grace's condition continues to deteriorate, and she is unable to live as she has in the past. In Dworkin's terminology, Grace has reached a stage at which she is incapable of actively advancing most of her critical interests (see chapter 5). She is no longer able to pursue her career, to practice her religion the way she did in the past, and to maintain her friendships. Furthermore, Grace's range of experiential interests has become extremely limited. She is incapable of playing the guitar, walking, eating as she used to, or visiting the theater. But Grace has a family, and she shows signs that her critical interest in having a family and enjoying their company is still present. Grace feels the love of her family. She appreciates them and enjoys the constant company and support of her parents and her other close relatives. From time to time she expresses her feelings by a smile or a sound.

In the past Grace voiced a critical interest in not sustaining her life upon reaching such a stage (for an discussion of critical interest, see chapter 5). When she was competent, Grace did not think that mere minimal communication with her family could constitute a worthwhile life. But her current behavior gives members of her family (and other people who care about her) the impression that their company in itself makes Grace's life worthwhile.

Dworkin does not consider the possibility of a conflict between two critical interests, one indicated in the past, the other alluded to in the present. He might say that demented patients cannot have critical interests. Further, Dworkin might not see Grace's present condition as a life that can be considered as an assignment, as a mission. Nevertheless, as far as people around Grace can judge, she finds some value in her life. Should we respect the critical interest that Grace voiced in the past in not sustaining her life upon reaching such a condition, or should we respect the other apparent critical interest that concerns Grace's family and their mutual love? Which critical interest should have precedence over the other? Moreover, are the family's critical interests of any relevance? That is, when physicians favor ending a life and the patient's loved ones object, are we to respect the family's critical interest in maintaining the patient's life?

In this situation, the family does not make Grace feel that she constitutes a burden. The family does not exert social pressure on Grace to die; the opposite is the case. If Grace were to feel that she constituted a burden on her family and on other people she loves, if she were to feel that her family would rather see her dead, then Grace might decide to opt for dying. But if those who care for Grace feel that her candle is still dripping (to use a metaphor that is frequently mentioned in halachic writings and that was adopted by the Israeli Supreme Court),[2] that, on balance, her life is still worth living, her pain is being controlled, and her smiles reinforce their support, then Grace would have no social incentive to terminate her life before she felt that her life was meaningless.[3]

This family is committed to Grace's care; they practically live their entire lives around her bed. Obviously, their commitment places some restrictions on their variety of options for action. But they do not view these restrictions as impediments on their freedom or autonomy. Members of Grace's family and others who care for her willingly accept the necessity of sacrifice, thereby expressing themselves, their sense of giving, of sharing, of love, and any other affective notion that is valuable for defining their world as autonomous agents. Many of us may have an interest in giving to others because the act of giving and the recognition that we make others happy contribute to our satisfaction, making us feel more humane, with a character that has been improved. Restricting ourselves in such circumstances does not go against our interests. Instead, it is conducive to promoting our position through the effort of contributing to others. We all have an interest in promoting egoistic motives, but for similar or other reasons, we also have an interest in furthering altruistic notions. Thus, we are willing to take on sacrifices and restraints. The endeavor of comforting a severely ill patient does not necessarily have to be regarded as an imposition. Many would prefer this demanding sacrifice to the alternative. Many of us feel that our character is improved when we do good for others. In this instance, egoistic and altruistic interests merge, and it is difficult at times to tell where one ends and the other begins.

A caveat has to be presented in this context. Not all families are like Grace's family. Sometimes partisan motives (financial considerations, rivalries within the family, etc.) may influence the family's position. It should not be taken for granted that the family truly cares for the patient in question. Sometimes other people (friends, colleagues, past and present lovers) care more for the patient than does the family. Someone has to verify that genuine interests are involved, and, I submit, that person should be the social worker assigned to the patient. The social worker is trained to inquire about familial circumstances and is qualified to make a judgment. I am not saying that the social worker should pry or listen in on confidential discussions. What is suggested is that the social worker have open and frank discussions with all those who claim to have close relationships with the patient so as to prevent or at least to minimize the possibility of abuse.[4] It is better to have these conversations than to leave the framework of relationships unexamined.

Sometimes the family is incapable of rational decision-making. Sometimes the strain on the family is too severe for its members to cope.[5] Evidence gathered during my extensive fieldwork in various hospitals in Israel shows that the closest ties are those between the patient and his or her parents.[6] Thus, whenever possible, it is preferable to ask for the opinion of not only the patient's spouse (when he or she has one), but also other members of the family, especially the parents.[7] Of course, parents are not immune to strain, and therefore it is advisable to enlarge the group of the loved ones who participate in the decision-making.[8] What I have in mind is a council of all those who step forward claiming to have close association with the patient, freely and openly discussing the future of their loved one, bringing forward all considerations for and against the continuation of life. This gathering would take place after physicians had expressed the opinion that available medicine could not cure the patient, that his or her condition would deteriorate, and that there was no hope for recovery. For a patient who was incompetent and had not named a proxy decision-maker, the medical staff would hold an open and candid discussion with this council and would try to reach a consensual decision with regard to treatment. If this were impossible due to conflicts within the council, the medical staff would act in a way that—to the best of their medical understanding and knowledge—would serve the patient's best interests.

Formal and Speculative Autonomy

The question of how we can (or should) protect a person's autonomy is of major importance. People who believe that rational patients should have the right to arrange their own deaths, with the help of willing physicians, often use the principle of autonomy as a justification for their position. Those who object to this idea, on the other hand, claim that people who really want to stay alive might be killed, maintaining that leaving the decision in the hands of the patient's family might negate patient autonomy. Here we have to distinguish between an implicit and an explicit desire to die, between formal and speculative autonomy. Formal autonomy is implemented when the patient actually made a decision. Speculative autonomy is what the patient would have decided if he or she had had the chance to make a decision. In assessing speculative autonomy, much attention is given to the opinion of the patient's guardian or proxy.

In 1990, the New York legislature enacted Article 29–C of the Public Health Law, entitled Health Care Agents and Proxies. This statute allows a person to sign a health care proxy for the purpose of appointing an agent with authority to make "any and all health care decisions on the principal's behalf." These decisions include those relating to the administration of artificial nutrition and hydration, provided the wishes of the patient are known. Accordingly, a patient has the right to hasten death by empowering an agent to require a physician to withdraw life-sustaining treatment.[9]

American courts prefer to rely on formal autonomy, in cases in which the actual consent of the patient to cease living in particular circumstances has been recorded. The standard to be satisfied is "clear and convincing evidence" that patient would have wanted to cease treatment. In the *Eichner* case, the court allowed the petition of Brother Fox's superior to terminate use of a ventilator, but only because eighty-three-year-old Brother Fox had clearly expressed the wish that this be done more than once, earlier, when he was competent.[10] In *Tavel*, the court authorized the removal of a feeding tube from an incompetent patient upon gathering evidence satisfying the "clear and convincing evidence" standard. The court said that when a person has clearly expressed his or her prior intentions about a course of treatment in the event of incompetence, those intentions should be respected.[11] In *O'Connor*, New York's highest court suggested that artificial life support could never be withdrawn without an explicit statement of the patient.[12] O'Connor had expressed her wishes not to be kept alive by artificial means in the past when family members and friends were dying of cancer.

The issue is further complicated when courts are forced to deliberate on patients' speculative autonomy, when the patients did not write advance directives or living wills. In such cases, the courts investigate what the patient would have wanted if he or she were able to pronounce an opinion. When the "clear and convincing evidence" standard is not satisfied, the courts are reluctant to authorize cessation of treatment. In *Wickel v. Spellman*, the request for removal of a nasogastric tube was denied because family had not established "by clear and convincing evidence" that the patient would have wanted to die.[13] In the *Storar* case, the New York Court of Appeals reversed a trial court order permitting termination of blood transfusions being administered to extend the life of a profoundly retarded fifty-two-year-old man with terminal bladder cancer.[14] The court explicitly rejected the substituted judgment test, enabling life-prolonging measures to be withheld from patients incapable of making decisions for themselves only if the patients had previously been competent and had expressed a wish not to receive such measures. In *In re Martin*, the petition of the wife of an incompetent but conscious patient to withdraw life-sustaining medical treatment was denied on the grounds that her testimony and affidavit did not constitute "clear and convincing evidence" of the patient's pre-injury decision to decline treatment in his current circumstances.[15] It should be noted that the patient's mother and sister opposed the wife's petition. In *Hayner v. Child's Nursing Home,* testimony of family and friends was insufficient to establish that the patient, while competent, had expressed "a firm and settled commitment to decline medical treatment in her current state."[16] In the *Cruzan* case (see chapter 5), both the Supreme Court of Missouri and the U.S. Supreme Court held that no sufficient reliable evidence was provided to support the parents' claim to exercise substituted judgment on behalf of Cruzan.[17] Guardians did not have the authority to order withdrawal of hydration and nutrition.[18]

In support of the courts' insistence on clear and convincing evidence, the empirical study by Jeremiah Suhl et al. showed that patient's surrogates were not able to predict the patient's wishes regarding forgoing life support in a range of commonly encountered medical scenarios. In fact, the surrogates under examination guessed no better than would have been expected from random chance alone. The amount of discussion between patient and surrogate regarding termination of treatment was the only identified factor that correlated with accurate surrogate decision-making.[19]

In the case of patients who had been incompetent since birth, the courts rightly insisted on having "clear and convincing evidence" regarding their medical condition. When no sufficient credible evidence was produced, the courts denied petition to terminate life-support treatments.[20]

Many times, the courts were asked to decide the fate of PCU patients. Often they held that guardians could direct termination of life-sustaining treatment, including nutrition and hydration, if the decision was "in the best interest" of the ward. In the *Quinlan* case, the Supreme Court of New Jersey, concerned with a patient in a state of persistent unawareness, recommended that Quinlan's guardian and family should decide "whether or not she would exercise it in the circumstances of the case before the court."[21] Quinlan's father was appointed her guardian, and, in accordance with his decision, her ventilator was disconnected.[22] In

In re Conservatorship of Wanglie the court ruled that the husband of an eighty-seven-year-old incompetent patient in PCU was the most suitable and best qualified guardian of his wife's interest, rather than a proposed court-appointed professional guardian.[23] In *In re Colyer*, the husband of an incompetent patient in a "chronic vegetative state" sought a court order to discontinue life-sustaining treatment. The court held that state interests in the preservation of life, protection of interests of innocent third parties, prevention of suicide, and maintenance of ethical integrity of the medical profession were not at odds with the removal of life-sustaining mechanisms from patients. The court maintained that the statute requiring a guardian to assert the rights and best interests of an incompetent person enables the guardian to use his or her best judgment and, when appropriate, to exercise the incompetent's personal right to refuse life-sustaining treatment.[24] In *Matter of the Guardianship and Protective Placement of Edna M. F.*,[25] concerning a guardian's petition to withhold artificial nutrition from an incompetent ward, the court insisted that the guardian could direct withdrawal of life-sustaining treatment, including nutrition and hydration, only if the incompetent ward was in a "persistent vegetative state" and the decision to withdraw was in the best interest of the patient.[26] I would suggest that the language of the court be qualified, taking into account the age of the patient, the causes of the condition, and the length of time in a state of unawareness (see chapter 2). In any event, in this case Edna M. F. was an Alzheimer's patient, and the only indication of her desires regarding treatment or lack thereof had been made at least thirty years previously and under different circumstances. There was not a clear statement of intent such that her guardian might authorize the withholding of her nutrition.

In *In re Fiori*, the mother of a PCU patient who lost consciousness in 1976 filed a petition requesting an order directing a nursing home to terminate treatment.[27] The Supreme Court of Pennsylvania held that a close relative acting as substitute decision-maker, with the consent of two physicians, could remove life-sustaining treatment from an adult PCU patient when the patient left no advance directives. It could be assumed that after so many years in this condition, the chances of some sort of improvement on the part of the patient were extremely slim. The court emphasized that close family members are usually the most knowledgeable about the patient's preferences, goals, and values, and that they have "an understanding about the nuances of our personality that set us apart as individuals."[28]

The conclusions of the U.S. President's Commission for the Study of Ethical Problems and Biomedical and Behavioral Research are relevant to the discussion. The commission argued in 1983 that "the family is generally most concerned about the good of the patient"; the family "will also usually be most knowledgeable about the patient's goals, preferences and values"; and the family "deserves recognition as an important social unit that ought to be treated, within limits, as a responsible decision maker in matters that intimately affect its members."[29]

Thus, family members or other guardians are permitted to decide on behalf of the patients on the basis of their acquaintance with them, believing that they know what patients would have chosen were they competent to make decisions. The substituted judgment test is intended to determine with as much accuracy as possible the wants and needs of the individual involved. The reasoning is similar to what John Rawls suggested in *A Theory of Justice*: "We must choose for others as we have reason to believe they would choose for themselves if they were at the age of reason and deciding rationally." Rawls maintained that trustees, guardians, and benefactors usually know the situation and interests of their wards, so they can often make accurate estimates as to what would have been wanted.[30]

Accordingly, when the substituted-judgment test is applied in order to determine whether an incompetent adult would refuse life-saving or life-prolonging treatment if he or she were competent, the decision of the patient's family and other loved ones, particularly where that decision is in accord with the recommendation of the attending physician, is of special importance. American law recognizes as valid a consent to treatment of an incompetent person given in a traditional manner by the family, next of kin, or a guardian for treatment of the person in question.[31]

If treatment can be terminated when a PCU patient left no advance directive, upon reliance on the statements of the patient's family, obviously it should be possible for treatment to be terminated when the patient has left directives. In *DeGrella v. Elston*, the mother of a PCU patient sought court authorization to order discontinuation of nutrition and hydration after the daughter had spent ten years in this devastating condition. The Supreme Court of Kentucky held that the mother could order life-sustaining treatments discontinued, in light of medical finding that her daughter's condition was irreversible and in light of the patient's statement, made when she was competent, that if she were ever to be in PCU, extraordinary measures to sustain her life should not be taken.[32] While the majority of the court recognized that nutrition and hydration were not "extraordinary measures," they stated that it would be unreasonable to require such a high degree of specificity on the patient's part while she was competent. The court concluded that Sue DeGrella's statements of choice were competent evidence upon which a surrogate decision-maker could exercise substitute judgment.[33]

In English law consideration is being given to the wishes of patients expressed prior to the onset of their persistent unawareness. The Court of Appeal stated in *Airedale NHS Trust v. Bland* that if the patient "had given instructions that he should not be artificially fed or treated with antibiotics if he should become a PVS patient, his physicians would not act unlawfully in complying with those instructions but would act unlawfully if they did not comply, even though the patient's death would inevitably follow."[34] In another case it was emphasized that such wishes are to be followed even if they are irrational in nature.[35]

Court Cases

The role of the patients' loved ones can be considered through a more detailed discussion of three precedents.

Saikewicz

The *Saikewicz* case law involves a sixty-seven-year-old patient who had been severely retarded since birth, whose I.Q. was equal to ten, and whose mental age was approximately two years and eight months.[36] He had never learned to talk and never had the capacity to form a view about his medical care. Saikewicz suffered from acute myeloblastic monocytic leukemia, for which chemotherapy was the only possible treatment. Despite the fact that most people in Saikewicz's position elect to suffer the side effects of chemotherapy rather than to allow their leukemia to run its natural course, a guardian *ad litem* (a special guardian, not a relative, appointed to represent him) recommended withholding the treatment, and his recommendation was accepted by the Massachusetts Supreme Judicial Court.

Justice Liacos, who delivered the opinion of the court, considered two factors in favor of administering chemotherapy: the fact that most people elect chemotherapy, and the chance of a longer life. These considerations were balanced against factors weighing against administration of chemotherapy. The court asserted that evidence that most people choose to accept the rigors of chemotherapy "has no direct bearing on the likely choice that Joseph Saikewicz would have made" (430). The guardian *ad litem* explained that if Saikewicz were to be treated with toxic drugs, he would be involuntarily immersed in a state of painful suffering, the reason for which he would never understand (430).

In addition to these two factors, the certainty that treatment would cause immediate suffering, and Saikewicz's inability to cooperate independently with the treatment, the court weighed four further factors against providing chemotherapy: Saikewicz's age (persons over age sixty have more difficulty tolerating chemotherapy, and the treatment is likely to be less successful than in younger patients); the probable side effects of treatment; the low chance of producing remission; and the doctors' opinion that a decision to allow the disease to run its natural course would not result in pain for the patient, and death would probably come without discomfort.

The *Saikewicz* ruling is highly problematic. Paternalism was disguised as action based on the premise of the autonomy principle. The court spoke of a "right of privacy" for incompetent individuals who cannot comprehend their situation and used the substituted-judgment doctrine to interfere with their privacy. The court recognized a general right of all persons to refuse medical treatment in appropriate circumstances, without knowing and without having the ability to know what Mr. Saikewicz would have wanted if he had been able to make a choice. The court for its own reasons chose to stress this general right, declining the fact that most people choose to accept the rigors of chemotherapy, by saying that this "has no direct bearing on the likely choice that Joseph Saikewicz would have made." The court contended that the recognition of that right to refuse medical treatment "must extend to the case of an incompetent, as well as competent, patient because the value of human dignity extends to both" (427). This has come to mean that the court should make that decision for the incompetent wards because they themselves are unable to make rational decisions and decide their fate. The court said that "the State must recognize the dignity and worth of such a person and afford to that person the same panoply of rights and choices it recognizes in competent persons" (428), although many would regard the continuation of life, rather than the discontinuation of life, as better protecting the dignity of incompetent persons.

The following statement encompasses many of the problems involved in the *Saikewicz* ruling: The court held that it believed the guardian *ad litem* should attempt "to ascertain the incompetent person's actual interests and preferences" and that the decision should be one that "would be made by the incompetent person, if that person were competent, but taking into account the present and future incompetency of the individual as one of the factors which would necessarily enter into the decision-making process of the competent person" (431). It is very difficult to understand what the court meant by this mumbo-jumbo formula. Saikewicz had been unable to express his preferences in the past. There is no plausible way to reconstruct his preferences from statements made at some earlier time, as there sometimes is for patients like those in the widely known *Quinlan* and *Cruzan* cases.[37] How can the court "ascertain the incompetent person's actual interests and preferences"? Furthermore, what is the purpose of trying to assess which decision "would be made by the incompetent person, if that person were competent"? It is obvious that the court did not really believe in this exercise, for Justice Liacos maintained that we should also take into account "the present and future incompetency of the individual as one of the factors that would necessarily enter into the decision-making process of the competent person." Justice Liacos had to maintain this position so as to rule in contradiction to the fact that most patients in Saikewicz's situation would elect to go on with chemotherapy. The self-deception finds expression in the concluding remarks, "that the patient's right to privacy and self-determination is entitled to enforcement" (435). This appears to mean that Joseph Saikewicz, who is incapable of understanding his situation or of making an informed choice, is entitled not to receive chemotherapy, and to die.

One crucial factor that is usually present in court cases concerning the right to die with dignity that is totally absent from this case involves the family. Justice Liacos mentioned in his ruling the guardian *ad litem*. He also said that two of Saikewicz's sisters, the only members of his family who could be located, were notified of his condition and of the hearing, but they preferred not to attend or otherwise become involved. Saikewicz had no one who loved and cared for him. If he had had a family, and the family had requested that he receive the chemotherapy, the case would probably not have reached the court. The absence of family decided, to a large extent, Saikewicz's fate. We can speculate that a caring family might have wanted to enjoy his company for as long as possible and might have ruled against the factors brought by the court to decide against treatment. Vulnerable, unwanted, and abandoned people may have to suffer the consequences of the *Saikewicz* ruling.[38]

The controversial *Saikewicz* ruling played a considerable role in another erroneous decision. The case law involved a minor diagnosed in a state of "irreversible coma." The Massachusetts District Court judge, substituting his own judgment for that of the incompetent child, found that, if competent, the child would choose not to be resuscitated by extraordinary measures. I cannot understand how he reached this conclusion. Does a competent child have the ability to comprehend such a tragic situation? The judge ordered that further ventilator treatment and resuscitative measures be withheld in the event the child suffered respiratory distress or cardiac arrest in the future. Because both of the child's parents were minors under the legal custody of the Department of Social Services, a guardian was appointed to represent the child, and this guardian sought relief from the District Court's DNR order. Finally, the case came before the Supreme Judicial Court. Abrams J. recognized that the child had not expressed any wishes from which it was possible to draw guidance. Still he held that evidence supported findings that the child would choose to decline resuscitative medical treatment in event of respiratory or cardiac arrest.[39] It is unclear what the "evidence" and "findings" were. He noted that the decision would have little if any impact on the child's family "because the family was never intact."[40]

Justice Nolan submitted his dissent. In a short and concise judgment, he rightly criticized this incoherent decision: "The court again has approved application of the doctrine of substituted judgment when there is not a soupcon of evidence to support it. The trial judge did not have a smidgen of evidence on which to conclude that if this child who is now about five and one half years old were competent to decide, she would elect certain death to a life with no cognitive ability. The route by which the court arrives at its conclusion is a cruel charade, which is being perpetuated whenever we are faced with a life and death decision of an incompetent person."[41]

It should be noted that the court said that the prognosis for the child, even if she received treatment, "would remain terminal because of the untreatable 'brain-dead' condition."[42] It is dubious whether the child's situation could adequately be described as "terminal," and it seems that the court did not really understand the difference between coma and brain death, lumping both conditions together as one and the same. It is a matter for speculation whether the court would have reached the same decision if the patient had had a loving family who would really seek to secure her best interests.

––––––––––

The family plays a crucial role in two other legal cases. In the *Spring* case, the family decided to terminate hemodialysis treatments of the patient, and the court concurred. The case raises doubts as to whether the role of the family should always be considered as crucial. The other case, *Gray v. Romeo*, clearly illustrates a situation in which the right to die with dignity should be respected.

Spring

This case involved an incompetent person whose wife petitioned the court for an order that hemodialysis treatments, which were sustaining the life of the ward, be terminated.[43] The court held that where it was established that it would have been the wish of the incompetent ward, if competent, to discontinue his dialysis treatments, the ward's life was essentially behind him, he was not a suitable candidate for a kidney transplant, his remaining days would be spent in an irreversible state of dementia, and the physician treating the ward supported the view of the ward's family that further treatment was inappropriate, the state's general interest in the preservation of life was not sufficient to warrant intervention in the treatment decision.

Justice Armstrong, who delivered the court's opinion, reviewed at considerable length the relationships between Earl N. Spring, the patient, and his family (495, 499). Mr. Spring had been married to his wife, Blanche, for more than fifty-five years. Their son, Robert, had lived for more than fifteen years across the street from his parents' house and had visited them virtually every day during that time. Mrs. Spring and Robert Spring had been active participants in caring for the patient's needs since the onset of his precipitous physical and mental deterioration. The court was convinced that this was a case of a close-knit family unit, with a long history of mutual love, concern, and support. In a footnote (499), Justice Armstrong addressed the issue of financial considerations and said that such considerations were not involved because the dialysis treatments were paid for by Social Security.

Justice Armstrong also emphasized the burden that Mr. Spring had imposed upon his family after he developed kidney failure. His wife and son had to transport him three times a week to a private kidney center in another town for five hours of dialysis treatment (495, 496, 500). Furthermore, Mr. Spring's physical deterioration was accompanied by mental disorientation. His behavior at home became somewhat belligerent and destructive, and he could no longer care for himself. Mr. Spring was diagnosed as having "chronic organic brain syndrome." Later his mental deterioration had progressed to the point at which he was unable to recognize his wife and son.

The crisis in the family had increased when Mrs. Spring suffered a stroke, temporarily losing her ability to speak. Robert Spring attributed the stroke to strain and exhaustion resulting from his father's behavior and condition. After some six months Mrs. Spring became well enough to be discharged from the hospital to her home, but she could no longer take care of her husband. She needed to devote all her energies to taking care of herself.

At that time Mr. Spring was in a nursing home. His disruptive behavior was controlled through heavy sedation. He had occasionally kicked nurses, resisted transportation for dialysis, and pulled the dialysis tubing from his body (496). Mrs. Spring and Robert Spring expressed the view that if Mr. Spring were competent to voice his opinion, he would wish to have dialysis discontinued, although that would result in his death. That view did not rest on any expression of such an intention by the patient (498). Nevertheless, the court accepted the view of the patient's family. The court held that in circumstances of a close-knit family unit "the decision of the family, particularly where that decision is in accord with the recommendation of the attending physician [as is the case here], is of particular importance, both as evidence of the decision the patient himself would make in the circumstances and, at a later stage of analysis, as a factor lending added weight to the patient's interest in privacy and personal dignity in the face of any countervailing State interests" (499).

While in the *Saikewicz* case the absence of a family may have been a factor in a decision not to order chemotherapy, in this case the presence of the patient's family was pivotal in the decision to terminate Mr. Spring's dialysis. However, while I strongly protest against the *Saikewicz* ruling and think the decision was wrong, I cannot hold the same for *Spring*.[44] This case raises a vexing moral dilemma.

Although the result, in which the interest of the state in the preservation of life is outweighed by other considerations, might be disturbing, it is nevertheless understandable. In a sense, the court was balancing the life of Mr. Spring against the life of Mrs. Spring. The situation as it developed had reached a point at which one life was being maintained at the expense of the other. The court gave more consideration to the one who had a better chance of living a meaningful life. In this crude situation of a zero sum game, the court had to weigh all interests and reached the decision that the best alternative was to cease treatment for Mr. Spring. The court held:

> When the treatments were initiated, it was hoped that they would restore the ward's ability to enjoy a relatively normal existence, subject of course to the burden of lengthy and uncomfortable treatments far from home three times a week, but otherwise permitting him the pleasure of life with his family in familiar and comfortable surroundings. Unfortunately, this hope did not and cannot materialize; he is, and must remain, institutionalized, heavily sedated to restrain his hostile impulses, uncooperative towards his arduous maintenance program, insensible of his family and his situation. There now obtains a very different set of circumstances from those in which the decision to undertake dialysis was made. (499–500)

One can infer from the data as described by the court that the Spring family was, indeed, a close-knit family unit. Indeed, one gets the impression that Mrs. Spring and Robert Spring loved Earl Spring. They found it terribly distressing to see the man they had shared their lives with for so many years fading away, failing to recognize them, acting brutally, and becoming a different person. They could not cope with this situation. The appeal to the court was made also to help them keep their own sanity, their own lives. It seems that Mrs. Spring and Robert Spring sincerely thought that by withholding treatment from Mr. Spring, they preserved his dignity. The question remains whether he himself would have preferred to die, as he gave no indication, while he was competent, that he would rather die in such a situation.

I struggled for a long time before concluding that the court was probably right in reaching its decision. Moving from the particular to the more general, even if we are convinced of the family's commitment to the patient, we should not see the family's position as obligatory in all circumstances. The family's role should be held as a prominent consideration, but we should take into account first and foremost the best interests of the patient. The family is not necessarily capable of rational decision making, and even if it is, its interests are not necessarily identical to the interest of the patient. Thus, against John Hardwig's contention that we should build our theory of medical ethics on the presumption of equality—the interests of patients and family members are morally to be weighed equally—my argument is that we should think in terms of hierarchy.[45] In some instances the patient's interests in the maintenance of treatment and in longer life may well be strong enough to outweigh the conflicting interests of other members of the family.

Gray v. Romeo

This legal case illustrates a case of familial decision-making on the right to die with dignity, which has to be cherished and respected, as the court indeed did rule.[46] Marcia Gray was forty-nine years old when, in January 1986, she developed a sudden and severe headache and lost consciousness. Surgical exploration established that Mrs. Gray had suffered a massive hemorrhage within her cerebrum and within the meninges, the membrane that covers the brain. There was a severe brain damage to the right cerebral hemisphere. She did not regain consciousness after surgery and was diagnosed as a PCU patient. With the consent of her husband, a gastrostomy was performed and a G-tube was inserted into the stomach by which nutrition and hydration were provided. A month later, Marcia Gray developed hydrocephalus, a buildup of excessive cerebrospinal fluid in the brain. Further surgery was performed at that time to insert a shunt to drain the fluid. Subsequently, four separate procedures were applied to correct malfunctions of the shunt. At some point, Gray developed an infection in the cranial wound that led to the permanent removal of the cranial bone plate (582). The consulting physician engaged by Mrs. Gray's family believed that there was no sensation and hence "no pain, thirst, or hunger recognition" (583). He agreed with the neurosurgeon who performed the craniotomy that there was no reasonable likelihood of her returning to a conscious state, and that there was "no chance" of Marcia Gray's recovery (583).

In May 1987, her family, including her husband, her two children, her mother, and her sister-in-law requested that her attending physician order that feeding be stopped and that Marcia Gray be permitted to die. Mrs. Gray's family was convinced that it would be her desire not to be sustained with artificial measures if her life were otherwise hopeless. The family relied on statements made by Gray explicitly asking not to be kept alive by artificial means should she ever be in PCU.

The court held that a person has a paramount right to control the disposition to be made of his or her body even if the decision results in that person's death. Marcia Gray's right to privacy encompasses the right to refuse life-sustaining medical treatment (586). The court was convinced by the evidence that Gray, if competent, would refuse treatment. Her right to self-determination outweighed competing governmental interests that include the preservation of life, the prevention of suicide, the protection of innocent third parties, and the integrity of medical ethics.

The court gave much emphasis to the role of the family. Justice Boyle, who delivered the opinion of the court, wrote: "the depth, quality, and reasoning of the family's prediction of Marcia Gray's intent is impressive. The family speaks with one voice and no apparent conflict of interest exists" (588).

This case raises no difficulties. It is an example of a family council, freely and openly discussing the future of a beloved relative who exhibited no conscious, cognitive, sentient responses, bringing forward relevant considerations for and against the continuation of life. This consultation took place after physicians expressed the opinion that there was no reasonable likelihood of Marcia Gray's returning to a conscious state or recovering. In this situation the patient's chances of recovery to a conscious state are "close to zero" (583), the patient expressed her desire several times in the past not to be maintained upon reaching such a state, and the members of her close-knit family, with a history of mutual love, concern, and support, exhibit a unified position that her dignity would be better served by letting her die. The court was right in honoring the family's request.

One useful mechanism is the loved ones' council. [47] The immediate family and the patient's other loved ones should make the treatment decision. A case that came before the Israeli Supreme Court illustrates this point.[48] It involved a two-year-old child, Yael Scheffer, who suffered from Tay-Sachs, an incurable degenerative neurological genetic disease. Yael's mother appealed to the court, asking to terminate treatment other than that designated to relieve her suffering. Specifically, the appeal asked that Yael not be connected to a ventilator and that she not be provided with drugs through transfusion.

Deputy President Menachem Elon, who delivered the judgment, rejected the appeal. Quoting the attending physician's testimonial, Justice Elon argued that Yael Scheffer did not suffer any pain. She was treated in a way that did not infringe on her dignity. Yael was kept clean, did not suffer from pressure bruises, and on the whole she did not cry. Yael cried, like any other child, when she wanted to be fed or when she suffered from stomachache, constipation, ear infection, and the like. Yael resembled a bright candle, said the Court. Under these conditions, the sanctity of Yael's life should be upheld, and this was the only value that determined the Court's decision. Any interference that ended Yael's life was contradictory to the values of Israel as a Jewish democratic state (para. 64).

Justice Elon ended his very detailed (150–page) ruling by addressing the role of the family. The plea to refrain from treating Yael Scheffer was made only by the mother. The father did not join the petition, nor did he appear before the court. The mother explained this by saying, "He hates publicity." Justice Elon noted the fact that the father was the person who treated Yael every day, while the mother rarely visited her daughter in the hospital. The mother explained this by saying that she devoted her time to take care of their other daughter, who was in a crisis. Justice Elon was not convinced that the father fully supported his wife's initiative. He said that in such matters concerning life and death, clear and explicit consent of both parents to the yielding of such a petition is required (para. 65). Indeed, this kind of examination is essential for estimating the role of the family, which is an important consideration for all cases, and of crucial importance when the decision concerns the lives of minors. In a case of disagreement between parents, it is better to err on the side of life and keep the child alive.[49]

Conclusions

In the United States, oral statements are conceived sufficient to remove or to withhold life-sustaining treatment.[50] The family may play a crucial role in deciding the destiny of their loved ones. In *In re Christopher*,[51] the court relied on a conversation that occurred ten years before the case between seventy-nine-year-old Anna Kushnir and her son to accept the son's bona fide refusal to consent to any procedure that would prolong the patient's life after she lost all cognitive functions and was in constant pain. The court conceived the surgical insertion of a feeding tube under these conditions as "futile and unnecessary."[52] Because of the weight that is accorded to the opinion of the patient's family, one of the medical staff, arguably the social worker, should review the relationships between the patient and the family to verify that the family does not hold partisan interests that run counter to the patient's best interests. Family members are not necessarily the patient's loved ones. We should try to ascertain that those who are truly beloved, truly caring for the patient, those who are around the patient's bedside, be included within the decision-making process together with the medical staff.

7 An Outsider's View of Dutch Euthanasia Policy and Practice

The Dutch experience has influenced the debate on euthanasia and death with dignity around the globe, especially with regard to whether physician-assisted suicide and euthanasia should be legitimized and legalized. A book about the right to die with dignity should therefore address the Dutch experience. However, review of the literature reveals complex and often contradictory views about this experience. Some claim the Netherlands offers a model for the world to follow; others believe the Netherlands represents danger rather than promise, that the Dutch experience is the definitive reason that we should not make active euthanasia and physician-assisted suicide part of our lives.

Given these contradictory views, fieldwork was essential to develop a more informed opinion. Having investigated the Dutch experience for a number of years, in the summer of 1999 I went to the Netherlands to visit the major centers of medical ethics as well as some research hospitals and to speak with leading figures in euthanasia policy and practice. This chapter reports the main findings of my interviews and provides detailed accounts of the way in which some of the Netherlands' leading experts perceive the policy and practice of euthanasia in their country.

The discussion begins with a review of the two major Dutch reports on euthanasia and the conflicting views and interpretations offered by the literature. Next, I provide some data about the interviews, and then analysis indicating that the Dutch guidelines on the policy and practice of euthanasia do not provide sufficient mechanisms against abuse. Virtually every guideline has been breached or violated. This finding reiterates Herbert Hendin's finding.[1] I conclude by recommending that the Netherlands amend its policy and remedy its troubling practice. The findings should compel us to conduct further investigation and research. The Netherlands should overhaul its policy and procedures to prevent potential abuse.

Background

Since November 1990, prosecution has been unlikely if a doctor complies with the guidelines on euthanasia and physician-assisted suicide set out in the nonprosecution agreement between the Dutch Ministry of Justice and the Royal Dutch Medical Association. These guidelines are based on the criteria set out in court decisions relating to when a doctor can successfully invoke the defense of necessity. The substantive requirements are as follows:

- The request for euthanasia or physician-assisted suicide must be made by the patient and must be free and voluntary.
- The patient's request must be well considered, durable and consistent.
- The patient's situation must entail unbearable suffering with no prospect of improvement and no alternative to end the suffering.[2] The patient need not be terminally ill to satisfy this requirement and the suffering need not necessarily be physical.
- Euthanasia must be a last resort.[3]

The procedural requirements are as follows:

- No doctor is required to perform euthanasia but if he is opposed on principle he must make his position known to the patient early on and help the patient get in touch with a colleague who has no such moral objections.
- Doctors taking part in euthanasia should preferably and whenever possible have patients administer the fatal drug to themselves, rather than have a doctor apply an injection or intravenous drip.[4]
- A doctor must perform the euthanasia.
- Before the doctor assists the patient, the doctor must consult a second independent doctor who has no professional or family relationship with either the patient or doctor. Since the 1991 *Chabot* case, if the patient has a psychiatric disorder the doctor must arrange to have the patient examined by at least two other doctors, one of whom must be a psychiatrist.[5]

- The doctor must keep a full written record of the case.
- The death must be reported to the prosecutorial authorities as a case of euthanasia or physician-assisted suicide, and not as a case of death by natural causes.[6]

In 1990, the Dutch government appointed a commission to investigate the medical practice of euthanasia. The commission, headed by Professor Jan Remmelink, solicitor general to the Supreme Court, was asked to conduct a comprehensive nationwide study of "medical decisions concerning the end of life (MDEL)." The following broad forms of MDEL were studied:

- Non-treatment decisions: withholding or withdrawing treatment in situations where treatment would probably have prolonged life;
- Alleviation of pain and symptoms: administering opioids in such dosages that the patient's life could be shortened;
- Euthanasia and related MDEL: the prescription, supply or administration of drugs with the explicit intention of shortening life, including euthanasia at the patient's request, assisted suicide, and life termination without explicit and persistent request.[7]

The study was repeated in 1995, making it possible to assess for the first time whether there were harmful effects over time that might have been caused by the availability of voluntary euthanasia in the Netherlands. It is still difficult to make valid comparisons with other countries, because of legal and cultural differences as well as because sufficient data are not available.[8]

The two Dutch studies were said to give the best estimate of all forms of MDEL (i.e., all treatment decisions with the possibility of shortening life) in the Netherlands as around 39 percent of all deaths in 1990, and 43 percent in 1995. In the third category of MDEL, the studies gave the best estimate of voluntary euthanasia as 2,300 persons each year (1.9 percent of all deaths) in 1990,[9] and 3,250 persons each year (2.4 percent) in 1995. The estimate for physician-assisted suicide was about 0.3 percent in 1990 and in 1995. There were 8,900 explicit requests for euthanasia or assisted suicide in the Netherlands in 1990, and 9,700 in 1995. Fewer than 40 percent were granted. The most worrisome data are concerned with the hastening of death without the explicit request of patients. There were 1,000 cases (0.8 percent) without explicit and persistent request in 1990, and 900 cases (0.7 percent) in 1995.[10]

In 1990, 30 percent of the general practitioners (GPs) interviewed said they had performed a life-terminating act at some time without explicit request (compared with 25 percent of specialists and 10 percent of nursing home physicians).[11] Performing a life-terminating act without explicit request occurred, on the average, with older patients than did euthanasia or physician-assisted suicide.[12] There were remaining treatment alternatives in 8 percent of cases in which a life-terminating act was performed without the patient's explicit request. The physician did not use these alternatives because the patient had indicated that it "only would prolong suffering," or because the expected gain was not sufficient to make the treatment worthwhile.[13] It should be noted that the level of consultation was significantly lower in life-termination acts without patient's explicit request compared with euthanasia or physician-assisted suicide. A colleague was consulted in 48 percent of the cases (compared with 84 percent in euthanasia and assisted-suicide cases). Relatives were consulted in 72 percent of the cases (compared with 94 percent in euthanasia and assisted suicide cases). In 68 percent of the cases, the physician felt no need for consultation because the situation was clear.[14] Paul van der Maas and colleagues note that this should be considered in light of the very brief period by which life was shortened.[15] In 67 percent of the cases, life was shortened by fewer than 24 hours. In 21 percent of the cases, life was shortened by up to one week.[16]

About a quarter of the one thousand patients had earlier expressed a wish for voluntary euthanasia.[17] The patient was no longer competent in almost all of those cases, and death was hastened by a few hours or days. A small number of cases (approximately fifteen) involved babies who were suffering from a serious congenital disorder and were barely viable; the doctor decided, in consultation with the parents, to hasten the end of life.[18]

The Remmelink Commission regarded these cases of involuntary termination of life as "providing assistance to the dying." They were justified because the patients' suffering was unbearable, standard medical practice failed to help and, in any event, death would have occurred within a week. The commission added that actively ending life when the vital functions have started failing is indisputably normal medical practice: "It deserves recommendation that the reporting procedures in place . . . will in the future also cover the active termination of life by a doctor in the framework of help-in-dying without an explicit request by the patient," except if it concerns a situation where there is "the beginning of irreversible, interrelated failure of vital functions." In this last case "natural death would very quickly occur even if the doctor did not actively intervene. . . . " The recommendation goes on to say that this is not the case with patients whose vital functions are still intact and who are subject to life-shortening treatment without explicit request. Such cases should be reported.[19]

On the basis of the 1995 report, the government decided to decrease the influence of the criminal law in cases of euthanasia by instituting regional review committees. These committees would review each case of euthanasia reported to the medical examiner and advise whether to dismiss the case or prosecute the physician involved. If this mechanism were introduced, the government thought, the willingness of physicians to report would increase.

Methodology

Before arriving in the Netherlands, I wrote to some distinguished experts in their respective fields: medicine, psychiatry, philosophy, law, social sciences, and ethics, asking to meet with them to discuss the Dutch policy and practice of euthanasia. Only one declined my request for an interview.[20]

The interviews took place during July–August 1999, in the Netherlands. They lasted between one and three hours each. Most interviews went on for more than two hours, during which I asked more or less the same series of questions.[21] During the interviews I took extensive notes that together comprise some two hundred densely written pages. Later the interviews were typed and analyzed.

Because I was interested in the problematic aspects of the euthanasia practice, after some general questions I addressed the troublesome aspects reiterated in the Remmelink report. This line of questions disturbed some of the interviewees, who wanted to know my own opinion on the subject matter before continuing to answer my questions. Others seemed eager to bring the interview to a close.

I was struck by the defensiveness expressed by some of the interviewees. Carlos F. Gomez also reported the notions of suspicion and guardedness on the part of his interviewees.[22] The attitude of some of my interviewees reminded me of my own initial reaction when I attended debates between post-Zionists outside Israel during the late 1980s and early 1990s. At that time I felt that our dirty laundry should not be aired; that the debate should be restricted to Israelis who were familiar with the intricate aspects of the debate, and that all who took part in the debates should show responsibility when they addressed the issue before non-Israelis and non-Jews, who might then exploit the information to harm Israel's interests. In the Netherlands I sensed that the interviewees did not like the idea of a foreigner asking these questions. Their attitude spurred me to call this chapter "An Outsider's View." Although many of my interviewees realized that the euthanasia policy was imperfect, they tried to defend it to the best of their abilities.[23] As a matter of fact, I was somewhat troubled by their lack of criticism and their readiness to accept the euthanasia procedure with all its flaws.[24] I presume some of the interviewees identified with their government's decision making to the extent of defending the system and suspecting foreigners like me, who pressed them with difficult questions. I also suspect that after the publications of Gomez, Keown, and Hendin,[25] they were not enthusiastic about cooperating with me. One interviewee was candid enough to tell me this directly. When I asked why he was willing to sit with me and answer my questions, he replied that he felt obliged as a researcher and scientist to cooperate and wanted his viewpoint to be heard.

Some of the interviewees were nominated by the Dutch government to conduct research on the policy and practice of euthanasia and to submit their recommendations for changes. Science commissioned by the state might be a tricky issue. The researcher might become identified with the project to the extent of becoming a spokesperson for the state and forgoing impartiality. It is preferable that research on controversial matters be funded by nonpartisan foundations rather than by an interested government.[26]

Breaches of the Guidelines

This chapter reports the answers to the questions concerning two breaches of the guidelines: lack of consultation and lack of reporting. My more extensive report of the answers to my fifteen questions can be found in *Euthanasia in the Netherlands* (forthcoming).

Consultation

I asked: "The physician practicing euthanasia is required to consult a colleague with regard to the hopeless condition of the patient. Who decides the identity of the second doctor?" I also asked about the common practice in small villages in rural areas where it might be difficult to find an independent colleague to consult. One prosecutor told John Keown that in the countryside there were towns with only two or three doctors. He asked rhetorically: "What's the use of asking one of those two or three to judge the handling of a euthanasia case by the other one? How objective can that be? I don't see it."[27]

The Dutch film *Death on Request*, presented on Dutch television in October 1994, showed a doctor performing the euthanasia who was careful to call a colleague to consult with him about his patient.[28] It is unclear why the GP picked this specific consultant. Was it because of his particular field of expertise or because the physician knew this doctor and assumed he would back his decision without too many questions? Were they acquaintances, on friendly terms? What worries me is that the requirement to consult could become a dead dogma, used only for paperwork, and that, in essence, one hand would wash the other: You approve euthanasia for my patients, and I will approve it for yours. And obviously, a doctor who approves euthanasia would not call on a colleague who was against it or was hesitant about the practice. Indeed, one study shows that the consultant was nearly always a partner in the practice or a locum. At least 60 percent of the so-called independent consultants giving the second opinion already knew the patient before the consultation. The family doctor sought a second opinion from a doctor he did not know personally in only 5 percent of the cases.[29] Another study showed, unsurprisingly, that almost all consultants regarded the request of the patient to be well considered and persistent, that there were no further alternative treatment options, and that almost all of them agreed with the intention to perform euthanasia or assisted suicide. In general, the GPs did not need to change their views or plans after consultation took place.[30] Two hypotheses may be offered to explain this finding, a positive one and a negative one. The positive one is that the GPs are very careful in their practice and agree to perform euthanasia only in clear-cut cases. The negative hypothesis is that the procedure is pro forma, consisting only of paperwork, and that the consultant does not take great care to examine the patient due to the consultant's reluctance to refute the GP's decision.

Consultation takes place in about 99 percent of reported cases of euthanasia and assisted suicide (of which only 41 percent of cases are reported). It is estimated that consultation takes place in 37 percent of unreported cases. In 88 percent of the cases the consultant had also seen the patient.[31] Physicians mainly consult colleagues of their own specialty. Recent research shows that familiarity and accessibility are very important factors in the choice of the consultant. Half the physicians who had been consultants more than once had previously been consulted by the same physician who consulted them in their most recent case. In 24 percent of these cases, the treating physician and the consultant had previously acted as consultants for each other. Physicians who previously consulted or had been consulted by the same physician agreed more often with the intended euthanasia or assisted suicide than physicians who did not (90 percent versus 80 percent).[32]

The interviews revealed sharply contrasting and contradictory opinions on this matter of consultation. I suspect that not all of the interviewees were completely candid in their answers, possibly because they were protecting the system and viewed me with suspicion as a foreigner.

My first interviewee, John Griffiths, said that the physician is supposed to discuss the matter with the patient's family and in his opinion should be required to explain in writing if this is not done. If the patient does not wish the family to be included in the deliberations, the doctor should be required to have the patient put that refusal in writing. According to current Dutch law, the nursing staff should be included in discussions of euthanasia. In cases of euthanasia performed at the patient's home, the patient usually has home nursing care, and the on-site nurse should be included in the decision-making process. As for the requirement to consult another doctor, Griffiths acknowledges that there are problems in the consultations of doctors with their colleagues. In rural areas it can be difficult to get hold of a colleague, especially an independent doctor, since doctors in rural areas are often members of the same covering group. In Griffiths's opinion, the consultation requirement should be adhered to more strictly than now appears to be the case, although the complexities of concrete situations require a rule that can be applied in a flexible and casuistic way, something that is difficult in the context of criminal enforcement. Currently the courts are rather lenient with doctors who do not comply, but the regional assessment committees seem to be trying to give the requirement more teeth.[33] In this context, Jacqueline M. Cuperus-Bosma et al. examined the minutes of the Assembly of Prosecutors General, and noting that if all requirements for accepted practice were met, except consultation, the physician was not prosecuted, but the case was usually referred to the health inspector. However, if there were doubts about other requirements for accepted practice being met, an inquest was held.[34]

According to Griffiths, among those prosecuted was a doctor who consulted another doctor, and then the consulted doctor, not the first doctor who asked for the consultation, performed the euthanasia. The guidelines say, however, that the physician who first recommended euthanasia, not the consulted doctor, should perform the euthanasia. When this reversal occurs, the case is usually not reported for fear of prosecution. Griffiths added that it is wrong to suppose that all unreported cases are unjustified.

Griffiths estimated that 10 percent of physicians in the Netherlands oppose the practice of euthanasia in principle, and a further 6 percent would not perform euthanasia themselves, but refer patients who ask for it to another doctor.[35] Griffiths further said that consultation on somatic cases is sometimes quite inadequate, being performed for example over the phone or by a busy specialist who stops by a hospital ward and notes on the patient's status sheet that he agrees with the attending physician. He argues that consultants should always see the patient, but the prosecution and the courts do not regard this as an absolute requirement. The Supreme Court should broaden the requirement of consultation in person to all patients, and not limit it to psychiatric patients only, as was the case at the time of interview.

Sjef Gevers reiterated the latter points in Griffiths's testimony. Until 1995, consultants were not required to see the patient. The Dutch Medical Association Euthanasia Guidelines of 1995 changed the picture, saying that the consultant needs to be an independent colleague, not part of the doctor's group, and must talk with the patient himself and be informed of the patient's medical situation. Consultation over the phone or by looking at the patient's file is insufficient. However, the courts do not insist that the consultant see the patient. Following the *Chabot* precedent, only in psychiatric cases is consultation required in person.

Several interviewees explained that in hospitals the general practice is to consult the whole medical team, including nurses, not just another physician.[36] Thus in hospitals consultants always see the patients; examining their medical files is conceived insufficient. In nursing homes, the standard procedure is to invite a consultant from another nursing home. As for GPs, many physicians have a trusted colleague whom they always consult in euthanasia cases. It was noted that it is important that the consultant not be from the GP's medical team or someone who fills in for the doctor on weekends. However, often GPs consult colleagues on their own team. The consultant is perceived to be independent because he or she is not directly involved with the patient, but of course that is not total independence from the perspective of the best interest of the patient. The common view is that the physician needs to hear and see the patient, examine him, feel him, listen to what the patient wants. However, there were incidents in which consultation was done over the phone without the doctor's seeing the patient. The interviewees accentuated that consultation might be a problem in small villages, where the GP may have to travel a relatively long distance to find an independent consultant, and that insisting on the consultant's independence is important in all euthanasia cases.[37]

On the other hand, Ron Berghmans and A. van Dantzig do not think that finding an independent doctor is a major problem. The Netherlands is a small country, and it is possible to find a consulting doctor who does not belong to the same medical team. Berghmans from Maastricht thinks the GP and the consultant might have other shared interests, but that they would not compromise the independence requirement. With regard to consultation over the phone, Berghmans contends that in the past too much respect was granted to maintaining privacy in physician-patient relationships, even to the extent of allowing consultation over the phone. This picture is now changing, and the new law requires that the consultant see the patient.

Paul van der Maas explains that "real consultation" means consultation with a colleague who is an expert in the field and who is able to verify that there are no available alternatives for treatment. The consultant should also verify that the patient really wants euthanasia, and that the decision-making process did not involve problems of transference and countertransference between doctor and patient.[38] Van der Maas maintains that he and his team train consultants to see patients and examine their condition firsthand. Similarly, van Dantzig argues that consultation involves seeing the patient, determining the motive for the wish to die, and exploring avenues of treatment. Seeing the patient in person is required, to verify that euthanasia is the only solution, and the most desirable solution.

G. F. Koerselman, who opposes the practice of euthanasia, was consulted in the past and objected to the practice. He testified that he felt pressure from his colleagues to sign the documents approving the euthanasia decision. At some point, his colleagues gave up on him and stopped consulting him. Now he is no longer consulted. Koerselman offered to serve as an expert witness in one court trial, but the court was not interested in hearing his expert testimony.

I asked the interviewees how much time is needed for a consultation. Arie van der Arend thought that a totally independent physician is unable to evaluate the condition of the patient within the customary half hour or hour of consultation. Ideally, the consulting physician should meet the patient several times. If there is only one short meeting, there may be a lack of communication. Van der Arend advised having three separate meetings before the consultant writes the report.

George Beusmans and Gerrit Kimsma, who practice euthanasia, do not share this view. According to Beusmans, after several meetings with the patient, he asks for the patient's request for euthanasia in writing. At a certain moment, when the patient says: "I can't deal with the suffering; you can do it," Beusmans asks: "When?" This discussion takes place when the patient is in the final phase of life, having only about two weeks left. When the patient insists that he wants euthanasia, Beusmans arranges for a colleague to come and see the patient. At this stage, Beusmans also contacts a pharmacy to arrange for the lethal drugs. The colleague is a general practitioner with whom Beusmans does not work. Beusmans has two colleagues with whom he cooperates on euthanasia matters, and these two colleagues also ask Beusmans to serve as a consultant for their euthanasia cases. The consultant sees the patient, speaks with him, and decides whether it is necessary to perform euthanasia. The consultant usually signs the papers after thirty minutes of conversation with the patient. Beusmans thinks thirty minutes is enough to verify that the patient qualifies for euthanasia.

Gerrit Kimsma also insists that the consultant see the patient. He thinks half an hour is enough when the consultant comes prepared with all the pertinent information. The consultant reads the patient's medical records, sees the patient, asks for the patient's view on his condition, and checks whether the patient knows why the consultant has come to see him. The consultant needs to see that the patient is of sound mind and is requesting euthanasia without pressure. He is required to verify that the guidelines have been fulfilled and that Kimsma's approval of the euthanasia decision was correct.

Kimsma testifies that he consults an independent colleague for whom he covers during the weekends. In his opinion, the independence requirement is not compromised because the main concerns are to examine the issues of transference and counter transference, and to determine that the GP has arrived at the decision to perform euthanasia without pressure and without identifying with the patient to the point of distorting his own medical judgment.

My interviews also included a meeting with the de Boer family, who experienced the euthanasia decision-making process. K. was a cancer patient who knew that death was inevitable. He could not adequately digest food and was very weak; he suffered great pain and consumed large doses of pain medication. K. felt that his life had no quality and filled out the papers he had obtained from the Voluntary Euthanasia Society, in which he expressed a will to die. He reiterated his request to his personal doctor and at a later stage became unconscious for a few days. The meeting with the consultant to approve the GP's decision was scheduled ahead of time, and on that day the consultant arrived an hour after K. woke up. K. was in a good mood and did not believe that he had slept for four days. The GP told K. that he had arrived to discuss K.'s euthanasia decision, and K. stated that he did not now believe the situation was that bad; he thought his family and the physicians had made this up. The consultant talked with K. about euthanasia, but K. found it difficult to comprehend why the consultant wanted to discuss euthanasia with him since he had had such a good sleep and was feeling quite happy. Clearly, the family testified, K. was not ready for euthanasia, though he still backed his euthanasia decision. I asked what the consultant decided after this confusing episode and was told that the consultant arrived again later and confirmed the decision in favor of euthanasia.[39]

Though K.'s family acted in a bona fide sincere manner, this episode is disturbing and demonstrates the intricacy of this issue. It is unclear why the GP and the consultant arrived that day. If K. had been unconscious for four days, the GP should have been aware of this. Surely, the consultant could not fulfill his responsibility if the patient was unaware and unable to communicate. The consultant here was not satisfied by the first visit, during which the patient clearly wanted to live, and felt an obligation to visit the patient again. In addition, it must have been quite a blow for K. to see his beloved family and the physicians, including his trusted GP, around his bed discussing his mercy killing at a time when he felt comparatively well.

Bert Keizer tells the disturbing story of a cancer patient who arranged to end her life, but during her last days of life became increasingly muddled. On the evening of her death, when she heard the doorbell, she let the doctor in, greeting him with some bewilderment: "And what brings you here tonight, doctor?" The doctor and the other people present at her home refreshed her memory, and later that evening the patient did take her dose. Before the doctor left he asked the patient's daughter: "This *is* what Mother wanted, isn't it?"[40]

Many interviewees spoke about the new SCEA project that began in Amsterdam and became a Dutch national project.[41] In 1997, the Support and Consultation of Euthanasia in Amsterdam (SCEA) project was initiated to provide all GPs working in Amsterdam with a support group of about twenty specially trained GPs for consultation or advice on euthanasia and PAS. The purpose was not only to make it easier for GPs to find an independent and knowledgeable consultant, but also to make the consultation more professional.[42] Physicians are required to contact SCEA consultants before they perform euthanasia, in order to make consultation as accurate as possible. Van der Wal says that most doctors do not like the idea that they do not select the doctor themselves, especially as long as euthanasia was officially illegal. They prefer to consult with someone they know. Gerrit Kimsma sees no problem in choosing the consultant himself or, for that matter, in allowing every GP to choose a consultant. He says that there is good faith among physicians.

Four of the interviewees (van Leeuwen, Kimsma, van Delden, and den Hartogh) are members of the newly established regional committees whose role is to review euthanasia cases and see that the rules of carefulness are observed. Evert van Leeuwen, a professor of philosophy and medical ethics from Amsterdam, testified that his committee did not review even one incident of consultation conducted over the phone. He thinks it is essential for the consultant to see the patient, to verify that he or she is competent and acting upon free will, and to review the patient's medical condition, by both physical examination and by examination of the medical files. The consultant usually spends thirty minutes with the patient during which he or she verifies that the patient wishes to die and that the medical condition is hopeless. Van Leeuwen thinks half an hour is sufficient for the purpose of consultation.

Govert den Hartogh, also from Amsterdam, explains that doctors who do not consult a colleague do not report to the regional committee. KNMG (Koninklijke Nederlandsche Maatschappij tot Bevordering der Geneeskunst, i.e., Royal Dutch Society for the Advancement of Medicine) advises consultants to see the patients, and the consultants have adhered to this requirement. The reports he reviewed said the consultation lasted one to two hours, but den Hartogh testified that he was unsure about this. He is certain that the time for consultation is often shorter, especially in hospitals.

The consultant should not be involved in the treatment of the patient. The consultant is required to visit the patient to determine that the request is voluntary and that the patient is helplessly suffering. Den Hartogh maintained that doctors in some islands in the south might find it difficult to find a consultant. In his comments on the first draft of this chapter he wrote that in August 2000 his committee reviewed a case of a doctor from one of those southern islands with an orthodox Protestant majority, in which the doctor had consulted his own associated partner. The physician explained that he had tried to find another consultant but had not been able to find one. So this does occur, although probably rarely.[43]

Den Hartogh further wrote in his comments that one unfortunate side effect of the fact that the rules for justifiable euthanasia are court-made, and rely on the defense of necessity, is that the matter of consultation for some time has not been given sufficient attention. As a result of KNMG policy and of the growing involvement of the government in the assessment of acts of euthanasia and assisted suicide, this matter has gradually been improved. In hospitals the report is often nothing but a short written note on the patient's state. But there is evidence that the SCEA project, which after becoming national is now called SCEN, already has had good effects on the quality of both consulting and reporting. Den Hartogh believes that the training of SCEN consultants and of doctors generally will be far more effective in shaping the Dutch practice than any possible form of legal regulation.

Since the installation of the review committees, the requirement is that the consultant should be independent, should see the patient in person, and should consider both the character of the request and the nature of the suffering. Den Hartogh clarifies that this does not mean that a doctor who failed to consult a colleague at all, or failed to consult an independent one, could not appeal on grounds of necessity. This appeal can be made even when the new law has formalized the new requirement.[44]

Johannes van Delden holds that the consultant should see the patient for one hour after examining the patient's medical files and speaking with the GP, inquiring whether the doctor tried other medical alternatives prior to the euthanasia decision. The consultant is required to explain his reasoning; simply writing "I agree" on the form is insufficient. Van Delden's committee asks for detailed explanations. The role of the committee is also educational, explaining that the reports should be informative.[45] According to van Delden's testimony, there was only one incident in hundreds of cases reviewed by his committee in which the GP consulted a colleague over the phone. The committee reported the case to the medical inspector. Van Delden does not think there is any problem with consultation in rural areas. Most doctors are willing to be involved in the practice of euthanasia, and it is not difficult to find an independent doctor.

Contrary to the testimonies of many medical and legal ethicists,[46] Dick Willems argues that the KNMG 1995 directives prescribe that the consultant must see either the patient or the files. He knows of cases in which consultation was done over the phone. The psychiatric guidelines are more detailed than the other medical guidelines because there are more doubts about patients' competence and because psychiatrists might identify too much with their patients. Willems himself thinks that the consultant should see the patients. Like some of the other interviewees,[47] he opposes the practice of looking at the medical files in lieu of examining the patient. Willems explains that the consideration of unbearable suffering is first and foremost on his mind, and physicians cannot verify that by only looking at the files. With regard to consultation in small villages in rural areas, Willems thinks doctors usually consult the physician next door. It is difficult for them to find someone who is totally independent as required.

Margo Trappenburg spoke of Sippe Schat, a physician who was viewed as "a God in his village," who did not consult colleagues, and who did everything alone without consultation. Eventually he was prosecuted and found guilty for not consulting a colleague prior to performing euthanasia.[48]

Egbert Schroten said that, to the best of his knowledge, most doctors consult their colleagues, and at least until the early 1990s the consultation was done over the phone. When I asked whether this is sufficient to warrant euthanasia, Schroten answered that doctors apparently think they can approve euthanasia without seeing the patients, believing they have enough information to decide the matter. Schroten, like many of my other interviewees, did not seem too concerned about this.

These testimonies are alarming. I question whether it is possible to conduct a reliable consultation over the phone. It should be obligatory to see the patient, to examine him or her, to confirm that the patient has freely decided on euthanasia, and that all options for treatment were exhausted before medical killing was deemed the last resort. At first I was astonished by the relaxed tone that interviewees used while speaking about consultation by telephone. In turn, they were somewhat surprised at my alarm.

H.J.J. Leenen does not think this way. He explains that during the 1980s, consultation was often conducted over the phone. Euthanasia was regarded in the same way as any other medical practice. Leading decision-makers and policy consultants, among them Leenen himself, said that euthanasia was, is, and should remain an exception. In consequence, a view emerged that euthanasia is not like other medical procedures that could be consulted about over the phone. Physicians now consult by looking at the medical files or by meeting patients in person. Although euthanasia is an exceptional medical procedure, Leenen does not think the consultant should always see the patient. In his view, consultation in person is often unnecessary, and he believes examination of the medical files is sufficient. Leenen does not agree with the 1995 KNMG directives that consultants must see the patients, because most of those asking for euthanasia are dying from cancer, and they can be evaluated by a review of their medical files. Many patients' families regard the consultation requirement as a beaurocratic stupidity, a redundant control mechanism. Leenen agrees that consultants need to see psychiatric patients, but feels there is no such need in what he terms to be "clear cases." He states that he trusts doctors and that his experience working with doctors for the past twenty-five years has been positive: "Doctors are morally decent and competent people." Leenen criticizes them for not spending enough time with their patients, "but their intentions are good."

Heleen Dupuis contests the views of most of her colleagues. Unlike Leenen, she thinks that because the wish of the patient and his/her medical condition need to be confirmed by a second opinion, consultation in person is absolutely required. She was puzzled by my question and remarked that "doctors want to help their patients, not to kill them." Doctors would jeopardize themselves by not consulting another doctor; they would compromise their duty by just sending the patient's medical files. Hence, consultation over the phone "is impossible." It is "not acceptable," and it "does not happen." As for the situation in rural areas, Dupuis asserted that those who request euthanasia are mainly cancer patients (who are examined by hospital doctors), and that this doesn't occur often. The requirement of independent consultation is not compromised, and if there is no independent doctor, euthanasia is not performed.

Lack of Reporting

Next I asked about the worrisome data on the lack of reporting: "Record-keeping of written requests for euthanasia has improved considerably since 1990; there are now written requests in about 60 percent and written record-keeping in some 85 percent of all cases of euthanasia. The reporting rate for euthanasia was 18 percent in 1990, and by 1995 it had risen to 41 percent. The trend is reassuring, but a situation in which less than half of all cases are reported is unacceptable for effective control.[49] What do you think? How could the reporting rate be improved?"

Most interviewees are worried about the lack of reporting and would like to introduce changes to increase the level of reporting. John Griffiths thinks the criminal law on euthanasia is ineffective and that noncriminal control would be more appropriate.[50] Evidently, doctors do not report abuse, and it is difficult to locate and identify incidents of abuse. Griffiths thinks that a different system is needed. In his view, the only way to improve the situation is to leave the issue within the realm of the medical profession. Griffiths suggests a three-tier system: medical committees to review euthanasia cases, medical inspectors, and disciplinary committees. Instead of five regional committees, Griffiths suggests a low level of control in which each hospital would have its own review committee to examine the circumstances of death. What is needed is effective control of the "whole balloon," in Griffiths's terms. Griffiths explains that pressing the balloon on one side would increase its size on the other side. By analogy, control of euthanasia might increase death as a result of pain relief and of not providing any treatment. Therefore, it is advisable to establish a committee in each hospital to review all cases of death and to refer questionable cases to medical disciplinary committees.[51]

Similarly, Bert Thijs and Dick Willems think the reporting rate will be improved if the threat of prosecution is lessened. They hope that the introduction of the regional committees will improve the reporting rate, because the committees are closer to the medical profession and don't have legal authority. Previously, all cases went to the public prosecutor, but now the committees serve as a buffer. The role of the public prosecution will decrease.[52] Another means for improving reporting is medical education. The ending of life should be discussed more in medical schools and in society at large. Thijs and Willems believe in increasing social control through education and communication.

Some interviewees thought that the major problem in the practice of euthanasia in the Netherlands was the low level of reporting.[53] They said that a reporting level of 41 percent was unacceptable. Several explanations for this finding were given: First, euthanasia still came at the time of the interviews under the Penal Code, and doctors feared possible prosecution. Second, there was a preference for secrecy, as part of the doctor-patient relationship. Physicians wished to maintain trust between themselves and their patients and felt that euthanasia was a private matter. Third, there was laziness on the part of doctors who wished to avoid paperwork. Finally, many physicians were also willing to lie at the patient's/family's request or for their own personal reasons.[54]

While trusting doctors, the view is that doctors need to report, because euthanasia should never become a routine action. Euthanasia should be considered an extraordinary measure to be employed in extraordinary circumstances. Doctors should discuss their conduct in the open and expose the practice of euthanasia to public scrutiny. Margo Trappenburg, Evert van Leeuwen, J. K. Gevers, Egbert Schroten, and Henri Wijsbek emphasized that doctors need not worry if they follow the guidelines. They think that the new proposal—a system of reports to the regional committees—might bring some improvement.

G. F. Koerselman does not share the optimism of others[55] about the positive role of the regional committees. He thinks the regional committees would not change much. He believes the organization is secondary, and it is the value system that is important. At this point, almost no one contests the vital policy decisions that were made. Koerselman added that even if the regional committees improve the level of reporting, a change in the climate is what is really needed.

Henk Jochemsen thinks the regional committees might improve the level of reporting, but like Koerselman he does not think this is the real issue. Physicians are now more aware of the guidelines, there is more pressure on them to report, and this pressure will probably continue. Jochemsen's impression is that the committees are and will continue to be tolerant of the physicians. The committees also educate physicians on the proper performance of euthanasia, and in his view, this will help to make euthanasia even more a part of society. Similarly, Chris Rutenfrans does not see great importance in the regional committees, since they receive only the politically correct cases, those performed according to the guidelines. There are many more cases in which the doctors do not follow the guidelines and do not report to the committees. Rutenfrans thinks the level of underreporting is quite high.

Arie van der Arend would be surprised if the regional committees did substantially increase the level of reporting. He expects the level of reporting by the end of the year 2000 to be around 50 percent. He thinks the committees will generate more paperwork, with few increased substantive positive results, and will not change the GP's inclination not to report euthanasia cases.

Many of the interviewees found it necessary to cite other countries, always apologetically arguing that the situation in the Netherlands is no worse than in those countries. The same line of apologetic tone can be found in Dutch publications authored by scientists who fundamentally agree with the policy of euthanasia. Consider, for instance, the concluding statement of an article compiling a very brief sketch of reports about incidence of euthanasia, assisted suicide and "actions intended to hasten a patient's death" in the Netherlands, Australia, Britain, the United States, Denmark, and Norway: "The conclusion is that EAS [euthanasia and assisted suicide] is occurring in medical care at the end of life in all countries studied. . . . Most worldwide surveys on incidence of EAS show lower figures than those reported in the Netherlands, where there is a lenient policy for prudent practice. Yet, in the Netherlands the actual incidence of EAS is lower than the number of requests received; more requests are refused than granted."[56]

H.J.J. Leenen, a noted jurist who has been instrumental in his efforts to change the penal code so as to permit voluntary euthanasia, said that outside the Netherlands no one reports. Doctors perform euthanasia, and the act is reported as a normal, natural death. If the Dutch want to conduct euthanasia in the open, it should be adequately controlled, and the reporting needs to be full and complete. The Dutch Medical Association accepted the new law proposal, which Leenen helped to formulate, stating that a physician who performs euthanasia but does not report it will be prosecuted for murder.

Although Leenen is skeptical about the work of the committees, he still thinks the number of reports is on the increase. He mentioned the SCEA project. According to Leenen's estimate, 70 percent of the Amsterdam cases were reported in 1999. Physicians knew they would not be prosecuted if they followed the guidelines. Jaap Visser of the Health Ministry also thinks there is an improvement in the level of reporting. However, he estimates that only 55 to 60 percent of the euthanasia cases are now reported.

Evert van Leeuwen and Govert den Hartogh provided insight about the regional committee of which they are members whose role is to examine whether the physicians observe the rules of carefulness, including reporting. Many interviewees feel these committees play a positive role in the policy and practice of euthanasia. In November 1997, the secretaries of justice and of health care, well-being, and sports published their intention to inaugurate five regional committees to supervise physicians in actively ending the lives of their patients. These committees have been functioning since December 1998 and evaluate retroactively the reported cases of euthanasia and physician-assisted suicide. The committees' members are a physician, a lawyer, and an ethicist, and their responsibility encompasses all cases in which a voluntary request has been made by a competent patient. Cases of physician-assisted death without such a request are sent directly to the prosecutor's office. The primary goal of having regional committees is to evaluate the prudence of the practice of physician-assisted death, with the intent of state control of a highly sensitive medical practice and moral issue. The secondary goal is to increase the number of reported cases and thus make public control more effective.[57] Van Leeuwen explained that the KNMG thought there should be a control body between the law and the practice. Until the early 1990s, the police investigated every incident of unnatural death. In some regions, the police came to both the home of the physician and the home of the patient; in other regions, the police came to the physician's home only. This was very disturbing, so those visits were stopped in the early 1990s.

Van Leeuwen, den Hartogh, and their colleagues go over the files and verify that the physician has made a careful judgment according to the guidelines. They assess the durable wish of the patient, the patient's willingness to undergo euthanasia and level of suffering, the GP's consultation with a colleague, and the use of the proper drugs to perform euthanasia. The committee provides moral support to physicians who conduct euthanasia in a moral way.

Each month van Leeuwen's committee examines fifty cases of euthanasia and physician-assisted suicide that took place in North Holland. In turn, den Hartogh's committee reviews forty to fifty cases per month. Other regions have thirty-five cases on average. Each regional committee meets once a month, and each of the committee members reads all cases before the meeting. They try to reach a consensus on every case. If euthanasia has not been done according to the guidelines, the committee asks the physician to provide clarification and more information. Each report should contain a declaration of will by the patient, the physician's report, a statement from the consultant, and the coroner's statement. Sometimes there is also a letter from the family.

Van Leeuwen emphasizes that the committee is not a prosecutorial body. Its aim is to convince physicians to report. In his opinion, euthanasia is not only a medical act; it is an extraordinary act that physicians should report to the public. However, there are physicians who think this is a private matter between themselves and their patients. The regional committees are trying to change this view. They also explain that if physicians perform euthanasia properly, there is no fear of prosecution. Members of the committees write letters to physicians, explaining the need for reporting and how they should perform euthanasia. However, the letters are sent to physicians who already do report, not to those who do not. The committee gets their names from the files.

The committee's verdict on each euthanasia case goes to the district attorney's office, where the prosecutor checks whether the committee examined the case thoroughly. There have been a few cases in which the DA disagreed with the conclusion of van Leeuwen's committee. Den Hartogh testified that there was no single case in which the prosecution overruled the decisions of his committee. Under the new law, the last word is given to the committees. Lawyers object to granting the committees the power to decide whether or not to prosecute because two thirds of the committee members are not lawyers (each committee is comprised of one lawyer, one physician, and one ethicist). Van Leeuwen expects there to be discussions on this issue in Parliament, and that this power will not be granted. He believes that Parliament will seek a way for the DAs to retain their freedom to prosecute.

Most of the reported cases were cancer patients (95 percent of the cases reported to den Hartogh's committee; 80 to 90 percent of the cases reported to van Leeuwen's committee). Den Hartogh said that cancer patients are the accepted group for euthanasia and speculated that doctors might not report euthanasia of noncancer patients because the committee might consider this conduct to be unusual and, therefore, might ask the doctor questions. This is an interesting speculation. Is it the case that most euthanasia involves cancer patients, or that physicians who provided mercy killing to noncancer patients did not report, and hence contributed indirectly to the data that associate euthanasia with cancer patients? This is a difficult and interesting question, which requires further empirical research and analysis.

Van Leeuwen's committee had reviewed some three hundred cases by the time of my interview with him, and in most of these cases the guidelines had been observed. In a small number of cases, from four to eight, the requests were very clear, the physicians could do nothing to help, and the patients were suffering, but were not on the verge of death; they still had four to six months to live. Van Leeuwen felt there were cases in which palliative care could have helped. This issue is something that still needs to be explored and developed. Govert den Hartogh testified that the problematic cases involved consultants who were not truly independent. Sometimes the patient did not form what den Hartogh terms a "categorical request" for euthanasia, or the practice was conducted too early. Nevertheless, the committee only "on occasion" asked physicians to clarify their actions, and only "rarely" concluded that the physician's action was not careful.

In his detailed comments on the first draft of this study, den Hartogh elaborated his explanation by saying that the cases in which his committee asked for more information and/or clarification, were not cases in which the guidelines had not been followed. Rather these were cases in which the information provided (by the doctor, the consultant, or both) was insufficient to make a reliable judgment on the issue. Such questions were asked in 15 to 20 percent of the cases. Den Hartogh added that other committees did it less frequently. In one or two percent of the cases members of the committee were not satisfied with the replies and invited the doctor for an interview. In one case the committee decided after the interview that "the patient had not made a relevant request, so the committee was not competent to decide the case, and the report was sent to the public prosecutor." In three or four cases the committee had some doubts concerning the condition of unbearable suffering, "but having interviewed the doctor we finally decided that his action met the criteria." In three cases the committee found that the requirement of independent consultation had not been satisfied. In three cases the committee's final judgment was that the doctor had acted carefully on the whole, but that during the procedure some mistakes had been made, either by him/her or by his/her colleagues, requiring the attention of the inspection of health care.[58] These last cases have all been scrutinized by the public prosecutor, but this did not lead to actual prosecution. The committee never recommended prosecution; it only recommended investigation by the health care inspection agency.[59]

Sometimes the committee saw from the report that the request for euthanasia, the consultation with another doctor, and the act of euthanasia had been performed on the same day. Den Hartogh explained that this happened when the patient was suffocating and suffering severely. Ordinarily, this rapid decision making should not take place. Nevertheless, these cases constituted, in den Hartogh's view, "unavoidable exceptions."

Den Hartogh mentioned religion as a significant factor that might hinder reporting. In the orthodox Protestant communities, doctors are more reluctant to perform euthanasia. Some would refuse, and others would refer patients to another doctor. And those who are willing to perform it would do it secretly, and would fail to report. Den Hartogh said that when the regional committees were established he had hoped their existence might lead to improved reporting. This has not happened yet; however, it may occur in the future.

Johannes van Delden is a member of a third regional committee. His response to my inquiry about his work was far more reserved. He said that almost all reported euthanasia cases "had something in writing," but he is "not allowed to say how many cases there were."[60] The documents clarified, among other things, that the patient had made the euthanasia request. Van Delden maintained it is too early to judge the regional committees' effectiveness. He explained that if the committees are too harsh on the doctors, they will not report. On the other hand, if the committees are too lenient, their work will have no real purpose. So the committees are required to preserve a delicate balance in their work. They tend to keep the process outside the realm of criminal law and to emphasize educating the doctors. If it appears that a doctor did not follow the guidelines, discussions will be held with him or her and, if required, with the consultant as well, explaining what was lacking and how their practice of euthanasia should be improved.

George Beusmans, who practices euthanasia in Maastricht, revealed that his experience with reporting (which involved calling a coroner) was not very good. He explained that the practice of euthanasia is an intimate moment between himself and the patient's family; and when an intruder (the coroner) arrives, that intimacy is destroyed. When the patient has a family, he tells them it is not necessary to call a coroner. However, Beusmans maintained that during the last few years he had been calling a coroner. Ten years ago, euthanasia was more the exception, but now it is practiced more often, and Beusmans has more experience now with euthanasia. He and his colleagues talk about it in their continuing education programs. Interestingly, Beusmans does not think the regional committees will make any difference.

Gerrit Kimsma, a bioethicist who also practices euthanasia in the Koog aan de Zaan area, said he did not report his first euthanasia case. He was convinced that he was doing the right thing and that the law lacked sensitivity. He claimed that his second case took place several years later and then he did report it. From then on Kimsma reported all his cases. He thinks physicians have a social role, with a professional obligation to society; hence the need to report. He believes it is unprofessional not to obey the guidelines, and doctors should not fear prosecution if they conform. With regard to the regional committees, Kimsma is unsure whether they would increase the level of reporting. He testifies from his experience as a member of one regional committee that of three to four hundred cases examined, there was only one case in which a physician was not careful enough in the euthanasia procedure.

Van Dantzig and Heleen Dupuis were sympathetic about the physicians' lack of reporting. They both said that physicians performing euthanasia do not want to be bothered with filling out forms and waiting months to find out whether they will be prosecuted. For this reason van Dantzig is worried about the need to report. He regards the institution of the regional committees as an improvement, a mechanism to be preferred over the criminalizing of euthanasia. Dupuis exclaims that lack of reporting is the consequence of legal ambiguity. Physicians who feel their behavior was moral do not see why they need to comply with the bureaucracy. Van Dantzig and Heleen Dupuis think euthanasia should be in the realm of the medical practice, not of criminal law.

Conclusions

I came to the Netherlands with mixed feelings and left the same way, but with greater anxiety. My study shows that there is room for concern. Furthermore, it seems that Dutch culture does not welcome a critical plurality of opinions regarding the legitimacy of euthanasia. Critics are regarded quite unfavorably.[61]

It was strange for me to discuss the issue of euthanasia in the Netherlands. Views that are extremely unpopular in other countries regarding euthanasia's place in society rule supreme in the Netherlands. These discussions were almost a mirror image of discussions I had in Israel, the United States, England, Canada, and Australia. What was striking in my discussions with the Dutch experts was the prevailing acceptance of the euthanasia procedure. There were only a few dissenters, people who were willing to go against the system. My first fourteen interviewees were, on the whole, in favor of the policy, and I felt a growing unease encountering such unanimity of opinion. This conformity worried me. Plurality and diversity of opinion are good for society, leading to a more comprehensive understanding of the issues, as well as a higher level of truth, as John Stuart Mill used to say.[62]

I found it troublesome that scholars and decision-makers support a system that suffers from serious flaws while the stakes are so high; after all, we are dealing here with life and death.[63] There were variants of opinion regarding specific questions and issues, but only a minority questioned the system itself. Many of the experts depicted a society in which it is the role of doctors to help patients. They did not question doctors' motives, and saw no reason that doctors would perform euthanasia without compelling reasons. They argued that, of course, criminals exist in every society, in every sphere of life, but that policy is not built around this small number of criminals. They believed there is a need to install control mechanisms against the possibility of abuse, but that the system's rationale is good: to help people in their time of need. They emphasized that the two major reports of 1990 and 1995 indicate there is no slippery slope, yet ignored the fact that there is already too much abuse. Many of the interviewees failed to recognize that the system does not work because all the guidelines, without exception, are broken time and time again.[64] It is not always the patient who makes the request for euthanasia or physician-assisted suicide. Often doctors propose euthanasia to their patients. Sometimes the family initiates the request. The voluntary nature of the request is thus compromised. On occasion, the patient's request is not well considered. There were cases in which no request was made and patients were nonetheless put to death. Furthermore, the patient's request is not always durable and persistent as required.

The guidelines speak of "unbearable suffering," a term that evokes criticisms because it is open to interpretation.[65] Are dementia patients, for instance, suffering unbearably? Was Chabot's patient in an unbearable state of suffering?[66] Was euthanasia the last resort for her? The guidelines instruct that a doctor must perform the euthanasia. There are cases in which nurses administered euthanasia. It is estimated that 10 percent of the nursing home physicians let nurses or even members of the patient's family administer the euthanasia drug.[67] Before the doctor assists the patient, the doctor must consult a second doctor. This guideline has been breached many times. The doctor must keep a full written record of each case and report it to the prosecutorial authorities as a case of euthanasia or physician-assisted suicide, and not as a case of death by natural causes. This guideline has also been violated.[68] Yet many interviewees were quite content with the guidelines.

The interviewees' answers can be grouped in this way:

1. Some interviewees believe that the option of euthanasia should be available for patients and are not willing to critically analyze the situation. They are avowed advocates of the system, no matter what. This group includes A. van Dantzig[69] and Heleen Dupuis.
2. The majority of interviewees defend the practice despite its major flows. Some of them work for government agencies and identify with the system. When the government commissions science, there is always a risk that the scientist will identify with the governmental policy to the point of compromising his or her critical capacity for impartial reflection. Other interviewees in this group are more critically open and think that some accommodations are needed, but that the system, on the whole, functions well. They think that euthanasia should be an option for patients in a liberal society and that, in

any event, the Netherlands cannot go back. The public largely supports the policy and wishes it to be continued.[70] This group consists of Paul van der Maas, Gerrit van der Wal, H.J.J. Leenen, Johannes van Delden, Jaap Visser, Dick Willems, J. K. (Sjef) Gevers, Ron Berghmans, Bert Thijs, Henri Wijsbek, George Beusmans, Gerrit Kimsma, Margo Trappenburg, Egbert Schroten, and Rob Houtepen.

3. There is a smaller group who recognize the flaws and would like to introduce changes, some of which are quite substantial: John Griffiths, Evert van Leeuwen, Govert den Hartogh, and Arie van der Arend. Like the two former groups, these people still support the practice.

4. Critics of euthanasia who would like to prohibit the practice are G. F. Koerselman, Henk Jochemsen,[71] and Chris Rutenfrans.

5. Ruud ter Meulen, Arko Oderwald, and James Kennedy recognize that the policy suffers from several serious flaws, some of which may not be correctable. They are struggling with the issue and have ambivalent views about the practice.

I was surprised during some of the discussions by the rosy pictures that were painted of the existing situation. I asked myself whether I was too cynical and suspicious, or my counterparts too optimistic; after all, they knew the situation in the Netherlands far better than I did. But the unanimity of opinion might suggest that there is not enough reflective thinking about this issue, that the practice of euthanasia is taken for granted; therefore, there might be greater room for abuse because those who wish to abuse would find it easy to do so given this high level of trust and lack of critical questioning.[72] Even issues that are acknowledged as problems are not conceived to be serious enough to press. The Dutch tend to argue and to accept highly troublesome contentions and to consider and allow euthanasia even in cases in which the guidelines are not satisfied. The culture surrounding euthanasia makes the practice accessible within the confines of what is permissible. This culture has a chilling effect on the open, critical debates.[73] In other parts of the world, under similar circumstances, in light of the justified critique, euthanasia would not be considered a viable option.

Some troubling questions have arisen as a result of my studying this Dutch phenomenon. The high number of unreported cases of euthanasia is alarming. The fact that some patients were put to death without their own prior consent is extremely worrisome. Society has to ensure ways that no abuse takes place and that the existing legal procedure does not open a window for abuse, or a way to get rid of unwanted patients. More research should be done on what outside the Netherlands is termed "passive euthanasia," the withholding or withdrawal of treatment. More attention should be given to patients suffering from dementia, newborns, and older children. The guidelines need to be clarified in detail, closing the door to possible misinterpretation that could lead to abuse.

I agree with most of the experts who contend that euthanasia should not be regarded as an integral part of the normal medical care. However, the fact that many physicians do not wish to be bothered with the procedures outlined in the guidelines is alarming. It shows that they have not internalized the idea that euthanasia is an exceptional medical procedure and, as such, requires social control. It is possible that the moral ambiguity surrounding the issue—allowing the practice while it was still prohibited under the Penal Code—made doctors feel that they had better conduct euthanasia in private, keeping it between the patients, their families, and themselves only. The understanding of euthanasia and its importance should be changed if it is to work without abusing the rules mandating carefulness.

I also think physicians should not suggest euthanasia to their patients as an option. By now, the Dutch people are fully aware that euthanasia is available. If patients wish, they can raise the issue themselves. Most of the euthanasia cases involve cancer patients, and at some time during the progressive course of their illness, they can take the initiative and discuss it with their physicians. If they do not, their physicians can assume that these patients do not wish to have euthanasia.

I believe the medical profession should not turn its back on patients who clearly request to shorten their lives. However, this issue should be open to a constant public debate. Wherever euthanasia is practiced, it should be subject to constructive criticism. I thought it was preferable to draft a better legal framework than that of the Netherlands during the time of research, which was ambiguous and presented an illegal-yet-tolerated model. The introduction of the new euthanasia law constitutes an improvement. The legal ambiguity ill served the policy and practice of euthanasia, confused physicians, and brought many of them to think that mercy killings should be conducted in secret, away from the public eye. Indeed, after the Dutch Parliament's positive vote on the euthanasia bill (104 votes pro, 40 against the proposal) on 28 November 2000, doctors spoke of the "psychological significance" of "no longer being guilty until proved innocent."[74] The Royal Dutch Medical Association (KNMG) also welcomed the vote. It has long argued for ending the "paradoxical legal situation" that doctors acting within strict criteria could still face criminal prosecution.[75]

Because the ending of patients' lives should be conducted in the light, not in shadowy areas where only selected people may enter, we should devise a better working framework to help patients in need.

Before I traveled to the Netherlands, I supported euthanasia and published some articles calling for the recognition of the need for euthanasia (in the active sense that is practiced in the Netherlands).[76] After my visit I changed my view. I no longer support euthanasia and restrict my plea for helping patients in need to physician-assisted suicide. This would give patients control over their lives and deaths until the very last moment and would provide a further mechanism to guard against abuse. At the same time, I am willing to concede the need for euthanasia in two circumstances: (1) the patient who asked for euthanasia is totally paralyzed, from head to toe, unable to move any muscles that could facilitate assisted suicide; and (2) the patient took oral medication and the dying process is lasting for many hours (see guidelines in the conclusions).

The majority of Dutch scholars do not share my view. They lump euthanasia and physician-assisted suicide together and even invented an acronym for this purpose: EAS. It should be noted, however, that in August 1995, in an effort to improve the control mechanisms, the KNMG refined its guidelines to recommend that assisted suicide rather than euthanasia should be performed whenever possible.[77]

I believe that the right to die with dignity includes the right to live with dignity until the last minute as well as the right to part from life in a dignified manner. There are competent, adult patients who feel that the preferable way for them to part from life is through physician-assisted suicide.

8 | The Oregon Death with Dignity Act

Proponents of physician-assisted-suicide (PAS) have been trying for over a decade to legalize some type of PAS at the state level.[1] They first attempted to use the traditional state legislative process.[2] Although they managed to get some bills introduced and considered, none of them were approved.[3] Consequently, in 1991 PAS proponents tried a new method, going directly to voters in Washington through the state's voter initiative processes.[4] When the measure was defeated in Washington, the legalization movement moved in 1992 to California, where a measure was again defeated.[5] The movement next moved to Oregon, which houses the national headquarters of the Hemlock Society and is the home of Derek Humphry, a prominent right-to-die activist. The politically independent sentiments of many Oregonians, combined with the state's history of progressive initiatives and health reforms, were instrumental in the passing of the Death with Dignity Act. Furthermore, Oregon has progressive advance directive laws and a long history of citizens using the initiative power as an instrument of legal and social change, sometimes in defiance of organized religion and external political pressures. John Pridnoff, executive director of the Hemlock Society in Eugene, Oregon, said, "Oregonians tend to be more open-minded to a wide variety of opinions."[6]

Oregon has an atmosphere that is conducive to the passage of legislation permitting physician-assisted suicide because of the main characteristics of its population. About 90 percent of Oregonians are white; research showed that whites are more likely than minorities (particularly African Americans and Hispanics) to support physician-assisted suicide.[7] In addition, Oregon is a relatively secular state where religious sentiments are not strong. This enables Oregonians to freely espouse moral views that do not necessarily coincide with majority U.S. religious norms. Chet Orloff, director of the Oregon Historical Society, explained, "This measure is in keeping with Oregon. Throughout history Oregon seems to be out there ahead of other states in testing things."[8]

Interestingly, in order to gain the support of most Oregonians, the activists of the Right to Die campaign distanced themselves from Derek Humphry and the Hemlock Society. The initiators of Measure 16 saw Humphry as a political liability, fearing that his controversial fringe views might scare away voters worried that the measure was the beginning of a radical campaign to help people kill themselves. Spokeswoman Barbara Coombs Lee explained that Humphry always criticized the bill for being too moderate. Measure 16 was not designed to satisfy "the fringe element on either side of this issue, not Derek Humphry and not the archbishop. It was designed to find the common ground with a moderate, rational and safe solution to a problem facing Oregonians."[9] At the same time, the campaign had quietly used Humphry's name to raise money across the country from right-to-die faithful. Humphry himself was very active in raising money for the campaign and contributed a large sum of money.[10]

In November 1994, the citizens of Oregon approved Ballot Measure 16, also called the Oregon Death with Dignity Act,[11] making Oregon the first and only jurisdiction in the United States to legalize PAS.[12] The act allows Oregon residents who are suffering from a terminal disease to receive prescriptions for self-administered lethal medications from their physicians.[13] *Terminal disease* is defined as "an incurable and irreversible disease that has been medically confirmed and will, within reasonable medical judgment, produce death within six (6) months."[14] It does not permit euthanasia, in which a physician or other person directly administers a medication to a patient in order to end the patient's life.[15] Implementation of the act was barred for several years by a constitutional challenge.[16] Passage of the act in November 1997, for the second time, not only legalized PAS in Oregon but also placed Oregon at the center of a national debate regarding PAS.[17]

The Oregon Death with Dignity Act requires that the Oregon Health Division (OHD) monitor compliance with the law, collect information about the patients and physicians who participate in legal physician-assisted suicide, and publish an annual statistical report.[18] This chapter discusses the history of the act from its passage in 1994 to the present, evaluates the strengths and weaknesses of the act, and analyzes the Oregon Health Division's reports on the consequences of the act. The act contains significant documentation and reporting requirements for every step of the procedure.[19] These provisions are designed to ensure that the patient is making a voluntary and informed decision. They help state agencies to monitor physicians' compliance with the act. This, in turn, helps safeguard patients' interests and protects against the risk of involuntary euthanasia.

While the act includes a number of safeguards that are intended to protect patients' interests and guard against the abuses that have occurred in the Netherlands,[20] there are still some flaws beyond the aforementioned weaknesses that do not necessarily advance the purpose of the act, which is to give a dying patient the right to request lethal medication to end his or her life in a humane and dignified way. The chapter proposes several improvements to the act, including modification to permit self-administered lethal injections in situations in which patients cannot take oral medications, additional reporting by pharmacists, mandatory psychiatric consultations for patients considering physician-assisted suicide, and enhanced control mechanisms. The meticulous set of guidelines will improve the implementation of the act and make patients less susceptible to abuse.

The reasoning behind the act recognizes that a person may face grave difficulties at the end of his or her life. The general argument offered by death-with-dignity advocates focuses on a special set of circumstances in which a capable person with a terminal disease has made the request to end his or her life voluntarily. According to the act, a person in this situation should have the autonomy to make the decision to end his or her life and to be able to do so in the most humane manner. This does not negate the principle that a person's life is always valuable at all times. Instead, the viewpoint is that although life is always valuable, patients' desire to control their manner of death and to die a more painless and/or dignified death should be given precedence over the value of their lives. The Oregon act specifies that this judgment should be made after a reasonable medical prognosis has given the patient only six more months to live.[21] To protect the individual's freedom to act, the right to autonomy and the right to choice in end-of-life issues are recognized. Both of these rights were cited by family members as extremely important reasons that patients chose PAS in its second year that it was legal in Oregon.[22]

History of the Oregon Act

The Oregon act passed in 1994 by a slight margin, with 51 percent in favor and 49 percent opposed.[23] The Oregon Medical Association (OMA) officially remained neutral on the act.[24] The Oregon Health Sciences University conducted an anonymous survey of all Oregon physicians eligible to participate in PAS in 1995. The OHSU survey results show that 60 percent of the 2,761 respondents believed that PAS is ethical and should be legal in some cases,[25] and 46 percent stated that they might be willing to write a prescription for a lethal dose of medication once the act went into effect.[26] The survey also indicated that the act may simply have legalized and expanded what was already being practiced by a small percentage of physicians: Of the 21 percent of OHSU survey respondents who said that they had been asked for a prescription for a lethal dose of medication within the year preceding the act, 7 percent admitted writing such a prescription although doing so was illegal.[27] Many physicians (86 percent) reported that legalization of PAS would have no effect on the way that they prescribe pain medication for terminally ill patients.[28] One interpretation of the statement that legalization of PAS would have no effect on the behavior of the majority of physicians is that providing a lethal prescription under the guise of pain management often has a so-called double effect, which most physicians agree is both ethical and legal.

Since the act initially passed by such a narrow margin, it is not surprising that it elicited a storm of protest and public debate.[29] The act was opposed by a coalition of religious groups, including the Catholic Church, that perceive PAS as disrespectful of God's gift of life, and the American Medical Association, which is afraid of altering physicians' traditional role of protecting and preserving life.[30] The most influential response was a lawsuit filed in federal district court by a group of physicians, residential care facilities, and other concerned Oregon residents challenging the act on constitutional grounds.[31] Citing the Fourteenth Amendment, the plaintiffs claimed that the act violated due process and equal protection rights by failing to protect vulnerable patients who might resort to assisted suicide because of undiagnosed depression or coercion.[32] In December 1994, the federal district court granted a temporary injunction, saying that serious questions were presented as to whether Measure 16 violated plaintiffs' freedom of association, freedom of religion, due process, and equal protection rights, and that balance of hardships favored plaintiffs. In August 1995, the district court struck down the act on equal protection grounds.[33] Judge Hogan made three complementary arguments: (1) provision of the Oregon act was not rationally related to any legitimate state interest for equal protection purposes; (2) provision of the act which established a subjective good faith standard of care for physicians and protected them from liability for actions taken in good faith was not rationally related to any legitimate state interest for equal protection purposes; (3) and the act was not rationally related to any state interest, as it did nothing to ensure that the decision to commit suicide was rationally and voluntarily made at the time of death.[34]

Although this decision was subsequently vacated for procedural reasons,[35] execution of the act was delayed yet again pending the Supreme Court decisions in *Washington v. Glucksberg* and *Vacco v. Quill*. In these decisions, the Supreme Court held that there is no constitutional right to PAS.[36] In addition, opponents of the act attempted to have it repealed.

The Act's Last Hurdles

For the first time in Oregon's history, a ballot initiative was voted on twice. In November 1997, Measure 51 (intended to overturn the act) was rejected by an even greater margin (60 percent to 40 percent) than had originally approved the act.[37] A plausible explanation for this much larger margin in support of the Death with Dignity Act is that by this decisive vote, voters expressed their anger at being forced to vote on the issue for the second time. It was the first time in state history that the legislature tried to repeal an initiative by referendum.[38] It is praiseworthy that the citizens of Oregon took an active part in the legislation process and that the law reflects the wishes of the majority of Oregonians. In that respect, Oregon serves as a model to be followed by other states and countries.

Some might object to this assertion, saying that legislation by referendum reduces complex public policy issues to TV sound bites, making it impossible for parties with differing views to reach mutual accommodation through legislative deliberation. On the contrary; discussions on issues decided by referendum are extensive, and the media provide ample opportunities to explore all relevant points of view. The statement that citizens hear only sound bites is oversimplified, exaggerated, and far from the truth. The deliberation process allows more than enough time to reach accommodation and, more fundamentally, the participation of the public at large in public affairs is of great importance. Democracy has a vested interest in securing feedback between citizens and their public representatives, and in stimulating discussion and public debate. It is so important and fundamental that liberals call the existing form of democracy "participatory democracy."[39] Legislation by referendum on a public matter that concerns the lives of all citizens is preferable to a decision-making process in a smoky room, where a small group decides for the people what they should do in an area that is intimate and personal: the right to die with dignity. The public has the right to decide on such an important private matter. Referendum is an excellent mechanism for the public to express its interests and goals.

The passage of the act yet again created a flurry of controversy not only in Oregon but also across the rest of the United States. On 30 April 1997, President Bill Clinton signed the Federal Assisted Suicide Funding Restriction Act of 1997,[40] which states that "Federal funds may not be used to pay for items and services (including assistance) the purpose of which is to cause (or assist in causing) the suicide, euthanasia, or mercy killing of any individual."[41]

Reacting to pressure from Senator Orrin Hatch and Representative Henry Hyde, the chairmen of the Senate and House Judiciary Committees respectively, Thomas Constantine, the administrator of the Drug Enforcement Administration (DEA), issued a statement to the effect that a physician who prescribed drugs under the Oregon act would violate the federal Controlled Substances Act, because the prescription would not promote a legitimate medical purpose. Constantine threatened that physicians who ignored his directive would risk losing their license to prescribe controlled medications.[42] The Oregon Medical Association counseled physicians not to write prescriptions until this threat was removed.[43] Many people worried that the DEA's threat would have the nationwide effect of deterring physicians from providing responsible and humane treatment to dying patients.[44]

Shortly after Constantine's statement, U.S. Attorney General Janet Reno contended that his statement had been issued without her permission.[45] She further stated that the Justice Department was in the process of reviewing the Oregon statute, and that the DEA should have waited for the findings of the review before issuing any warnings to physicians.[46] Following its review of the statute, the Justice Department determined in June 1998 that the DEA does not have the authority to discipline physicians who write prescriptions in accordance with the Oregon act.[47]

In response to this announcement, the Lethal Drug Abuse Prevention Act was presented to the House and Senate in 1998.[48] When this bill did not make much progress, its scope was narrowed to exclude drugs for sedation and to focus only on analgesics (painkillers) and was introduced as the Pain Relief Promotion Act of 1999.[49] The bill would authorize the DEA to enforce prohibitions on the use of controlled substances for assisted suicide in any state, regardless of state law. The bill also prohibits the attorney general from giving force and effect to state laws permitting assisted suicide or euthanasia.[50] This would seriously impede Oregon's assisted-suicide law and would practically preclude other states from passing new assisted-suicide laws.[51]

In addition, the bill defines a safe harbor for physicians to prescribe increased amounts of painkillers for palliative purposes, even if doing so increases the risk of death. The measure directs the Health and Human Services Department to create a program to study pain management and dispense that information to public and private health care programs and providers, medical schools, hospices, and the general public. The bill also authorizes $5 million for grants to train health professionals in the care of patients with advanced illnesses. The DEA would have authority to interpret and enforce physicians' compliance with the guidelines for permissible or illegal uses of controlled substances.

Despite the national American Medical Association's endorsement of the Pain Relief Promotion Act of 1999, twelve state AMA chapters have opposed the bill.[52] Moreover, many physicians are uncomfortable with the AMA's support of the bill and are concerned that the bill may not create a clear and adequate safe harbor, but would instead expose them to the risk of DEA enforcement, creating the very chilling effect on the use of palliative measures that the bill is intended to avoid.[53]

In addition to having the endorsement of the American Medical Association, the bill is supported by other organizations, including the National Legal Center for the Medically Dependent and Disabled, the National Hospice Organization, and Physicians for Compassionate Care.[54] The organizations opposing the bill include the American College of Physicians, the American Society of Internal Medicine, the American Society for Clinical Oncology, the Oregon Medical Association, the American Pain Foundation, the American Cancer Society, and the American Pharmaceutical Association.[55] These groups oppose the bill primarily because they believe it will reduce physicians' ability to prescribe sufficient pain medication and will reduce patients' privacy. The Oregon Medical Association said the law would do more harm than good for treatment of terminally ill patients and would expose doctors to investigations and possible loss of their license to write prescriptions.[56] Justice Department spokeswoman Gretchen Michael stated that the administration "ultimately opposes the bill as 'an unwarranted expansion of federal authority.'"[57]

The bill passed the House on 27 October 1999 by a vote of 271 to 156. It was read and referred to the Senate Committee on Judiciary on 19 November 1999.[58] In December 1999, the Oregon's assisted-suicide law suffered another blow when the American Medical Association voted to continue backing federal legislation intended to prevent doctors from prescribing lethal doses of drugs to 'terminal' patients who want to die.[59]

On 26 October 2000 the Congress passed the Pain Relief Promotion Act. Derek Humphry commented on the passing of the bill: "This legislation is a sad day for civil liberties in America. It is a sneaky way of closing down the Oregon assisted suicide law which has been in operation for almost three years." Humphry maintained that if the president signed this bill—which apparently he could not because it was attached to a tax bill of which he did not approve—then assisted suicide for the dying "will be driven even further underground than it is currently. It will remain the secret crime of the deathbed instead of a honest, cautious, voluntary procedure."[60]

Implementation of the Act

On 26 February 1998, the Oregon Health Services Commission voted (ten to one) to add PAS to the list of medical procedures paid for entirely by the Oregon Health Plan for low-income patients.[61] Complaints were heard that Oregon's Medicaid scheme paid for physician-assisted suicide but not for caregivers to provide sufficient home care to enable elderly and disabled people to live independently.[62] Other commentators were bothered by the fact that the commission attempted to reduce coverage of antidepressant drugs at the same time that it added coverage for PAS.[63]

Several other bills that would restrict the act are currently being considered by the Oregon legislature. The bills include proposals to increase restrictions on where and from whom a patient suffering from a so-called terminal disease can receive PAS services, and increased methods for ensuring that all physicians participating in PAS follow the detailed guidelines.[64] One bill would permit health care facilities to forbid physicians to participate in PAS at their facilities and to punish physicians who disobey. This bill would also restrict sites for PAS to health care facilities, physicians' offices, and private residences.[65] Another measure proposes that a patient must have reasons other than age or disability to participate in PAS and would require physicians to state the purpose of PAS on prescriptions for lethal doses of medication.[66] Although the Oregon legislature has yet to approve any of these measures, it did approve a bill making minor changes to the statute in May 1999.[67]

Analysis of the Oregon Act

In this section we analyze the Oregon act in detail. First, we explore what the act allows by reviewing the terms and definitions. Second, we discuss the set of procedures that define how the act would be implemented. We then discuss the documentation and reporting requirements that formalize the act's safeguards, critiquing the current procedures and oversight rules and showing where improvements are needed.

Terms and Definitions

The Oregon Death with Dignity Act allows Oregon patients who suffer from a terminal disease to receive prescriptions for self-administered lethal medications from their physicians. The act legalizes only physician-assisted suicide, stating that "nothing in this act shall be construed to authorize a physician or any other person to end a patient's life by lethal injection, mercy killing or active euthanasia."[68] It permits a capable, adult Oregon resident[69] diagnosed with a terminal disease to "make a written request for medication for the purpose of ending his or her life in a humane and dignified manner."[70] Physicians who write such prescriptions in good-faith compliance with the act are shielded from civil or criminal penalties and professional discipline.[71]

Procedures

In response to concerns about inadequate safeguards, the authors of the Oregon Death with Dignity Act provided detailed procedures that patients and physicians must follow.[72] The patient who is suffering from a "terminal" disease must first make an oral request, then a written request,[73] and last an additional oral request before the "attending physician" may assist.[74] The written request must be signed and dated by the patient, and witnessed by at least two individuals, one of whom must not be a relative, an heir, or the owner or operator of a health care facility where the patient is receiving treatment or is in residence.[75] Neither of the witnesses shall be the patient's attending physician.[76] The requirement of both oral and written requests encourages patients to consider their condition and the significance of the decision, thus serving their own best interests. It also provides physicians with a record of patients' wishes, to safeguard them from liability. In order to ensure that a patient's request is not a result of familial pressure, the doctor or another member of the medical team should be obliged to conduct conversations with patients and relatives to determine whether their motives are genuine, aiming to serve the patient's best interests.

Physicians must also allow patients to withdraw their request at any point and are required to explicitly offer patients the opportunity to change their minds before prescribing a lethal dose of medication.[77] Like the requirement for both oral and written requests, these requirements provide additional safeguards to ensure that patients are making voluntary, informed, and cautious decisions. They likewise protect the best interests of patients by encouraging them to reconsider their choices and provide prescribing physicians another indication that patients are not making rash decisions or deciding under coercion.

Once a patient makes the first oral request, the physician must inform the patient of the diagnosis, prognosis, potential risks, and probable result of taking the prescription, as well as alternatives, including pain management and comfort and hospice care.[78] This ensures that the patient is being given the pertinent information with which to make a reasoned and informed decision. It gives the patient an opportunity to arrive at a decision in view of the available choices.

The physician must wait at least fifteen days after the patient's first oral request before writing the prescription,[79] arguably too long for a patient who is on the verge of death. Although it is important to allow sufficient time for patients to contemplate their decisions and for physicians to assess the patients, a fixed waiting period may prevent a patient closest to death from utilizing PAS before a natural death can occur. In comparison, the annulled Northern Territory law in Australia required a cooling-off period of only nine days.[80] It was argued that a substantial fraction of the Oregon patients have died during the mandatory fifteen-day waiting period between their initial request and the date that they would have received medication to end their lives.[81] According to Linda Ganzini, 20 percent of the patients who requested assistance with suicide died during the waiting period.[82]

During the waiting period, the attending physician must refer the patient to a consulting physician[83] for confirmation that the patient is suffering from a terminal disease, mentally capable, and acting voluntarily[84] and must ask the patient to notify next of kin regarding the decision.[85] The referral to a consulting physician prevents one physician from making a unilateral decision to prescribe lethal medication. It also allows an important additional evaluation of the patient's illness, prognosis, and mental soundness. A specialist who is not dependent on the first doctor, either professionally or otherwise, should provide the second opinion. It is important that the consultant be able to form an opinion without being pressured in any way by the attending physician, the patient, or the patient's family. The consultant should not work in the same practice, be a trainee, relative, or friend, or have any other compromising relationships with the attending physician, and should not be or have been a coattending physician of the patient.[86] To avoid the possibility of arranging deals between doctors ("You will consult for me regarding Mr. Jones, approving my decision, and I will consult for you regarding Ms. Smith, approving your decision"), it is advisable that the identity of the consultant be determined by a small committee of specialists nominated by the state of Oregon that reviews requests for physician-assisted suicide. In this regard, Oregon may learn from the lessons of the Support and Consultation of Euthanasia in Amsterdam project that was launched in 1997. All GPs from Amsterdam can turn to a group of about twenty specially trained GPs for consultation or advice on euthanasia and PAS. The Royal Dutch Medical Association (RDMA) and the Amsterdam Association of GPs initiated the project because of their interest in quality improvement through consultation and because GPs felt a need for information and advice on euthanasia. The project is intended not only to make it easier for GPs to find an independent and knowledgeable consultant, but also to provide professional consultation.[87]

An attending or consulting physician who believes that the patient is suffering from a psychiatric or psychological disorder must refer the patient to a counselor.[88] Although this requirement is in the patient's best interest, it provides insufficient protection, because attending and consulting physicians are not trained to identify and treat patients with psychiatric or psychological disorders, and therefore may not be competent to determine whether the patient needs a counselor in the first place. Twenty-eight percent of the 2,761 physicians in the OHSU survey reported that they were not confident that they could recognize depression in a patient who requested a prescription for a lethal dose of medication.[89] Linda Ganzini and colleagues report that 20 percent of the patients had symptoms of depression.[90] In light of this information, it is even more important that attending or consulting physicians be required to refer patients to a psychiatrist or psychologist for further assessment. Since the act prohibits the dispensing of lethal medication to an "incapable" person, the act should be revised to include a mandatory referral to a psychiatrist to assess patients' mental capabilities and to determine whether they suffer from depression.

The Oregon Health Division Reports
The following discussion reviews the reports on the results of the act since it came into effect. First, we cover the findings of the reports in detail. Second, we discuss several implications and conclusions that can be drawn from the reports' results. The analysis uncovers several weaknesses in the act, and proposes further ways to amend the act to eliminate those weaknesses.

Findings of the First Report
On 18 February 1999, the Oregon Health Division issued its report on the effects of the Death with Dignity Act during its first year.[91] Since no prescriptions were written under the act for most

of 1997, the report contains data only about the number and character-istics of Oregonians who received medication to end their lives between November 1997 and December 1998. The study was conducted as part of the required surveillance and public health activities of the Oregon Health Division and was supported by division funds. In formulating its report, the division relied exclusively on physicians' perceptions of care at the end of life, and physicians' perceptions of patients' experi-ences.[92] Patients and their families were not interviewed.[93] Because the report is not a firsthand account, it may be invalid to draw definitive conclusions about the first year's experience with legalized PAS in Oregon.[94]

Another important consideration in the assessment of the data is that, although physicians are required to report the writing of all prescrip-tions for lethal medications to the Oregon Health Division, the division could not know whether physicians provided assistance with PAS with-out reporting it.[95] The division's report contains no data on the percentage of doctors suspected or known to have participated in PAS without re-porting to the state.

Despite these methodological weaknesses, the findings do suggest some interesting preliminary conclusions. The division matched each case patient (a patient receiving a prescription for a lethal dose of medi-cation) to up to three control patients (forty-three control patients in all) who died from similar illnesses but did not receive prescriptions for lethal medications.[96] In addition to the similarity of the underlying illness, the control patients were matched according to age (within ten years of the case patient's age) and date of death (within thirty days of the case patient's death). Only control patients who would have met the requirements of the Death with Dignity Act were included in the study. The data on control patients and case patients were obtained by the same methods—that is, by studying death certificates and interviewing physicians.[97]

The first annual report on assisted suicide indicates that only twenty-three patients had invoked the Oregon act. They received legal drugs to end their lives under the provisions of the law. Of these twenty-three, fifteen had actually used the drugs and died; six others had died from their illnesses, and two were still alive as of 1 January 1999.[98] Physician-assisted suicide accounted for five of every ten thousand deaths in Or-egon. The median age of the fifteen patients who died after taking lethal medication was sixty-nine years; eight were male, and all fifteen were white. Thirteen of the fifteen patients had cancer.[99] The report holds that finances and fear of pain did not appear to be critical considerations in the choice of physician-assisted suicide. Instead, persons who chose physician-assisted suicide were primarily concerned about personal autonomy and control over the manner in which they would die.[100] The fact that a significant number of Oregonians die under hospice care may provide a possible explanation for the relatively few patients who requested physician-assisted suicide.

The report was quickly hailed by advocates of doctor-aided dying as evidence that the law had not led to abuses, botched suicides, or a widespread rush among the sick or suffering to move to Oregon for the right to be put to death, as many critics of the law had contended would happen. Peter Rasmussen, a cancer specialist in Salem, Oregon, who said he has been present for at least two occasions of physician-assisted suicide, said that it was a very positive experience to have people gather around the patient, reminisce, and say their final good-byes: "One of the potential advantages is, you can plan it—people who have relatives far away can gather everybody together."[101] On the other hand, a group opposed to assisted suicide criticized Oregon's report on the Death with Dignity Act, saying that the study's conclusions were unfounded.[102]

Findings of the Second Report

In February 2000 information on patients who received prescriptions for lethal medications in 1999 was reported to the Oregon Health Division. The report compiles the data of the second year's experience with legalized physician-assisted suicide in Oregon. The patients who received prescriptions for lethal medication were identified through the regulation that requires doctors to report this. Health Division epidemiologists collected additional information using physician interviews and death certificates. Unlike the case of the first report, here family members were also interviewed to understand better why some patients requested physician-assisted suicide. According to the report, thirty-three prescriptions were written in 1999 for lethal doses of medication, and twenty-seven died after using this medication; twenty-six of these patients obtained their prescription in 1999 (nine of the ten thousand deaths in Oregon during the period in question) and one in 1998. Five of the 1999 prescription recipients died of their underlying illness, and two were alive at the end of 1999. The median age of the twenty-seven patients who took the lethal medication was seventy-one. Sixteen were male, twenty-six were white, and twelve (44 percent) were married. Seventeen patients had end-stage cancer, most commonly lung cancer. Four had chronic lung disease, and four had amyotrophic lateral sclerosis (Lou Gehrig's Disease). All patients had health insurance, and twenty-one were in hospice care before death.[103]

Findings of the Third Report

In 2000, the number of terminally ill patients in Oregon who chose physician-assisted suicide remained small. Oregon physicians wrote 39 prescriptions for lethal doses of medication, as compared with 24 in 1998 and 33 in 1999. Twenty-six of the 39 patients who received prescriptions died after ingesting the medication, 8 died from their underlying disease, and 5 were still alive on 31 December 2000. During 1998 and 1999, 16 and 27 patients, respectively, died after ingesting the medication. One patient who received a prescription in 1999 died in 2000 after ingesting the medication; another patient who received a prescription in 1999 was still alive on 31 December 2000. Physicians were present at 14 of the 27 deaths (52 percent).[104]

The twenty-seven patients who ingested lethal medications in 2000 represent an estimated rate of 9 per 10,000 deaths in Oregon, as compared with a rate of 6 per 10,000 in 1998 and 9 per 10,000 in 1999. Twenty-one of the patients had cancer. Thirty-three enrolled in hospice. The demographic characteristics of the patients who chose physician-assisted suicide in 2000 resembled those of 6,981 Oregon residents who died from similar underlying illnesses in 1999, with a single exception: As their level of education increased, their likelihood of choosing physician-assisted suicide increased (thirteen of the twenty-seven patients were college graduates. Only two patients did not complete high school).[105]

The median age of the twenty-seven patients was sixty-nine. Fifteen of them were women; twelve men. Patients with a college education were more likely to choose physician-assisted suicide than those without a high-school education; patients with postbaccalaureate education were even more likely to choose physician-assisted suicide. The patients in 2000 were demographically similar to those in previous years, except that they were more likely to be married. Eighteen of the patients were married; six widowed, and three divorced.[106]

One of the twenty-two physicians who had prescribed the lethal medications was reported to the Oregon Board of Medical Examiners for submitting an incomplete written-consent form. For the first time, the Health Division reported a doctor for not fulfilling a requirement of the law. On the patient's written request for a lethal prescription, the doctor obtained a signature from only one witness rather than the required two. The Health Division contacted the doctor and learned that a designated second witness had forgotten to sign the document. The witness subsequently signed it. Katrina Hedberg of the Health Division, who wrote the report, said she does not expect that the doctor would be disciplined.[107]

Physicians continued to report that the patients who chose physician-assisted suicide in 2000 had multiple end-of-life concerns that contributed to the patients' requests for lethal medications. Losing autonomy came in first (93 percent), followed by decreasing ability to participate in enjoyable activities (78 percent), losing control of bodily functions (78 percent), and being a burden on family, friends, and other caregivers (63 percent). Concern over pain was cited by just under a third of the twenty-seven individuals who went through with a physician-assisted suicide in 2000, the highest percentage so far. In the first year, only 12 percent of those who completed an assisted suicide had told their physicians that pain was a concern. Pain is on a standard list of issues used by Oregon to gain insight into why patients request suicide aid. Worry about the cost of treatment came in lower than pain this year. In the previous two years, no one cited it at all. That is not surprising, because most of the patients over the three years had insurance.[108]

As in previous years, most of the patients who used PAS in 2000 (twenty-three) were enrolled in hospice care, compared with twenty-one patients in 1999 and eleven patients in 1998. Of the three who declined hospice, two patients felt they did not need it, and one patient did not wish to stop treatment (a requirement for hospice). Almost all patients died at home. No patient died in an acute-care hospital.[109]

Susan Tolle, director of the Center for Ethics in Health Care at Oregon Health Sciences University, reacted to the report by saying: "To me the most profound thing about the process is that after three years of being legal in Oregon, it is still an option that less than one in 1,000 people in this state uses."[110] George Eighmey, executive director of Compassion in Dying of Oregon, commented: "The three-year cumulative report to me proves what we said during our campaign—that this will be used very rarely, and when used, there are very few complications, if any."[111]

Implications of the Reports' Findings and Suggestions for Improvement

The three published studies provide a clearer picture of the workings of the Oregon Death with Dignity Act, through which seventy people have ended their lives in the last three years. Twenty-two physicians prescribed lethal medication to thirty-three patients in 2000 and also in 1999. Six of the physicians had also prescribed such medication in 1998. The majority of the twenty-two physicians were in family practice or internal medicine (thirteen in 2000; fourteen in 1999), five were oncologists, and three were in other specialties (four in 2000; three in 1999). In 2000, physicians were present in fourteen of the twenty-seven cases (52 percent) compared with sixteen of the twenty-seven cases in 1999 (59 percent) and eight of the sixteen cases in 1998 (50 percent).[112] The presence of physicians at the patients' bedside is important for three reasons: First, it could enhance the trust between patients and physicians, welcoming physicians to the patients' private homes during the intimate moments of dying, sharing with them as well as with the patients' loved ones the last moments of the patients' lives.[113] Patients are thus reassured that their physicians will stand by them until the very last moment.

Second, the wide variations in the times between the administration of medication and actual time of death support the assertions that physicians should be required to be present when patients die. According to the 1998 report, the median time from ingestion of the lethal medication to unconsciousness was five minutes (from three to twenty minutes) and the median time from ingestion to death was twenty-six minutes (from fifteen minutes to 11.5 hours).[114] In comparison, according to the 2000 report, the median interval between ingestion and unconsciousness was nine minutes (from one to thirty-eight minutes), and the mean interval between ingestion and death was thirty minutes (from seven to seventy-five minutes).[115] In turn, according to the 1999 report, the median interval between ingestion and unconsciousness was ten minutes (from one to thirty minutes) and the mean interval between ingestion and death was thirty minutes (from four minutes to twenty-six [!] hours).[116] During a prolonged process of dying, the physician may provide much needed counsel and explanation to the patient's loved ones.

Third, the physician's presence may be required to finalize an agonizing process of death. Restricting the act to include only self-administered oral medication is problematic, because such medication may not end the patient's life and/or may prolong the patient's suffering needlessly. Oral medication may be difficult or impossible for many patients to ingest because of nausea or other side effects of their illnesses. Studies of lethal oral medications have found that death may take hours or may never occur. In the Netherlands, physicians who intend to provide assistance with suicide sometimes end up administering a lethal medication themselves because of the patient's inability to take the medication or because of problems with the completion of physician-assisted suicide.[117] It was argued that lethal prescriptions of oral medications are ineffective 25 percent of the time.[118] Fifty percent of physicians in the OHSU survey reported that they were not sure what they would prescribe if they decided to comply with a patient's request for a prescription of lethal oral medication.[119] This widespread uncertainty about the effectiveness of orally administered drugs and dosages raises serious concerns that family members might face a situation in which their loved one is forced to endure an unsuccessful suicide attempt or a protracted death. To date, there are no known failed suicides in Oregon, but families should be counseled on the possibility, which is not slim, of a protracted death. Possible alternatives for patients who are incapable of taking oral medication are lethal injection, which is proscribed in the Oregon Death with Dignity Act, and self-administered, lethal intravenous infusion, which may not be prohibited.[120]

In the second year, the number of patients who died after ingesting lethal medication increased, as could be expected given the growing public awareness of the availability of PAS. It remained the same (twenty-seven) in the third year. The number of PAS remained small in relation to the total number of persons in Oregon who died during these years.[121]

Many patients who sought assistance with suicide had to ask more than one physician for a prescription for lethal medication. The act states that no health care provider is under any obligation to participate in the dispensing of medication to a patient who desires to end his or her life. Any health care provider who is unable or unwilling to assist the patient with such a request is required to send the patient and the patient's records to another health care provider.[122] Only eight of the twenty-seven patients in 1999, and eight of sixteen patients in 1998 were able to initiate the prescription process with the first physician they approached.[123] The other patients had to request a prescription from a second or third physician. According to the physicians' reports in 1999, ten patients asked one other doctor, and eight asked two or three physicians. Information on one patient was not available.[124] These data show that many physicians in Oregon were still reluctant to provide assistance with suicide during the second year. The picture somewhat changed during the third year: Eleven of the first-asked physicians (44 percent) wrote lethal prescriptions.

Ganzini and colleagues reported that physicians grant about one in six requests for a prescription for a lethal medication and that one in ten requests actually results in suicide.[125] A recent study shows that fourth-year medical students in Oregon are significantly less willing than other medical students in the United States to provide a patient with a lethal prescription.[126] In the OHSU survey, less than half of physicians stated that they would be willing to write a prescription for a lethal dose of medication once the act went into effect.[127] Moreover, the study indicated that physicians practicing in rural communities were less likely to be willing to participate in PAS because of greater threats to confidentiality, lack of anonymity, and social disapproval. Considering that 62 percent of Oregon's population resides in rural communities, many patients are likely to be transferred at least once.[128] Patients may have a difficult time finding assistance. Each transfer to another health care provider creates a delay during which the patient may deteriorate further and may continue to suffer.

Obviously it is not proposed that physicians should be forced or pressured to participate in PAS. Physicians should not be compelled by the state to take part in a medical activity, especially an activity that many find morally repugnant or religiously offensive, unless the state has a compelling interest, which is not the case here. Granted that PAS should be a voluntary act by both the patient and the physician, physicians should be open and candid about their views on PAS and should express their reservations about the act, if they have any, so patients can know what to expect from them near the time of their death. Physicians should be required to alert patients to a blanket opposition before subjecting them to the time and expense of assessments, which may have to be repeated by other physicians.

Particularly troubling findings in the first report were that persons who were divorced were 6.8 times more likely to choose PAS than married persons, and persons who had never married were 23.7 times more likely to choose PAS than married persons. Although these findings do not necessarily lead to the conclusion that patients choosing PAS are more socially isolated than the norm, there is often a direct correlation between marital status and level of familial support and care. At a minimum, these findings indicate that the psychological makeup and life circumstances of the patients choosing PAS should be studied further, because they may be facing an even more difficult situation because of weak family support.

The low proportion of married persons in 1998 was not found in the second and third reports. In 1999, twelve of the patients who died by PAS were married, six were widowed, eight were divorced, and one never married. This issue should continue to be observed in the coming annual research studies. Reduced family support may exacerbate patients' fears of loss of autonomy and loss of bodily control that were reported as important motivating factors for choosing PAS. The higher risks associated with the unmarried status of some patients and the fact that only five of the sixteen patients had undergone psychological consultation in 1998 indicate the need for increased psychiatric and/or psychological assessments of patients and support the recommendation that the act could be improved by requiring psychiatric consultations for all patients, as did the Australian Northern Territory Right of Terminally-Ill Act.[129] The second-year report says that ten of the patients who died by PAS in Oregon in 1999 (37 percent) were referred for psychiatric evaluation. This is a slight increase compared with 1998 (31 percent of the patients who died by PAS).[130] In comparison, in 2000 there was a sharp decrease in the number of patients referred for psychological evaluation: only five (19 percent).[131] The report does not state the time spent on the consultations. This point should be explored and pondered.

Most patients in the three reports said that they chose death because of a fear of loss of autonomy (75 percent in 1998; 78 percent in 1999; 93 percent in 2000) and decreasing ability to participate in activities that make life enjoyable (69 percent in 1998; 81 percent in 1999; 78 percent in 2000). Other major concerns were losing control of bodily functions (56 percent in 1998; 59 percent in 1999; 78 percent in 2000) and being a burden on family, friends, and caregivers (12 percent in 1998; 26 percent in 1999, and a sharp increase in 2000: 63 percent).[132] In the Netherlands, fear of loss of dignity and of being a burden, rather than pain, are the impetus for most requests for assistance in dying.[133] In Oregon, eight patients in 2000, seven patients in 1999, and only two patients in 1998 expressed concern about inadequate pain control. These findings may reflect advances in palliative care in Oregon, which ranks among the top five states in per capita use of morphine for medical purposes.[134] Other studies have shown that pain is not prominent in oncology patients' attitudes toward PAS. Ezekiel J. Emanuel and colleagues found that patients actually experiencing pain were more likely to find euthanasia or physician-assisted suicide unacceptable.[135]

On the other hand, the findings that only two patients in 1998 and a more significant number of patients in 1999 and 2000 expressed concern about inadequate pain control may indicate only physicians' opinions that they are capable of managing pain. It might also be the result of poor communication between cancer patients (the majority of patients who asked for lethal drugs) and physicians. This hypothesis is strengthened when one looks at interviews with family members, conducted in 1999. The most frequently cited reasons by family members for the patient's decision to request assistance with death were concern about loss of control of bodily functions (68 percent), loss of autonomy (63 percent), and physical suffering (53 percent).[136] Ganzini and colleagues report that pain was an important consideration for 43 percent of patients who requested prescription for a lethal medication.[137]

Moreover, studies showed that pain control for cancer patients is often inadequate and that physicians typically underestimate pain. Patients with significant pain caused by cancer visit their physicians and frequently leave with as much pain as they came with because their pain was never discussed or treated. Impediments to adequate pain treatment include health care providers' fear of inducing physical or psychological addiction, misconceptions about pain tolerance, and assessment bi-ases.[138] Furthermore, communication about pain often depends on the patients' complaining of it. Patients, however, are often reluctant to re-port pain for a variety of reasons, including wanting to be a "good" (noncomplaining) patient, concern about having to take strong painkill-ers, or worries that talking about pain might take too much time and distract the physician from dealing with the disease itself.[139] Moreover, many patients seek pain relief from complementary therapies. Often they feel that these methods offer a holistic approach that is lacking in the traditional allopathic model.[140] It is advisable that doctors examine whether the prescribed pain control is adequate. Palliative care is able to prevent or at least to ease most manifestations of physical pain.[141]

In addition to the dearth of data regarding patient perspectives on PAS, insufficient data exists on the level of underreporting by physi-cians.[142] The Oregon Health Division is not only responsible for collecting information under the Death with Dignity Act; it is also obligated to re-port any cases of noncompliance with the law to the Oregon Board of Medical Examiners. According to the division's report, its responsibil-ity to report noncompliance makes it difficult, if not impossible, to de-tect accurately and comment on underreporting. Furthermore, the reporting requirements, as written in the Oregon act, can only ensure that the process for obtaining lethal prescriptions complies with the law. "[The division] cannot determine whether PAS is being practiced out-side the framework of the *Death with Dignity Act.*"[143]

One way to decrease the chances of underreporting, which is a ma-jor problem in the Netherlands,[144] is to require reporting by pharmacists who dispense lethal prescriptions in addition to requiring reporting by physicians. Indeed, recent changes in the act require pharmacists to re-port separately all prescriptions. If physicians knew that pharmacists were also required to report all prescriptions for lethal medication, thus pro-viding a check on physicians' reporting, they would be more likely to comply with the act's reporting requirement. Although some pharma-cists might be less willing to fill prescriptions for lethal medication if they knew that their names would be associated with the procedure, ad-ditional reporting requirements would help protect the state and the public's compelling interest in monitoring PAS and would ensure that safety procedures were followed. The Health Division could guarantee the confidentiality of pharmacists, as the division currently guarantees the confidentiality of the reporting physicians.[145] Furthermore, the Or-egon Medical Association should establish a committee that will inves-tigate the underlying facts accounted for in the reports as well as whether there were so-called mercy cases that were not reported and/or did not comply with the act. Licensing sanctions would be used to punish those health care professionals who violated the required procedure.

The wide variations in patients' time to death support the assertions that physicians should be required to be present when patients die. For those patients who are unable to ingest oral medication, a mechanism can be introduced by which they need only activate a lethal injection administered by a qualified physician. Alternatively, patients may administer lethal intravenous infusion. When patients who took the oral medication are lingering for an unusually long period, such as twelve hours rather than just minutes, the physician should be allowed to administer a lethal injection.[146]

On the positive side, many of the Oregon Health Division's findings refute arguments commonly voiced by the public and by opposition groups on the dangers of PAS. For instance, the division's studies provide no evidence to support the common fears that PAS will be disproportionately chosen by or forced on patients who are poor, uneducated, uninsured, or afraid of the financial costs or pain of their illness. The 1998 case patients and the larger group of 5,604 Oregon residents who died from similar underlying illnesses in 1996 did not differ statistically with respect to age or education. Moreover, the case patients did not differ from the matched control patients in age, race, sex, level of education, and rural or urban residence. Finally, neither the case patients nor the control patients expressed concern about the economic costs of their illness.[147] Similarly, the 1999 report indicates that poverty, lack of education or health insurance, and poor care at the end of life were not important factors in patients' requests for assistance with suicide.[148] And in 2000, only one patient was concerned about the financial implications of treating or prolonging illness.[149] Although these results are based on a relatively small number of patients, and ongoing supervision is needed, these findings suggest the conclusion that PAS will not be disproportionately chosen by or forced on unwilling, uneducated, and/or socially and economically disadvantaged individuals. Judging from the reported motivations of the patients examined in the reports, PAS seems to be associated more with the desire for autonomy and control than with fear of intolerable suffering or devastating financial consequences.

Conclusion

Although polls have consistently shown for over a decade that a majority of Americans, from 60 to 70 percent, support making assisted suicide legal for patients who are mentally competent and have less than six months to live,[150] Oregon remains the only state to legalize assisted suicide, and the future of Measure 16 is uncertain.[151]

Physical and mental pain and suffering, as well as the loss of dignity and autonomy resulting from patients' lack of bodily control due to a degenerative disease, are strong arguments supporting Oregon's Death with Dignity Act. Although it is important to allow patients the right to decide when to end their pain and suffering, it is also important to protect their best interests and ensure that their lives are not being ended involuntarily. Although the Oregon act already includes many safeguards that serve the best interests of patients, incorporating greater protections will help ensure that all patients receiving lethal medications are truly making an informed and voluntary choice.

Several improvements to the act were proposed, including modification of the act to include self-administered lethal injections in situations in which oral medications cannot be taken, additional reporting by pharmacists, consultation by an independent specialist assigned by a medical select committee, and additional mandatory psychological or psychiatric consultations for patients considering PAS. Adoption of these suggestions will serve three primary purposes: First, it will help ensure that patients are not motivated by depression to choose PAS.[152] Second, it will enable researchers to distinguish between the perceptions of patients and physicians. This information will allow a more informed public debate on the controversial issue of PAS and will create a more knowledgeable and empathetic culture surrounding dying patients and their families. Finally, it will help ensure that patients for whom taking oral medication is difficult or impossible will also have the ability to choose PAS.

There is always the risk that patients and doctors might view a proposal for increased regulation as too paternalistic and unjustifiably intrusive. Although the proposals do create more regulations and will be viewed by some patients and physicians as unnecessary increases in bureaucratic red tape, these regulations are necessary to protect the best interests of patients, and thus to ensure the effectiveness and longevity of the act. Implementation of the proposals will strike a better balance between the need for information and monitoring and the need to protect the privacy and confidentiality of those involved. Despite its flaws, the Oregon act is a significant step toward establishing a patient's right to autonomy and choice in deciding end-of-life issues. Strengthening its weak areas will assure that the act achieves its laudable purpose, to ensure that competent, adult Oregon residents have the right to exercise control and autonomy in end-of-life decision-making, including the right to die in a humane and dignified manner.

In general, the studies from Oregon portray the people opting for assisted suicide as well educated, well insured, often in hospice care, and very concerned about loss of independence. The most frequently cited reasons for PAS were loss of autonomy and an inability to participate in activities that make life enjoyable. Worries about money played almost no role in the patients' decision. There is no evidence that the poor, uneducated, mentally ill, or socially isolated are disproportionately seeking or getting lethal prescriptions for drugs under Measure 16.[153]

Based on the Dutch experience, the Oregon experience, and the Northern Territory abolished act, the next chapter formulates specific guidelines for physician-assisted suicide. The argument for physician-assisted suicide is a circumscribed one, sensitive to the needs and the wishes of patients, aiming to consider carefully the wishes of the patient without creating an opportunity for abuse or coercion.

Conclusions

A Circumscribed Plea for Voluntary Physician-Assisted Suicide

The concept of death with dignity does not automatically imply a desire to die; it certainly does not mean to put someone to death in a dignified way. Organizations that support euthanasia speak of the right to die with dignity, and this terminology has become a euphemism used to promote euthanasia. I believe in the concept of death with dignity and recognize that some prefer death over the continuation of tormented living. Some organizations are so dedicated to the idea, however, that they conceive of themselves as missionaries whose role is to educate and advance society in what they believe is the right direction, and sometimes they do not make judgments and decisions carefully.[1] They become too eager, and their strong motivation overshadows the need for utmost caution. It is imperative not to be simplistic or ambiguous in considering this delicate issue.

In a discussion with an Israeli attorney who specializes in representing patients who wish to die and who is active in the right-to-die organization in Israel, I asked him about his prime concern. His answer was the patient's expressed will to die. I further pressed the issue and questioned him about various scenarios: What if your client needs some emotional support? What if your client is unaware of all the relevant considerations relating to his or her disease? I wanted to understand to what extent the attorney was sensitive and cognizant of the possibility that some patients/clients might change their mind if things were explained to them in a different manner. The attorney's answers clearly showed that this did not matter to him. For him the client's desire to die was sufficient. His attitude seemed to imply a lack of compassion for his clients.

Our first obligation is to place the issue in its proper context and to emphasize that most patients seek to preserve life. With this proviso in mind, I support the right to die with dignity in certain cases. I will do my best to describe these cases clearly, without being overzealous, and without offending the people involved. Life should not be seen as a virtue to be preserved at any cost, regardless of the patient's will; at the same time, euthanasia should not be supported without reservation. In this context there are grounds for the criticism of Dr. Jack Kevorkian's campaign for euthanasia and the utilization of his Mercitron. Kevorkian may not be considered seriously by bioethicists, but his deeds deserve serious consideration. From 1990 until his arrest in 1999, Dr. Kevorkian, a retired pathologist, helped dozens of people to die. Kevorkian recognized a specific need that is not met adequately by society, and he entered this lacuna with a missionary vigor. His campaign is the result of failures of the medical system in caring for patients with intractable or chronic problems. He has forced society to think harder than before about medical mercy and assistance at the end of life, and to find suitable answers so that Kevorkian's ministrations may be made irrelevant.

The *Eyal* case, which took place in Israel in 1990, serves as an illustration of the fact that on some occasions physician-assisted suicide may be allowed. In such instances, the patients' autonomy would be sustained and their dignity better served by helping them to die. It is not always true that keeping a person alive is equivalent to treating this person as an end. In the case of some incurable conditions, we respect the dignity of patients in agony when we help them to cease living. My justification for helping such patients fulfill their request rests on the assumption that they freely and genuinely have expressed their will to die, and that they persist in expressing that desire.

The Benjamin Eyal *Case*

In 1990, the magistrate court of Tel Aviv received an appeal made by a patient named Benjamin Eyal, who suffered from amyotrophic lateral sclerosis (ALS), the same disease that attacked Sue Rodriguez in Canada. Eyal, aware of the expected progressive deterioration of his condition, asked not to be attached to a ventilator when he could no longer breathe spontaneously, but to be allowed to die. He expressed this wish in an affidavit, on a videocassette as well as verbally. The specialist who testified before the court said that his commitment to care for Eyal "does not include a duty to prolong life of unimaginable suffering by committing an intrusive act that could be avoided by following the will of the patient."[2]

In considering Eyal's motion, Judge Uri Goren emphasized two principles: the "sanctity of life" principle, and the "decent death" principle. Judge Goren articulated that the first principle should be employed when medical treatment could save life or improve the medical state of patients. (However, Jewish law does recognize the need not to afflict dying people, taking into consideration human suffering and pain.)

Judge Goren explained that in this case, no doubts arose with regard to the wishes of the patient. Eyal clearly manifested his wish not to be connected to a ventilator when the time came and no other alternative was available to keep him alive. In addition, there were no doubts that Eyal was competent and clear-minded upon voicing his request, knowing its obvious consequences. In his testimony before the court, the director of Lichtenstaedter Hospital, Dr. Nachman Wilensky, explained that Eyal was a longtime patient, well known to the hospital officials, and that he was thoroughly convinced that Eyal's intentions were sincere and that his decision had been freely made.

Judge Goren decided to accept the appeal. He emphasized that such a decision concerning life and death should be made by a senior director, either by the director of the hospital or by the head of the chronic-care department. This was because the decision involved medical expertise, moral values, religious issues, and ethics.[3]

The *Eyal* case stimulated extensive debate in Israel. Rabbinical authorities were asked their opinion regarding this situation. The major difference between the halachic view and the liberal view is that many halachic commentators do not endorse the autonomy principle. From their perspective, human beings are not masters of their lives. Life is given to us as a gift from the Creator, and we should not destroy it.[4] Human life is intrinsically good irrespective of its condition. Rabbi Elyashiv, a well-known *posek halacha* (halachic arbiter), said that when medical treatment may only prolong transient life and involves additional suffering, a patient may refuse to accept it. The physicians, he decided, would be allowed to terminate treatment when the last stages of Eyal's disease were reached. Rabbi Israel Meir Lau, currently the Ashkenazi chief rabbi in Israel, also endorsed this view.

In a letter concerning the *Eyal* case, Rabbi Lau wrote that his determination was limited to the case in hand and to the specific circumstances as described to him. He contended that the halacha did not require, and sometimes prohibited, the administering of exceptional treatment that only prolonged the patient's suffering without healing the cause of the pain. Eyal's disease was said to be incurable, and the disputed treatment would not sustain his life in any meaningful sense. So, when the time came, the attending physicians should be allowed to act upon Eyal's request and refrain from connecting him to a ventilator. Rabbi Lau maintained that, in any event, regular medical treatment should continue. That is, Eyal should be provided with nutrition, and all means should be taken to relieve his pain.[5]

Benjamin Eyal died of complications before his disease had reached its final stage and before a ventilator was necessary. Thus, the physicians at Lichtenstaedter did not have to act upon the court's decision. For the sake of argument, however, let us suppose that the final stage had been reached, and the physicians refrained from connecting Benjamin Eyal to the ventilator. Would it be humane to witness Eyal suffocating to death? I asked one of Eyal's senior doctors if it would be possible for him to stand idly by while his patient was choking to death. The doctor replied, "I would give Eyal something to shorten his suffering."

I think that this is a humane answer, in harmony with the morals of humane medicine. Any other answer, principally opposed to active intervention, would be inhumane and cruel. Under such circumstances, there are strong reasons to consider physician-assisted suicide. If the patient is obviously suffering and expresses the will to die, and his doctors admit that they are unable to cure the illness and that they can ease only the physical and not the emotional pain, there is no substantial difference between voluntary passive euthanasia and voluntary physician-assisted suicide.[6] The term *voluntary* refers both to the request of the patient and to the act of the doctor. The patient should have the right to decide for himself about his fate, and the doctor should not be compelled to implement the decision, but should participate in this process only if she feels that physician-assisted suicide is the appropriate, dignified, and kind medical measure.

Those who oppose assisted suicide will say that there is no need to reach the stage at which we have to consider such termination of life. Benjamin Eyal could have been given medication to stop his suffering. The responsibility rests with the doctor to give medicine to patients, even if the medicine shortens their lives. This is allowed because the purpose is to care for the patients and decrease their suffering, not to bring about their death.

The double-effect doctrine serves both spiritual leaders and careful healers as a way out of dealing directly and sincerely with the question of mercy termination of life (see chapter 1). Undoubtedly the doctrine provides a better solution than does letting people like Benjamin Eyal die slowly in agony. In everyday medical practice in hospitals, doctors' actions often have a double effect: Their intention is to alleviate pain and suffering, not to kill the patient, but the result is the death of the patient. However, I suspect that there are enough cases in which partisan interests rather than the patients' best interests come first and foremost in the doctor's eyes, and the double-effect doctrine serves as a convenient guise for pursuing those partisan interests.

This is not to say that permitting merciful medical assistance for ending life, in cases in which the patient's condition is irreversible and the patient lacking autonomy seeks assistance to fulfill his or her desire to die, is a precedent for the killing of patients in other instances. On the basis of these assumptions it might be argued that people in PCU cannot possess dignity because they are not autonomous. Thus the argument might be that in order to safeguard their dignity we might be required to help them cease living. Justice Haim Cohn writes in this context: "In a conflict between human life and human dignity, it is for the human being to make the choice, and, failing his or her declaration to the contrary, he or she is always presumed to choose human life in preference to human dignity: it is only where human life is reduced to a phantom or chimera of human life that human dignity must prevail to bring about at least a dignified death."[7]

But sometimes a patient whose human life is reduced to "a phantom or chimera of human life" might progress and improve. It is only when we are certain that no progress may be made (as in cases of severe, irreversible damage to the brain described as whole-brain death) that we can speak in definite terms of a shadow of life rather than a life. Physicians are convinced that, for all practical purposes, the identification of brain death means that the patient is dead. As things stand now, in the case of brain-dead patients, human dignity must be perceived as of paramount importance, to bring about at least a dignified death. The case is different regarding PCU patients in whom the cerebral hemispheres of the brain are damaged. There are reported cases of PCU patients who showed progress in their condition.[8]

The question becomes more complicated when PCU patients, who are by definition not brain dead, demonstrate no signs of improvement. Then the question of how we can (or should) protect a person's autonomy becomes one of the major considerations. Among the criteria to be examined are the view of the patient's loved ones regarding the fate of the patient concerned and whether the patient has left prior directives regarding treatment in the event that he or she becomes incompetent (for further discussion, see chapter 2).

The Doctor's Role

A troubling question is whether or not it is within the doctor's responsibility to terminate life. Obviously, when patients are competent and able to commit suicide they can assist themselves and seek death in various ways without having the need to involve doctors. The case is different when the patients are unable—physically or mentally—to commit suicide. These patients seek doctors' assistance.

Doctors who are opposed to active euthanasia and physician-assisted suicide find no dignity in killing a patient, and express anxiety about the character of a society in which doctors assume such a responsibility.[9] Charles Sprung describes doctors' consent to perform euthanasia as "unethical."[10] Avraham Steinberg writes in his criticism of this study that the doctor's role does not include killing. If society accepts the need for active euthanasia, then any person can commit such an act. The doctor's role is to heal, to help patients and to relieve their suffering. Society must not assign its doctors the additional task of execution.

Although my plea is limited, in favor of physician-assisted suicide and not active euthanasia, I resent the use of the term "execution" in this context. Support for active euthanasia is not necessarily associated with the acceptance of capital punishment in society. One of the doctor's roles is, indeed, to ease patients' suffering. Daily practice in hospitals demonstrates that sometimes the only way to achieve this objective also shortens the patient's life. We are dealing with a population of patients with motivations, drives, and wills. The failure to consider these things would lead to gross paternalism: an unjustified action that takes the responsibility from the patient. Such behavior is unjustified because (1) the person for whom the doctor acts paternalistically is competent, and (2) the conduct in question is involuntary and coercive. Is it the task of a doctor to keep a person alive against that person's will? How do we answer that small group of patients who have lost their will to live and beg their doctors for help? Steinberg and others think that it is not among the doctor's responsibilities to perform mercy killings. The question is whether another professional body exists in society that could take responsibility for this troubling task. Is it conceivable to ask another association (trained paramedics) or social group (for example, the patient's loved ones) to assume this responsibility? The answer is conclusive. It is impossible to act properly on matters of health without a qualified medical opinion. Only a trained physician equipped with the data about the particular disease and about the process of dying is qualified to evaluate the patient's condition. As John Hardwig contends, the physician could provide a rich source of information about death and about strategies for minimizing the trauma, suffering, and agony of death, both for the dying person and for the family.[11] I see no escape from including doctors in the decision-making process, but Steinberg wishes, in his words, "to keep the doctor outside the killing circle," and does not want to consider active intervention as an option. I seek an answer for all patients, including those who wish to die, but Steinberg ignores those patients who suffer from incurable diseases and express their wish to die. Obviously Steinberg and others who are opposed to physician-assisted suicide should not be expected to commit an act that is contrary to their beliefs or violates their conscience; that would be as paternalistic as ignoring the patient's will. However, there are doctors who agree with this line of reasoning and who do not necessarily regard such medical intervention as contrary to their medical and moral conscience.

One major objection to the circumscribed argument evinced here for limited physician-assisted suicide holds that the action is irreversible in the sense that it curtails the possibility of medical "miracles." Medicine is not a precise science, and doctors do not know everything. Often when the body responds differently from what was expected, contrary to the prognoses, contrary to the statistics and to recorded probabilities, explanations are given in a vocabulary that expresses humility regarding human knowledge and ability to comprehend. The popular press often terms such positive responses as "miraculous." Physician-assisted suicide precludes any chance for such so called miracles and the possibility of reevaluating a misdiagnosis. There is also the fear of abuse, of killing patients against their will; thus there is a need for safety valves and for installing control mechanisms.

The Need for Safety Valves

The warnings presented here are well founded, so we should strive to minimize the possibility of errors taking place. Because most patients wish to live irrespective of their condition, this discussion is relevant to only a small number of cases, like those of Benjamin Eyal and Sue Rodriguez.

To minimize the danger of misdiagnosis, a separate prognosis should be provided by at least two independent experts. One should be patients' attending physician(s), who is/are in charge of their treatment and know(s) their cases better than other doctors. Where none of the attending doctors really knows the patient well, the decision-making process should involve the entire medical team. Competent patients should be advised of the doctors' doubts and hesitations about the nature of their illness, if such doubts exist. The patients should be informed, in language they are able to understand, of the existing knowledge about their illnesses, to what extent it is based on data or speculations, and the margins of error. When the patients are incompetent, their family members and other loved ones should be told about the prognoses and the doctors' opinions.

As to the claim that physician-assisted suicide unnecessarily shortens life: Many of the patients who ask to die do so not because they want to live another day, another week, another month, but because life has become a burden they are better off without. People like Benjamin Eyal no longer wish to explore just how constrained such a life might be. The argument in favor of circumscribed physician-assisted suicide relates only to people at the end of their lives, when their medical situation has been diagnosed as incurable, and when patients reiterate their request to die several times over a certain period of time. This formulation would exclude physician-assisted suicide for patients for whom helpful medicine could improve their condition. The argument would also exclude physician-assisted suicide for patients who might suffer depression and who might come to life again after the depression has lifted.

Fear of Sliding Down the Slippery Slope

A serious objection to both active euthanasia and physician-assisted suicide concerns sliding down the slippery slope toward total disrespect and contempt for human life. The argument holds that it is preferable to keep active euthanasia and physician-assisted suicide illegal so as to speak out clearly regarding the value and importance of human life and to force physicians to think hard when they assume the responsibility of shortening life. This argument contains several warnings: First, people who are weak and easily manipulated, who are unable to protect themselves, could be severely harmed if active euthanasia and physician-assisted suicide were allowed. Sweeping interpretations of laws allowing active intervention to terminate life could bring about the ending of lives of the poor, the neglected, the unwanted (see the discussion of the *Saikewicz* case in chapter 6). Justice Menachem Elon's decision in the *Scheffer* case is germane to this discussion: "When we begin to estimate and to consider the worth of human life, these 'evaluations' and 'weightings' will lead firstly to permission to kill people whose minds and bodies are severely defective, then to the killing of those who are defective a bit less, and with time there will be no measure as to how limited the defect would have to be."[12]

Second, there is a danger that pressure will be applied on patients to die. This pressure could stem from various causes. The patient might be exploited by family members who are after the patient's money and consequently welcome his or her death. In fact, this claim raises suspicion about doctors who do not always act in accordance with the best interests of the patient and hence allow room for family exploitation.[13] There is also a danger of exploitation by the establishment—that is, by hospitals and medical centers that often operate under circumstances of scarce resources and budget cuts. The argument is that, in an atmosphere permitting active intervention to end life, human life might become less important, and thus it might be in jeopardy when there are serious budgetary pressures and limited bed space.

Warnings against a slippery-slope process that might result in the deaths of some who wish to continue living are valid. The rationale for creating ethical directives for doctors, from the Hippocratic Oath to hospital ethics committees, arises from the recognition that doctors might abuse the power they possess. Such fears can be avoided by paying careful attention to the fine details when concepts and regulations are formulated, and by using explicit wording that does not allow abusive interpretations. The fear of abuse and the desire to grant patients control over their lives until the very last moment are my prime motivations in restricting my plea to physician-assisted suicide and in refraining from advocating active euthanasia as well. From the Netherlands and Oregon we learn that most patients who opted for death were cancer patients. It can be assumed that they were capable of activating a lethal needle administered by a qualified doctor. The claim made by some Dutch physicians that active euthanasia is preferable to physician-assisted suicide can be rebutted.[14] In the Netherlands, unsuccessful physician-assisted suicide happened because physicians administered oral drugs that were not always effective. In the scheme offered here, the lethal medication would be provided by injection, and it is the patient who would operate the suicide mechanism.

Fear of the slippery slope should not lead to an unequivocal rejection of active involvement of physicians in the termination of lives, but to a commitment to create clear and definitive guidelines. We must examine the will of the patient, her condition, the extent of her suffering, and the doctors' prognoses regarding the possibility of improving her condition.[15] At the same time we should punish abusers to prevent them from committing further wrongdoing and to deter others who might contemplate abuse. The fear of abuse in itself, however, does not constitute a strong moral ground that overrides the autonomy interests of patients.

Conscientious commentators, while aware of the possibility of the slippery-slope argument, that allowing mercy killing in some cases might lead to allowing this act in other cases, nevertheless argue that in specific circumstances mercy killing (often active euthanasia and physician-assisted suicide are lumped together) does not go against the patient's

interests but conforms with them.[16] Such an act is conceived as not offending against the intrinsic value of human life but rather as affirming
its convictions, its sense of integrity, and its dignity. Where PCU patients
are concerned, their best interests are said to include factors that concern their dignity and the avoidance of so-called futile treatment.

There are a number of warnings concerning possible negative ramifications for society at large. Some critics claim that licensing mercy killing and physician-assisted suicide in certain cases will lead to an increase
in violence and in indifference to human life in general.[17] The slippery-
slope argument does not state that active euthanasia and physician-
assisted suicide are wrong or immoral, but that permitting them might
have negative consequences. The argument emphasizes what could happen to society if we indulge a request of a certain patient, but to a certain extent it disregards the patient. On the contrary, we should not ignore
the individual in need, and each case should be considered in its own
right. Moreover, the slippery-slope argument focuses the attention on
what might happen in society as a result of granting a certain patient
her wishes, but it ignores the present misery of the patient. The individual patient should be the central consideration of any analysis of this
problem. Voluntary physician-assisted suicide conducted out of an honest
and true motivation to provide relief from suffering is a humane act that
respects the patient. Allowing physician-assisted suicide under clearly
specified terms could increase sensitivity to human suffering and dignity, rather than contributing to the devaluation of human life. The consequences of voluntary physician-assisted suicide for society may be
positive.

We will be in danger of continuing down the slippery slope if we
allow the present situation to continue. It is my feeling that we have
been sliding down the slope for some time. As a result of the common
use of supposedly simple terms (discussed in chapter 1) such as those
referring to "terminal" patients, life "devoid of quality," "futile" treatment, "vegetative" patients (or simply "vegetables") and the double-effect
doctrine, the shortening of life—not always for sincere motives geared
to serve the best interests of the patients—is a common practice in hospitals. Patients will be better off if those terms are replaced by long explanations describing their diseases and by elaborate discussions about
their medical prognoses and about the knowledge available to help them
cope with their illnesses. Catchphrases and obscure Latin words serve
the interests of doctors, not of patients. They facilitate an atmosphere
that does not really help to relieve patients' insecurities and anxieties.[18]
In addition, physicians often are hard to reach, are not sufficiently at-
tentive to patients and their families, are too impatient to explain things

in detail, and prefer or are compelled to cut consultations short in order to do other things. As R. Anspach shows, this inattentive attitude leads medical staff to refrain from using the consent model; rather, they obtain "assent," or agreement, to decisions to terminate life support already made by the staff.[19] Passive euthanasia, practice of the double-effect doctrine, and discrimination against weak groups such as aging patients and PCU patients are taking place in hospitals around the globe without the use of sufficient mechanisms of control in order to ascertain that the patients' best interests are being served.

Many of the fears that are voiced against allowing active euthanasia and physician-assisted suicide are concerned with the possible misbehavior of doctors, yet the people who express these fears are content with the present situation, with its gray areas for doctors' maneuvering. Gray areas will apparently always remain. The question is whether we should be content with the present situation or look for ways to reduce these areas. It is time to change the procedures used in the present situation, because they do not address the genuine needs of some patients who raise a clear and agonizing plea to die; because we should not consent to the amount of abuse that is already taking place;[20] because the responsibility for terminating patients' lives lies with doctors, not with the patients' families,[21] and because society cannot allow free-riders to terminate patients' lives without proper control (see the forthcoming discussion on Kevorkian). What is suggested is a two-tier process: (1) to open a public debate about patients' rights and doctors' duties, educate the citizens about the existing state of affairs, put the key concepts on the public agenda, speak openly about the conflicting considerations, and mobilize the media to address these issues; then (2) to ask the public whether the institution of guidelines is preferable to the present situation. It might be the case that the public would feel that clear and specific guidelines would limit doctors' flexibility and better serve the interests of all patients, those who wish to live and those who wish to die. Society should address these troubling questions in a common endeavor to specify the roles and duties of doctors, as well as the rights of patients, including their right to ask for a dignified death. This two-tier process is preferable to leaving the situation as it is, when various interested parties might act in ways that may not coincide with the best interests of the patient.[22]

Fear of Overzealousness

The overzealous promotion of medical active termination of life may create the impression that dying with dignity is more important than living with dignity. The guiding rule must be to preserve and maintain life. The termination of life must be the exception. Caution is necessary, both morally and professionally. The prime example of overenthusiasm for the shortening of life concerns the innovation called the Mercitron.

The Mercitron is a suicide machine invented by Dr. Jack Kevorkian, who has led the campaign for assisted suicide and has become a folk hero in the United States and throughout the world.[23] From 1990 until September 1998, Kevorkian helped at least sixty-five women and twenty-eight men to die.[24] During the 1990s, in a nine-year battle against the medical, legal, and religious authorities in Michigan, Kevorkian was acquitted three times by juries in Oakland and Wayne Counties in the assisted-suicide deaths of five people. A fourth trial in Ionia County ended in a mistrial. In those trials, Kevorkian relied in his defense on evidence about the pain and suffering of people he was charged with helping to die.[25]

On 4 August 1993, Thomas Hyde, age thirty, of Novi, Michigan, who suffered from amyotrophic lateral sclerosis, inhaled carbon monoxide. He was the seventeenth (some say the twentieth) person to die in Kevorkian's presence. In May 1994, Kevorkian stood trial for the first time for his involvement in Hyde's death and was acquitted. After the trial, a juror commented, "He convinced us he was not a murderer, that he was really trying to help people out." A second juror said, "Dr. Kevorkian had acted principally to relieve Mr. Hyde's pain, not to kill him, and that is an action within the law."[26] One month later, Kevorkian's medical license was revoked on the grounds that he had been disciplined by the Michigan Board of Medicine, and that he had assisted five patients to commit suicide.[27]

In March 1996, Kevorkian stood trial for the second time on the charge of causing the deaths of Merian Frederick, who suffered from amyotrophic lateral sclerosis, known as Lou Gehrig's disease, and of Ali Khalili, who suffered from bone cancer. Kevorkian said that Frederick and Khalili had caused their own deaths by removing the clip on the tubing to allow poisonous gas to flow from a small black tank into their plastic masks. Kevorkian further claimed that he encouraged both of them to remove the mask if they changed their mind at the last moment. Frederick's and Khalili's relatives testified that they appreciated Kevorkian's help and compassion in ending their loved ones' suffering. The prosecutors suggested that Kevorkian did not fully explore other options with Frederick and Khalili and made hasty decisions about their conditions without consulting their doctors. The jury, however, was not convinced; they felt that Kevorkian's purpose was merely to relieve the patients' suffering, not to cause their death; hence he was found not guilty.[28]

One of the first patients who asked for Kevorkian's assistance in dying was Janet Adkins, an Alzheimer's patient in the first stages of the disease. Aware as she was of the deterioration of human characteristics as a result of this terrible disease, Adkins wished to die while she was still competent and able to be in charge of her actions. Kevorkian assisted in her suicide, although Adkins apparently had quite a few months left to live during which she could have functioned more or less autonomously. Her private doctor thought that Adkins had at least another year before losing her ability to think clearly, and Kevorkian agreed that she was not a "terminal patient."[29] He estimated that Adkins had four to six months before becoming incompetent.[30] If Adkins's mental health was intact and she "was not the least depressed over her impending death," as Kevorkian testified,[31] the question arises: Why the rush? The criticism concerns the doctor's neglecting his obligation to preserve life. Clearly it would have been possible to perform this assisted suicide at a later more advanced stage of the disease. Similar charges were brought against Kevorkian at his second trial.

The case of Janet Adkins exhibits the need to change the legal system to accommodate physician-assisted suicide. If patients knew that physician-assisted suicide would be available to them as an option, they would not need to seek physicians like Kevorkian to end their lives prematurely. The existing situation brings patients to forgo life earlier than they should in fear of helpless degeneration into a prolonged, painful, and degrading dying process.

Kevorkian's third trial was concerned with the assisted suicide of Marjorie Wantz and Sherry Miller. Wantz (fifty-eight years old) suffered from excruciating pelvic pain; Miller (forty-three years old) suffered from multiple sclerosis. Chief prosecutor Larry Buntig characterized Kevorkian as a "reckless agent of death." Referring to Wantz, whose subsequent autopsy showed she was unlikely to die from her illness, Buntig said she "needed mental health treatment, not a bottle full of poison."[32] Here as in the previous trials the jury remained unconvinced and acquitted Kevorkian.

In December 1997, Kevorkian challenged Michigan lawmakers to pass a law banning assisted suicide, declaring at a news conference that he would no longer "sneak around" in his assisted suicide campaign, and that he would starve himself to death in prison if he were convicted of the offense. Kevorkian vowed, "We shall not submit to that tyranny." At a news conference with his associate in the latest killings, Dr. Georges

Reding, a retired psychiatrist, Kevorkian maintained that a ban on "patholysis" (Kevorkian's term for assisted suicide), "is sorely needed to clear the air. . . . The ban itself will then be put on trial, because we fully intend to challenge it to facilitate a so-called trial—so-called because any trial mandated by an immoral law is nothing if not a lynching."[33] Kevorkian also said that the convictions of himself and his colleague would help future, more enlightened societies gauge the darkness of our plutocratic and theocratic age.[34] When repeatedly pressed by reporters to name the number of people whose suicides he had attended, Kevorkian would not be specific. But he did place the number at "somewhere between 80 and 100."[35]

My impression from an examination of Kevorkian's deeds is that his acts are tainted with overenthusiasm. In his book *Prescription: Medicide*, Kevorkian describes in detail his obsession with assisted suicide: how he came to the decision to help patients end their lives; his efforts to convince his colleagues that his conduct is justifiable; the process of building his suicide machine, and the efforts to receive recognition for his newly adopted profession ("obitiary," in his words, a term derived from the Latin word *obitus* and from the Greek word *iatros*, meaning "a doctor who helps patients meet death").[36] The efforts to find a place to perform Adkins's suicide were described as "Herculean."[37] Kevorkian states that he does not help patients who are confused and are not of sound and coherent mind.[38] The first patient that Kevorkian considered treating lost his ability to think clearly before the appointed date for treatment. Kevorkian described what had happened as a "near miss . . . The patient unexpectedly slipped into babbling incoherence. That eliminated him as the first candidate for my services."[39]

Kevorkian's acquaintance with most of those patients who sought his help through his suicide machine, the Mercitron, was superficial. He did not know the patients who approached him, nor did he take pains to study their medical history. He knew Janet Adkins for only two days. The decision to nominate her as his first candidate for his suicide machine was made after a few telephone calls and after he had read through her medical file, without ever having met her face-to-face.[40] Adkins's doctor strongly opposed her killing and refused to cooperate with Kevorkian. Kevorkian himself coldly describes their meeting in a businesslike manner. He writes, "After getting acquainted through a few minutes of conversation, the purpose of the trip was thoroughly discussed."[41] Kevorkian did not invest effort in convincing those who turn to him to reconsider their situation, and perhaps to opt for life. He did not insist that the request to die be consistent, expressed several times over a certain period of time, so as to make sure that the patients were convinced they reached the right decision. For him, as for the Israeli attorney I mentioned before, the important thing was the expressed will of the autonomous patients to die. The doctor supplied a service that honored their request.

However, the emphasis in Kevorkian's book is not on the patient who asks to die but upon the doctor who takes the action. Janet Adkins, Thomas Hyde, Sherry Miller, Marjorie Wantz, Merian Frederick, Ali Khalili, and the other dozens of patients whom Kevorkian helped to die are but a means to convey his message to the world. The first patient who experienced the Mercitron, Janet Adkins, served in his book as no more than a secondary actress in a tragedy he wished to mount on any possible stage to diffuse his cold ideas, which lacked human compassion. I confess that I found it difficult to read his book. The concept of the right to die with dignity, which is, in my opinion, a concept worthy of the most serious and painstaking consideration and study, becomes distorted there.[42] His book is an easy target for those who oppose euthanasia and assisted suicide; a battering ram against those who side with the right to die with dignity.

Kevorkian's respect for the individual's right to decide autonomously about his or her destiny (for some reason, Kevorkian mainly helped women) was extreme. He posed the virtue of respect for the patient's autonomy as the most important consideration, overshadowing other concerns. Because he was unqualified and apparently uninterested in examining his patients and verifying their cause of illness, he assisted in the suicide of some patients who were misdiagnosed. Kevorkian did not care very much. These people wanted to die, and all he did was help them fulfill their desire.

Kevorkian and his attorney, Geoffrey Fieger, insisted that the retired pathologist had assisted in the suicides only of people with terminal illnesses—including, by Kevorkian's definition, the late stages of Alzheimer's disease and multiple sclerosis—or severe, chronic pain. But of the forty-four people Kevorkian had acknowledged helping die in Oakland County, Dr. Ljubisa J. Dragovic said eleven were terminally ill, twenty-nine had chronic conditions, and four others had no signs of disease. Dragovic, the coroner who examined the bodies, has classified nearly all of the forty-four deaths linked to Kevorkian as homicides.[43] Among the controversial deaths were those of Margaret Garrish, seventy-two, of Royal Oak (26 November 1994), who suffered from rheumatoid arthritis. Kevorkian kept his promise to help her die if doctors did not provide better pain medication. Judith Curren, forty-two, of Pembroke, Massachusetts (15 August 1996), had chronic fatigue syndrome and suffered from depression.[44] Loretta Peabody, fifty-four, of Ionia (30 August

1996), had multiple sclerosis. Her husband remarried shortly after her death. Janet Good was Kevorkian's assistant (26 August 1997). She had pancreatic cancer, but the coroner said she would have lived at least six months before eventually succumbing to the disease.[45] Deborah Sickels, forty-three, of Arlington, Texas (7 September 1997), suffered from multiple sclerosis and other medical ailments. Her family said she was mentally unstable and accused Kevorkian of being irresponsible for helping her die.[46] Rebecca Badger was a thirty-nine-year-old woman who was diagnosed as suffering from multiple sclerosis, but Dragovic says autopsy findings revealed a robust, physically fit young woman.[47] Roosevelt Dawson, a twenty-one-year-old quadriplegic college student from Southfield, Michigan (26 February 1998), was paralyzed from the neck down and had relied on a ventilator to breathe since a virus infected his spinal cord.[48]

The assisted suicide of young Dawson energized Kevorkian's critics. They charged that the retired pathologist has slowly evolved his practice from terminal patients to all comers. Not Dead Yet, a national disabled-rights group fighting the legalization of assisted suicide, contended Kevorkian was slowly conditioning people to view death as the logical alternative to life with a disability. During a August 1990 court proceeding in Oakland County, Kevorkian made this chilling statement: "The voluntary self-elimination of individual and mortally diseased or crippled lives, taken collectively, can only enhance the preservation of the public health and welfare." Kevorkian's associate Dr. Georges Reding, who attended Dawson's death, was quoted as saying that anyone can choose assisted suicide because "we are all terminal."[49]

However, this case was not a case of assisted suicide. Dawson was completely incapacitated before his death and could not have operated the Mercitron. No wonder that right-to-die activist groups distanced themselves from Kevorkian. Carol Poenisch of Merian's Friends, a Northville-based group working to legalize assisted suicide, said that according to Kevorkian "we are cowards because we want to document things and do it in a proper fashion. . . . [Dawson's] case would need much more careful study before he would qualify under Merian's Friends' guidelines. He may not have qualified."[50] Indeed, for Kevorkian a person's choice to live or die should depend on how they view their quality of life.

In June 1998, Kevorkian harvested the kidneys of Joseph Tushkowski, a Nevada man who died with his help. By this act he wanted to attract more media attention and to inflame the debate. The medical authorities refused to accept the organs. The national transplant organizations and area hospitals said that Kevorkian's conduct did not meet their criteria. Dave Wilkens, a spokesman for the University of Michigan Medical Center in Ann Arbor, commented that Kevorkian's act was nothing that any kind of responsible institution would participate in. Joel Newman, spokesman for the United Network for Organ Sharing—a private company in Richmond, Virginia, with a federal contract to match organ donors with recipients—said regulations require detailed medical and social histories and that procedures are carried out by surgeons in a hospital setting.[51]

In November 1998, Kevorkian further radicalized his campaign. Throughout his crusade he had been dictating the moves, provoking public debate, pressing harder and harder on the issue of assisted suicide and the right of people to choose the time of their death, forcing the legal authorities to address the questing and calling upon them to prosecute him. On 22 November 1998, the *Detroit News* reported that Kevorkian actively euthanized Thomas Youk, who was suffering the advanced stages of Lou Gehrig's disease. By that time, it was estimated, Kevorkian had been responsible for more than 130 deaths.[52] On this occasion, Kevorkian publicly admitted that he had administered the lethal poison and, furthermore, submitted videotape to CBS's *60 Minutes*.[53] Derek Humphry commented on this development:

> I think that Dr. Kevorkian was absolutely right, in human terms, to help Mr. Youk to die by lethal injection. Not to have helped him die just because he could not do it himself would have been the worse kind of discrimination. But I part company with Kevorkian in that active voluntary euthanasia should only take place under a new law, with strong guidelines. He seems to think the medical profession can be trusted, and be willing to hasten deaths in this manner; I think the people should—if a majority want it—pass a careful law permitting both physician-assisted suicide and active voluntary euthanasia for a competent, terminally ill adult. But he's made the point very effectively. I have been making the same arguments (accompanied by a plea for a new law) for the past 20 years. Kevorkian—and CBS TV—have moved the educational process forward hugely this Sunday evening.[54]

After the showing of the *60 Minutes* episode, which documented Kevorkian administering a lethal injection to Thomas Youk,[55] a public poll was conducted asking, among other things: "Did the experience of watching tonight's '60 Minutes' segment on Jack Kevorkian influence you to be more supportive of assisted suicide or more opposed to assisted suicide?" The results were:

6 percent much more supportive of assisted suicide

31 percent somewhat more supportive of assisted suicide

13 percent somewhat more opposed to assisted suicide

38 percent much more opposed to assisted suicide

12 percent undecided/don't know.[56]

The majority of those polled testified that the program made them feel more opposed to assisted suicide. So Kevorkian's initiative granted him huge publicity and served his interest in provoking public debate, but it did not further public support for his mission.

Ellen Goodman, a *Boston Globe* columnist, wrote that Thomas Youk was little more than a prop for Kevorkian's act, a dead body he could use in challenging authority. It is scarcely surprising that Kevorkian upped the ante, moving to active euthanasia. Assisted suicide no longer caught the spotlight. Goodman expressed the opinion that Kevorkian was the wrong role model to cast for the lead in the movement for a more merciful death. Kevorkian forced the issue of assisted suicide and active euthanasia onto the public stage, but he also polarized that public audience. Goodman maintained: "Nor would I wish him at my deathbed offering these last words of comfort: 'We're going to inject in your right arm. OK? Okey-doke.'"[57]

In the videotape, Kevorkian said that he explained to Thomas Youk that euthanasia was preferable to physician-assisted suicide because it provided "better control," meaning that the physician performing euthanasia had better control over the process of medical killing. It did not occur to him that it is desirable that the patient, not the doctor, should have "better control" until the very last moment, a strong claim for physician-assisted suicide denoting the difference from euthanasia. Euthanasia may be allowed only in exceptional cases (see guideline 11 below).

By videotaping himself giving a man a lethal injection, bringing the tape to the CBS News program *60 Minutes*, and daring prosecutors to charge him with murder, Kevorkian was trying to move the legal system further and faster than most Americans were ready to accept. The Michigan prosecutor could not remain indifferent to this blunt breach of the law. Kevorkian stood trial on charges of first-degree murder and delivering a controlled substance for injecting Youk with lethal drugs. This time, the jury could not ignore the explicit videotape and the language of the law. A not-guilty verdict would have nullified the law on murder and left Kevorkian free to continue his death campaign with a quick-to-inject syringe. Kevorkian was found guilty of second-degree murder, and of delivering a controlled substance.[58] He was given a jail sentence of ten to twenty-five years on the second-degree murder conviction, and three to seven years on the controlled-substance conviction. Judge Jessica Cooper emphasized in her verdict that the trial was not about the political or moral correctness of euthanasia. Instead, it was about lawlessness: "It was about disrespect for a society that exists because of the strength of the legal system. No one, sir, is above the law. No one." Judge Cooper told Kevorkian: "You had the audacity to go on national television, show the world what you did and dare the legal system to stop you. Well, sir, consider yourself stopped."[59]

Interestingly, Kevorkian announced that he objected to showing *Final Exit*, a do-it-yourself suicide videotape, on television. In this thirty-four-minute program, Derek Humphry lists various drugs that will hasten death, and demonstrates how to crush pills with a spoon and mix them into applesauce. Tea and toast beforehand help the body absorb the drugs, and using a shot of vodka to wash them down makes them deadlier. For those who cannot obtain drugs through a prescription, Humphry demonstrates how to end a life using over-the-counter sleeping pills and a plastic bag over the head to end it all.[60] Through his lawyer, Kevorkian said that he was appalled at the videotape and instead urged the ill to seek aid from a doctor. In his opinion, the videotape is risky because it might get into the hands of teenagers and others who are not as well intentioned as members of the Hemlock Society.[61] Humphry responded by saying that the videotape opens by imploring people to see their doctors first.[62] Recently it was reported that shortly after the televising of *Final Exit* in Hawaii (for some reason it was shown twice within four days), two depressed people—a woman in her forties and a man in his sixties—committed suicide in Honolulu using plastic bags. Neither of them was chronically ill.[63] The airing of such a videotape raises a vexing question in the field of media ethics. Media decision-makers should think about the consequences of airing such a program and not simply air anything that is likely to attract audience because of the sensational character of the material.[64]

Both *Final Exit* and Kevorkian's deeds put the issue of death with dignity on the public agenda and compel American authorities to invest some effort in finding a solution to the problem Kevorkian poses. If adequate solutions are not found then, one should not be surprised to find more Kevorkian-like doctors who will come to the help of patients. Indeed, the Reuters Agency in Pontiac, Michigan, reported that Dr. Georges Reding, who began an apprenticeship under Kevorkian in December 1997, helped a thirty-five-year-old San Francisco woman suffering from AIDS to die.[65] Reding became an active participant in some other cases of assisted suicide until he was charged with first-degree murder in the August 1998 death of Donna Brennan, a fifty-four-year-old multiple sclerosis patient who died of an overdose of the sedative pentobarbital. In January 2000 it was reported that Reding had fled to Europe, and that the authorities did not know where he was.[66]

Kevorkian's missionary vigor, like any unqualified vigor, betrays the best interests of patients and ill serves the interests of society. The United States as well as other democracies should devise ways to stop Kevorkian and like-minded doctors, to think creatively to comply with the genuine desires of all patients in this modern, technologically advanced era of medicine, and to help doctors who feel that sometimes termination of life is necessary. Doctors need not disguise or hide what they are doing to help their patients in fear of criminal prosecution. It is time to face the existing reality in a sincere and direct way and find adequate answers to pressing moral dilemmas. Openness, clarity, and sincerity serve the best interests of all parties concerned: patients, their loved ones, and medical staff.[67]

Conclusions

The right to die with dignity includes the right to live with dignity until the last minute and the right to part from life in a dignified manner. There are competent, adult patients who feel that the preferable way for them to part from life is through physician-assisted suicide. We must ponder the following considerations on their behalf:

Guideline 1. The physician should not suggest assisted suicide to the patient. Instead, it is the patient who should have the option to ask for such assistance. Initiation by the physician might undermine trust between patient and physician, conveying to the patient that the doctor has given up, and values the patient's life only to the extent of offering assistance to die. Such an offer might undermine the will to live and to explore further avenues for maintaining quality of life. Many Dutch physicians do not see this issue as significant. Some of them think it is important for them to raise the issue when it seems that the patient does not dare to raise the issue upon his or her own initiative. However, undoubtedly all people in the Netherlands are aware of the availability of active euthanasia and physician-assisted suicide in their society. Any reluctance the patients show with regard to this issue should be honored and respected.

Guideline 2. The request by an adult[68], competent patient who suffers from an intractable, incurable and irreversible disease for physician-assisted suicide must be voluntary.[69] The decision is that of the patient who asks to die without outside pressure, because life seems the worst alternative in the current situation. The patient should state her wish several times over a period of time.[70] We must verify that the request for physician-assisted suicide does not stem from a momentary urge, an impulse, a product of passing depression. This emphasis of enduring request was one of the requirements of the abolished Northern Territory law in Australia,[71] and is one of the requirements of the Oregon Death with Dignity Act,[72] and of the Dutch guidelines.[73] We must also verify that the request is not the result of external influences. It should be ascertained with a signed document that the patient is ready to die now, rather than depending solely on directives from the past. Section 2 of the Oregon act requires that the written request for medication to end one's life be signed and dated by the patient and witnessed by at least two individuals who, in the presence of the patient, attest to the best of their knowledge and belief that the patient is capable, is acting voluntarily, and is not being coerced to sign the request.[74]

A person can express general attitudes regarding euthanasia, in an informal discussion made in a social setting. She might say that she would not want to live on if she had to rely on the mercy of others, if she had to depend on them, and if she were unable to function alone. Such hypothetical observations do not constitute reliable evidence of the patient's current desires once an actual illness is in progress. This is especially true if the wish was stated when she was young and healthy. The younger people are, and the further they are from serious disease, the more inclined they are to claim that in a hypothetical hopeless, painful, and degrading state, they would prefer to end their lives. At the other end of life, there is a tendency to come to terms with suffering, to compromise with physical disabilities, and to struggle to sustain living, and this tendency grows as the body weakens. Many people change their minds when they confront the unattractive alternatives. Many prefer to remain in what others term the "cruel" world, and continue the Sisyphean struggle for their lives.

Guideline 3. At times, the patient's decision might be influenced by severe pain.[75] In this context, the role of palliative care can be crucial. Ganzini and colleagues report that as a result of palliative care some patients in Oregon changed their minds about assisted suicide.[76] The World Health Organization defines palliative care as the "active, total care of patients whose disease is not responsive to curative treatment," maintaining that control of pain, of other symptoms, and of psychological, social, and spiritual problems, is paramount.[77] The medical staff must examine whether by means of medication and palliative care it is possible to prevent or to ease the pain.[78] The Oregon Death with Dignity Act requires that the attending physician inform the patient of the feasible alternatives including comfort care, hospice care, and pain control.[79] Bill proposals to legislate PAS in Illinois, Hawaii, Maine, Michigan,

Vermont, Washington, and Wisconsin explicitly required the attending physician to review with the patient options for palliative care including hospice and/or pain control options.[80] If it is possible to prevent or to ease the patient's pain, then we may not fulfill the patient's wish, but instead prescribe the necessary treatment. This is provided that the informed patient (i.e., a patient who was advised by the medical staff about the available palliative care options) does not refuse to receive the pain-killers, and that when the pain goes so does the motive (or one of the main motives) that caused the patient to ask for assisted suicide. If the patient insists on refusing all medication, doctors must try to find the reasons for this insistence before they comply.

At times, coping with pain and suffering can demand all the patient's emotional strength, exhausting her ability to deal with other issues. In cases of competent patients, it must be determined that the patient is capable of making decisions. The assumption is that the patient understands the meaning of her decision. A psychiatric assessment of the patient could confirm whether she is able to make such a meaningful decision concerning her life. A meeting with a psychiatrist should confirm that the decision is truly that of the patient, expressed consistently and of her own free will. The Northern Territory Rights of Terminally Ill Act required that the patient meet with a qualified psychiatrist to confirm that he or she is not clinically depressed.[81] It is worthwhile to hold several such conversations, separated by a few days. The patient's loved ones and the attending physician should be included in at least one of the conversations.

Guideline 4. The patient must be informed of his situation and the prognoses for both recovery and escalation of the disease and the suffering it may involve. There must be an exchange of information between the doctors and the patient.[82] Bearing this in mind, we should be careful to use neutral terms and to refrain from terms that might offend patients and their loved ones (see chapter 1).

Guideline 5. The patient's decision should never be a result of familial and environmental pressures. At times, the patient may feel like a burden to loved ones. It is the task of social workers to examine the motives of the patient and to see to what extent they are affected by various external pressures (as opposed to a true free will to die). A situation could exist in which the patient is under no such pressure but still does not wish to be a burden on others. Obviously we cannot say that the feelings of a patient toward loved ones are not relevant to the decision-making process.

Guideline 6. The diagnosis must be verified. To minimize misdiagnosis, and to allow the discovery of other medical options, the decision-making process should include a second opinion provided by a specialist who is not dependent on the first doctor, either professionally or otherwise.[83] The patient's attending physician, who supposedly knows the patient's case better than any other expert, must be consulted. All reasonable alternative treatments must be explored. The Oregon Death with Dignity Act requires that a consulting physician examine the patient and all relevant medical records and confirm, in writing, the attending physician's diagnosis that "the patient is suffering from a terminal disease," and verify that the patient is capable, is acting voluntarily, and has made an informed decision.[84] The Dutch guidelines require that the physician consult a colleague.[85] The Northern Territory Rights of Terminally Ill Act required that the patient be examined by a physician specializing in treating terminal illness.[86]

Guideline 7. To avoid the possibility of arranging deals between doctors, it is advisable that the identity of the consultant be determined by a small committee of medical specialists (as in the "Support and Consultation of Euthanasia in Amsterdam" project)[87] that will review the requests for physician-assisted suicide.

Guideline 8. Sometime prior to the performance of physician-assisted suicide, a doctor and a psychiatrist are required to visit the patient, perform an examination, and verify that this is the genuine wish of a person of sound mind who is not being coerced or influenced by a third party. The conversation between the doctors and the patient should be held in private without the presence of family members and other people so as to prevent familial pressure. A date for the procedure should then be agreed upon.[88] The patient's loved ones should be notified so they may be present until the performance of the act, making the day an intimate occasion.

Guideline 9. The patient can rescind the request at any time and in any manner. This was stipulated under the Australian Northern Territory Act,[89] and is stipulated under the Oregon Death with Dignity Act.[90]

Guideline 10. Physician-assisted suicide may be performed only by a doctor and in the presence of another doctor. The decision-making team should include at least two doctors and a lawyer, who will examine the legal aspects involved. An insistence on this demand would serve as a safety measure against possible abuse. Perhaps a public representative should also be present during the entire procedure—the decision-making process and the actual performance of the act. This extra caution should ensure that the right to die with dignity does not become a duty. The doctor performing the assisted suicide should be the one who knows the patient best, has been involved in his treatment, has taken part in the consultations with him and with his loved ones, and has verified through the help of social workers, nurses, and psychologists or psychiatrists that PAS is the wish of the patient.

Guideline 11. Physician-assisted suicide may be conducted in one of three ways, all of them discussed openly and decided by the physician and the patient: (1) oral medication; (2) self-administered, lethal intravenous infusion; and (3) self-administered lethal injection. Oral medication may be difficult or impossible for many patients to ingest because of nausea or other side effects of their illnesses (see chapter 8). In the event that oral medication was provided and the dying process continues for many hours, the physician is allowed to administer a lethal injection.[91] There is also a need for euthanasia in the event that the patient who asked originally for assisted suicide is now totally paralyzed, unable to move any muscles that could facilitate assisted suicide. These are the only two exceptions for allowing euthanasia.

Guideline 12. Doctors may not demand a special fee for the performance of assisted suicide. The motive for physician-assisted suicide is humane, so there must be no financial incentives and no special payment that might cause commercialization and promotion of the death operation.

Guideline 13. There must be extensive documentation in the patient's medical file, including the disease diagnosis and prognosis by the attending and the consulting physicians; attempted treatments; the patient's reasons for seeking physician-assisted suicide; the patient's request in writing or documented on a videotape recording; documentation of conversations with the patient; the physician's offer to the patient to rescind the request; documentation of discussions with loved ones, and a psychological report confirming the patient's condition. This meticulous documentation is meant to prevent exploitation of any kind: personal, medical, or institutional.[92] Each physician-assisted suicide report should be examined by a coroner.[93]

Guideline 14. Pharmacists should also be required to report all prescriptions for lethal medication, thus providing a further check on physicians' reporting.

Guideline 15. Doctors must not be coerced into taking actions that contradict their conscience and understanding of their role as physicians. This was provided for under the Northern Territory Act.[94]

Guideline 16. The local medical association should establish a committee whose role will be not only to investigate the underlying facts that were reported, but to investigate whether there are so-called mercy cases that were not reported and/or that did not comply with the guidelines.

Guideline 17. Licensing sanctions should be taken to punish those health care professionals who violate the guidelines, who fail to consult and to file reports, or who engage in involuntary euthanasia without the patient's awareness or consent, or who euthanize patients lacking decision-making capacity. Physicians who fail to comply with the guidelines should be charged, and procedures to sanction them should be opened by the disciplinary tribunal of the medical association. The maximum penalty for violation of the guidelines should be the revoking of the medical license. In the event that this penalty proves insufficient in deterring potential abusers, there should be room to consider further penalties by approaching the courts: heavy fines and prison sentences.[95]

What is presented here is a closely reasoned argument for physician-assisted suicide in limited cases, intended to help a designated group of patients who require help in departing from life and who deserve to get such help from the medical profession to meet their wish. The detailed procedure is required to prevent abuse. After all, human life is at stake. This procedure should at first be adopted for a trial period of one year, after which an examination should be conducted to determine whether the consequences justify implementation of the policy for a longer time. During this one-year trial period, feedback between physicians, ethicists, and the public at large in reviewing the policy and practice of physician-assisted suicide should be welcomed and encouraged. If the proposal fails (for instance, because physicians do not adequately report incidents of physician-assisted suicide), all the data should be brought before a reviewing committee to closely study both policy and practice. Members of the committee should issue a report recommending or advising against continuing the practice, amending the guidelines, or abolishing physician-assisted suicide. Preferably, the final decision should be made with the participation of the public at large in a referendum, as in Oregon.

With regard to more complicated situations that do not satisfy these criteria presented earlier (free, voluntary, persistent and enduring requests for assisted suicide made by a competent patient who suffers from an incurable and irreversible disease), I urge expanding the circle involved in the decision-making process, discussing these cases in ethics committees and in the courts. The issue is urgent and real, and people from various walks of life and with different perspectives—medicine, law, philosophy, psychology, social work, religion, and others—should take part in the decision-making process, enriching the discourse with their insights.

Finally, although these guidelines refer only to competent patients, I would like to note that in the case of minors, their parents serve as their guardians. The parents decide on behalf of their child after consulting the attending physicians. We must insist, as Justice Elon did in the *Scheffer* case, that the decision must be made by both parents (assuming that the minor has two parents), and not by only one of them.[96]

Appendix

Ethical and Financial Considerations in Allocating Health Care Resources

"The enjoyment of the highest attainable standard of health is one of the fundamental rights of every human being."

Preamble to the Constitution of the
World Health Organization

In most liberal societies, basic health is seen as one of the necessary conditions for the exercise of personal autonomy. It is generally acknowledged that individuals have a right to health care. The prevalent assumption is that this right generates an obligation or duty on the part of the state to ensure that adequate health care is made available and that further requires that equal access to available health care is provided through public funds. The state itself has no obligation to provide a health care system, but the state does have the obligation to ensure that such an adequate system is provided. Basic health care is now recognized as a "public good" rather than a "private good" that one is expected to buy for oneself.[1] The Constitution of the World Health Organization states: "The enjoyment of the highest attainable standard of health is one of the fundamental rights of every human being without distinction of race, religion, political belief, economic or social condition."[2]

The constraints on the financial resources allocated for care of the ill force us to consider, in an honest and serious manner, the tension between the ideal and the real. Currently, challenges to our health have medical solutions, albeit sometimes partial, that were unimaginable in the previous century. The new technology is very costly, and some have claimed that saving lives is not a goal that should be achieved at any cost.[3] Costs and benefits must be examined and priorities determined so as to invest resources only in "worthy cases." The term *worthy cases* is often juxtaposed with the term *quality of life* (see chapter 3). The claim is that expensive technology should be used to help patients who are likely to maintain a certain quality of life. When there is a low quality of life, it is preferable to exercise discretion as a society and to reserve our finite resources to treat patients who are more likely to lead autonomous lives.

This appendix examines the financial issues surrounding the provision of medical care and the manner in which resources should be allocated. Financial resources are obviously limited, and the national budget must be prioritized according to various needs: technology, security, education, culture, health, housing, food, transportation, science, the legal system, environmental protection, and so on. The debate about how to allocate health care resources revolves around three basic concepts: duty, ability, and rights. The central questions are: Does a democratic society have a duty to provide optimal health care for every citizen? Can the state provide optional health care for every citizen? Do citizens have a right to demand such a commitment from their government?

Every discussion on the allocation of resources is bound to reveal the tension between the macro and the micro, between the needs of society and the needs of the individual. The tension is inescapable, and the work of establishing the appropriate balance is delicate. Emphasizing the needs of society might inevitably result in ignoring the needs of some individuals. In the liberal tradition, the individual, rather than the society, is the starting point. Liberals conceive the shift of emphasis from the individual to society as a dangerous move.

Health Care Costs

The cost of health care is high and continues to grow as technology develops and knowledge advances. In the Western world as a whole, the health sector employs between 5 and 10 percent of the workforce, and has a crucial bearing on the production, exports, and imports of medical commodities and services.[4] A closer examination of the relevant data in the United States, Canada, Britain, and Israel reveals a constant rise in the cost of health care in the last three decades. In the United States, Medicare expenditures in 1967 were $4.5 billion. In 1975, the total was $15.6 billion, and in 1982, Medicare costs were $50.9 billion. The U.S. Health Care Financing Administration (the agency responsible for Medicare) reports that for fiscal year 1998, the U.S. budget for Medicare benefits was $210 billion, and for fiscal year 1999, the U.S. budget for such benefits was $222 billion.[5] The total public expenditures on health care were \$104.8 billion in 1980, \$284.4 billion in 1990, \$389 billion in 1993, and \$483.1 billion in 1996.[6] An examination of the percentage of the health package in the Gross National Product shows that in 1929, 3.5 percent was spent on health; in 1950, it was 4.4 percent; and since the 1960s, the figures have continued to rise steadily.[7] In 1987, total medical expenses reached 11.5 percent of the national American budget, and in 1992, the total medical expenses reached 14 percent.[8] The latest available information compiled by the U.S. Centers for Disease Control show that U.S. health care costs constituted 13.6 percent each year for 1993, 1994, 1995, and 1996.[9]

By comparison, Canada's total health expenditures were 9.2 percent of GDP for 1996, and Canada's medical insurance gives its citizens more extensive coverage than America's medical insurance gives its citizens.[10] In 1990, the United States spent an average of \$2,556 on medical care for every citizen, whereas Canada spent an average of \$1,770 (U.S. dollars) per person on medical expenses.[11] Despite this exorbitant U.S. governmental expenditure, between 37 and 42 million American citizens still do not have any form of medical insurance. Approximately 70 million citizens do not receive proper medical care.[12] These numbers suggest that there are some basic moral and practical flaws in the American health care system, which is too detached, impersonal, and uncaring. The American health care model exposes the fallacies of crude capitalism. There are better ways to strike a balance between societal concerns and individual needs. The American model for health care is simply not a good model, especially considering how much money is spent and the fact that large parts of the American public still receive poor treatment.

Great Britain spends 6 percent of its gross domestic product, GDP, on health care.[13] Its National Health Services (NHS), financed by income taxes, came into existence on 5 July 1948. It was the first health care system in any Western society to offer medical care to the entire population. Resources for the NHS have increased year after year in real terms. The average annual increase since 1978–1979 has been 3.3 percent; and it has been 3.6 percent since 1986–1987.[14] The NHS budget was £644 million higher in 1980–1981 than it was in 1975–1976, which represents an increase of 9.3 percent.[15] According to Great Britain's Government Statistical Service, National Health expenditures were £33,044 billion for 1996–1997 and £34,688 billion for 1997–1998.[16]

Many researchers express concern regarding this phenomenon of increasing medical expenses due to technological development. Those researchers claim that no society can afford to spend such large sums of money. Some of the researchers raise concerns about our social responsibility not to cater to the needs of certain patients. These arguments are made most often with regard to patients whose quality of life is seen by these researchers as particularly low. Emphasis is placed on the high costs of care for these patients, the psychological and economic burdens on the patients' families, and the financial constraints of operating hospitals.[17] The focus of these researchers' analysis shifts from the individual to society, as exemplified by John F. Kennedy's famous remark: "Ask not what your country can do for you. Ask what you can do for your country."

One function of liberal democracy is to promote the prosperity of individuals even when they are ill. Democracy has an obligation to preserve individuals' rights; namely, it recognizes that certain demands of its citizens are legitimate and should be satisfied within the framework of society. The right to life is recognized as a first priority. Some (most notably John Locke) call it a natural right, in the sense that it is the consequence of nature, a right that precedes the state.[18]

The rationale of this study is grounded in the liberal tradition. It places the individual at the center of concern, and attempts to fortify the individual's basic right to health care. Assuring health care to citizens is perceived as one of the basic duties of every democracy. Recognizing that decisions are influenced by the reality of scarce resources, this appendix examines various approaches to resource allocation, suggesting a just approach for democracies. The approach combines components of the contract theory that deals with the state's commitment to its citizens. The approach also takes some components of the insurance basis plan to allow the execution of a fair and just health care plan.

Approaches to Allocation

In recent years some interesting discussions have been published on rationing, justice, and the allocation of resources.[19] The following general approaches will be examined: the compassionate approach; the contractarian approach; the socialist approach (also called the comprehensive social responsibility approach); the approach based on income tax and insurance; and the utilitarian or cost-benefit approach.

The Compassionate Approach

This approach states that all individuals must do whatever is in their power to help people in need. It emphasizes the principles of mercy, concern, and respect for others, envisioning people in the Kantian tradition as ends rather than as means. Its critics consider it to be unrealistic, claiming that people must recognize that the modern world has limited resources and that society cannot possibly provide for the needs of all citizens. At times, the costs of medicine and the obligation to choose among different people competing for the same scarce resources will result in insufficient treatment for the ill and sometimes even in the prevention of care altogether. A realistic outlook necessitates the separation of the ideal from the actual and an acknowledgment that inadequate treatment may be common.

The Contractarian Approach

This approach follows a different logic based on the idea of fairness, not of compassion, although it seeks results that are similar to those offered by the compassionate approach. The contractarian approach holds that a contract exists between the state and its citizens. This contract must not be violated, especially at the time when people are in distress and in need of state aid. The contract involves the promise that just as citizens are prepared to make sacrifices for their state, so the state is prepared to make sacrifices for its citizens. This approach emphasizes the principles of justice, fairness, human rights, and equality. The criticism of this approach is similar to that voiced against the compassionate approach: A line must be drawn between what exists and what is desirable. It is difficult to maintain the contract in the face of a reality of limited resources.

The Socialist Approach

This is also referred to as the comprehensive social responsibility approach. This approach promotes a version of the Marxist idea, which holds that all citizens contribute according to their abilities in return for services corresponding to their needs. The assumption is that society must aid all citizens. Each individual will pay for services according to ability, and this is how the state will be able to afford care for all citizens. People who are able to pay more for the services they receive will also pay for those who cannot afford to pay the full price for the same health care services. In other words, the affluent people pay both for themselves and for the needy.

Critics of this approach believe that in our materialistic world, the altruistic belief in helping others is difficult to sustain in a reality of scarce resources and increased expenditures.

Approach Based on Income
Tax and Insurance

Supporters of this approach claim that it is realistic because it requires the state to provide only the minimum necessary for the preservation of its citizens' health. Only in exceptional cases does the state facilitate access to costly treatments and subsidize them. For example, in Great Britain, where the system is planned, organized, and financed by income taxes and not by insurance, the National Health Service limits access to new high-tech costly treatments. A tight supervisory system exists that carefully verifies that expensive treatments are allocated only to those who are deemed to truly need them and to those who cannot cover the costs via private insurance systems. As a result, there are long waiting lists for elective operations (as opposed to emergency life-saving operations) aimed at improving quality of life and diminishing pain. Patients who require such operations are likely to wait on lists for as long as three years.[20] Dialysis is provided to the most needy, and some claim that the rationing of dialysis treatment has resulted in the death of people whose lives could have been sustained if they had been given the appropriate care.[21] There has also been limited access, monitored by GPs, to diagnosis by means of advanced and costly equipment such as MRI.

The implementation of the NHS in Great Britain has achieved a decrease in death and sickness, but the British public express dissatisfaction with the standards of medical care. The proportion of the public declaring themselves to be dissatisfied with the NHS rose from 25 percent in 1983 to almost half the population, 46 percent, in 1989.[22] Dissatisfaction with the health care system is higher than dissatisfaction with flaws in the employment market or in the educational curriculum.[23] The NHS continues to ration not so much by restricting its scope as by limiting access to the available services, and the process of rationing tends to be largely invisible. The rationing process is diffused among the clinicians who decide which patient is going to be treated and who determine the methods of treatment.[24] Those in Great Britain who can afford private insurance purchase such insurance to shorten the waiting period for operations and other costly treatments.

In 1980, there were 154 private hospitals in Great Britain with 7,000 beds. By the end of the decade, there were 216 hospitals with almost 11,000 beds. The British government encouraged the development of private medical insurance. The growth of the private sector reflected frustrated access and a demand for consumer control over the nonmedical aspects of treatment: personal privacy, the timing of an operation, and the right to insist on being treated by a consultant. This expansion also reflected the expansion of the insurance market. In 1980, only 6.4 percent of the population was covered by private insurance plans. By the end of the decade, the proportion had risen to 11.5 percent, and the figure was much higher still among professionals (27 percent) and employers and managers (23 percent).[25]

The 1980s saw little or no change in the nature of the demand for private health care. Demand remained predominantly for the treatment of conditions requiring elective surgery, for which there were long waiting lists in the NHS. The private sector continued offering treatment to improve quality of life rather than dealing with life threatening conditions in the population as a whole.[26]

Traditionally, the British allocate less of their resources to health than do the North Americans. While technological progress has increased the portion of American and Canadian health packages in their total national budgets, in Great Britain the percentage of the budget allocated to health has hardly changed. In 1980, 5.8 percent of the budget was spent on health. In 1987, 6.1 percent was spent on health, which is a very moderate increase, indicating that expensive treatments are usually obtained only by those who can afford them or by those who live long enough to make their way to the top of the waiting list.[27] This fact reflects the long-standing social class division that has prevailed in Britain.

The Canadian model seems preferable to the British one. In Canada, the concept of class division is considered offensive.[28] Under the Canada Health Act (R. S. C., 1985) health care delivery is governed by five principles: public administration, comprehensiveness, universality, probability, and accessibility.[29] The guiding principle in Canada holds that all citizens should have access to an equal level of care, regardless of their financial situation. The Canada Health Act ensures that all citizens have access to treatment considered "medically necessary for the purpose of maintaining health, preventing disease or diagnosing or treating an injury, illness or disability."[30] The principle of equality underlies the Canadian health insurance, which covers all hospitals and all doctors; it is given to all Canadian citizens regardless of income and assures open access to health services. Most of the cost of health insurance is covered by the taxpayers. No separate health service tax exists in Canada. Canadian citizens pay for health services indirectly by means of income tax, taxes on sales and businesses, and through various government plans meant to enlarge the health budget. No penalty exists against citizens in need of frequent health services. A citizen requiring expensive medical treatments is not asked to pay more than a citizen who does not need such treatments. The doctors determine to what extent certain medical care is required. They act within the restrictions placed upon them by the hospitals. They decide how to divide their time among patients, keeping in mind the hospital resources at their disposal.

Canadian health insurance does not provide access to all medical treatments. The government provides for 75 percent of the health budget. The citizens of Canada cover the remaining 25 percent, either directly or via complementary health insurance policies.[31] Many Canadian employers provide group insurance policies that cover expenses, such as purchasing corrective eyeglasses, costly medication, dental treatments, and various health aids that are not included in the governmental scheme. The Canadian national health system has many inadequacies, yet Canadians still receive a high quality of health care.

Costs must be examined when society seeks benefit from expensive technological treatments. We must realize that it is unrealistic to expect the government to pay for the most expensive treatments. The question of the extent to which the public is willing to finance the most expensive treatments should be raised in public forums. The state should provide several insurance alternatives that would suit citizens' varying capacities to pay for health services: the higher the premium paid, the more inclusive the medical treatment that citizens would enjoy.[32]

The Utilitarian or Cost-Benefit Approach

This approach seeks a policy that will bring the greatest number of advantages to the largest number of citizens. Recognizing that it is not possible to provide for the health care needs of everyone, some seek a different criterion that would eliminate some of the expenses for everyone. Under this approach the affluent people would find the means to care for themselves, so this approach deals with most of society, not all of it.

This approach has two main versions. The first excludes some patients. A decision is made in advance to exclude certain categories of people from receiving treatment. For instance, elderly people over a certain age may be excluded. Treatment is equal for those who do not fall into the excluded category and for those who cannot afford more expensive medical insurance. The rationale suggests that it is preferable to invest in the young, who have a better chance of recovery as well as a better chance to live longer and more quality-filled lives than the elderly.

The second version excludes certain illnesses from the health care package because their treatment is especially costly. Equal treatment is to be given to those who suffer from most, but not all, illnesses. The equality principle is expressed as a common minimum assured to all. The treatment to be provided is not necessarily the optimal treatment. Once again, we can assume that the affluent will insure themselves against all sicknesses, thereby undermining the equality principle. The Oregon Health Plan (henceforth the Oregon plan) is an example of this version.

The following discussion criticizes the different versions of the utilitarian approach while accepting the insurance-basis plan along with certain components of the contract approach as the guiding rationale. Daniel

Callahan, one of the main representatives of the age-rationing approach, suggests using old age as a valid criterion for limiting medical care. Callahan's approach is too cold and detached. Ultimately, age should not serve as the decisive criterion. Criticism of this criterion is based on two different lines of reasoning: the medical and the moral-contractual. From the medical perspective, although age is an important variable in determining a patient's medical condition, there are other—no less important—factors that influence one's health. Young people who suffered a grave emotional trauma or barely survived a road accident might find themselves in a much worse physical condition than an eighty-year-old person who leads a healthy and active life. The age criterion is too simple, too general, too sweeping. It provides too convenient an answer to a tough and troubling question.

From the moral-contractual perspective, democracy should not neglect its elderly citizens at the time of their greatest need. There is an unwritten contract between the state and its citizens that should be maintained and preserved. As the state expects its citizens to contribute to its maintenance, so the citizens expect their state to assist in their own maintenance. The contract is mutual, not one sided.[33] It is based on the principles of justice and fairness. Despite that, in a constrained reality that does not assume that all needs will be provided, people are forced to recognize that optimal health care for all is an unrealistic expectation. Prioritizing becomes unavoidable, and there is a need for the state to offer citizens a number of insurance alternatives.

Allocation of Resources, Individual Responsibility, and Social Responsibility

I opened this essay with a quotation concerning the right to achieve the highest level of health. At first glance, this declaration of intention is quite compelling, and it could serve as a worthy cause for the World Health Organization. But the concept of rights should be further examined, and the question of whether we are dealing with a right that is shared by all needs to be answered. Different people can choose different paths for their lives, and the liberal state seeks to respect the autonomous decision of each person as long as he or she does not harm fellow citizens. The state sees it as its prerogative to intervene when someone hurts another to promote his or her goals.[34]

The question that arises is how the state should treat those who choose to harm themselves. One must examine the concepts of self-responsibility, social responsibility and the relationship between them. Idealization of one of these concepts might lead to neglect of the other. These two concepts are important, and one cannot come at the expense of the other. The concept of social responsibility should be promoted, but it should not be seen as an all-encompassing substitute for individual responsibility. A view of society that assumes responsibility for everybody might lead to the collectivization of the individual, who might consequently disappear within the collective mass.

The concept of social responsibility cannot be applied equally to those who assume responsibility for themselves and to those who shirk it. In the case of an individual who becomes addicted to drugs, cigarettes, or alcohol, there is room in democracy for a certain amount of paternalism, but this does not include the power to force this person to stop drinking or smoking. Liberal society may assist alcoholics and drug addicts to overcome their addiction, but it cannot coerce them to quit and act without their consent. The question is whether the state has an obligation to provide identical health care rights to people who look after themselves and to others who deliberately ruin their bodies. Health cannot be conceived as a concept that is stripped of individual responsibility. To a great extent, individuals possess the liberty to destroy their health. Does the state have an obligation to invest its limited resources in people who do not undertake the basic responsibility to preserve their health?[35]

Individuals have basic medical rights, but it does not follow that the state has a duty to protect the health of those who harm themselves in various ways. The state has an obligation to warn us of dangers. The individual has the liberty to take risks. The state can offer schemes for rehabilitation from addiction. When the individual knowingly takes serious risks, such as consumption of hard drugs or alcohol, and does not show a genuine desire to find a way out of this situation, the state's duty loses all significance.[36] It is neither fair nor possible to make the health of one person the duty of another. The state may accordingly decide that assuming responsibility for one's life can serve as a criterion for the allocation of resources. Consequently, certain groups should not receive the care for which they are prima facie eligible. Society must declare loudly and clearly that people who refrain from taking responsibility for their own health cannot expect equal attention in the distribution of limited medical goods. These people have brought about their own exclusion from the right to receive health services. As Joseph M. Boyle believes, a person who lacks responsibility in achieving "human good" undermines his or her ability to take an active part in the community and weakens his or her claim on social resources.[37] The need for medical treatment does not, in and of itself, ensure our right to receive medical treatment. The need should be rooted in the concept of rights only when it is accompanied by personal commitment to the preservation of health and to the promotion of social good. A person as a moral agent who lives in a society is obligated not to neglect his or her health if he or she wants to be equally deserving of medical care.[38]

This does not mean that medical care should be denied to smokers. They should receive care, but the state cannot compel them to take treatment to quit their addiction. When there is no will on the part of the smoker, the treatment is bound to fail. Similarly, when the doctor sets as a precondition to cease smoking for the success of lung treatment and the patient is not willing to make the commitment, the treatment is bound to fail, and there is no reason to invest valuable resources in that patient. Resources, which are always limited, should be invested in patients who are willing to make the commitment and who, therefore, have a better chance to succeed in overcoming the disease.

At the center of this perception lies the concept of responsibility. Responsibility is a personal concept, internal to people and subjective in essence, requiring self-awareness and a certain amount of self-sacrifice. Of course, personal responsibility does not exclude the possibility that we may ask for assistance and advice from people whose experience and expertise we appreciate. People can ask for the opinion of doctors, family members, and friends to consider and reconsider options concerning their health. But after reaching a decision, we must be held accountable for our resolution. Responsible people recognize and know that they must pay, whether in monetary or other terms, for their (mis)conduct. People who do not take responsibility for their lives thus manifest lack of responsibility for their surroundings and society at large and alienate themselves from the existing social contract. The contract is a mutual one between the individual and society. There is no way to force people to be free when they fail to uphold their side of the contract. They must not make demands on society as long as they do not uphold their basic obligations to it. An ongoing, open social discussion will determine the boundaries of social accountability resting on the shoulders of every individual and the commitments of the state to its individuals. The boundaries are fluid and nonpermanent, and they are open to discussion and argument.[39] This is not a matter of the state shirking its responsibility toward certain populations. The state must offer those people chances for bettering their situation and must rehabilitate them by helping them overcome their addictions; however, the state may not impose means of correction to force them "to be free."

Although there is logic in withholding care and resources from those who fail to care for themselves, I find it difficult to agree with those who suggest withholding resources according to criteria that are beyond individual control. The concept of individual responsibility is relevant to the allocation of resources to drug addicts, but it is meaningless with regard to the elderly. Age is an arbitrary concept, existing regardless of the conduct and condition of any individual.

Determining Boundaries for Medical Treatment: The Place of Old Age in Society

Daniel Callahan examines the place of old age in our lives. He predicts that the shortage of resources and the growing expenses of modern medical treatment will force us to determine a limit for deserving and obtaining access to medical treatments. Callahan opposes the idea that life must be prolonged as much as possible. He suggests accepting old age as a part of life and not as an obstacle or a medical challenge to be overcome. In his opinion, limits must be placed on governmental health care expenditures. He addresses his book *Setting Limits* to people of his own age group and invites them to ponder his ideas on allocation of scarce resources in health care, aiming to change their thinking and expectations about old age and death.[40] Callahan suggests the concept of a "full biographical life span," meaning the point at which it can be said that a person has lived a complete, fulfilling, whole life. He does not determine a specific age but suggests a range, from the late seventies to the early eighties, which in his opinion is equivalent to a natural, complete life cycle.[41] Callahan claims that today medical technology can extend life beyond the point that he believes is sensible and worthwhile. He examines what can be done to avoid such a result.[42]

Callahan does not clearly locate the point at which life stops being worthwhile, nor does he say how that point can be determined, nor by whom. According to his perspective, however, not all life is worthwhile. Callahan thinks that there is an objective scale of worthwhile life, and that it is possible to determine when other people's lives cease to be worthwhile. Callahan makes gross generalizations about scales that, in his opinion, should convince any logical individual of their veracity. For Callahan, age is such an objective scale.

Callahan's statements must be placed within a given historical context. The average life expectancy in Western countries is not static. People live many more years today than in the past. The health care system is improving; the ability to cope with many formerly incurable illnesses has increased. Awareness of hygiene and cleanliness is much higher than it was a century ago; for example, the introduction of Western medicine had a profound effect on Israel's occupied territories after the 1967 Six Day War. In 1967, the average life expectancy for inhabitants of the territories was forty-eight years. By the 1980s, the average life expectancy had risen to sixty-two years, and the figure is still rising.[43] There are various places worldwide that demonstrate similar results due to increased awareness of cleanliness and hygiene and the introduction of modern Western medicine. In Canada, the life expectancy of women rose from 70.9 years in 1951 to 81 in 1991. In the same period, men's life expectancy rose from 66.4 to 74.6 years.[44]

Had Callahan written his book in the 1950s, he might have set the critical age at sixty. In the twenty-first century, life expectancy is higher, so that Callahan's assumption needs to be updated. The age criterion, therefore, cannot be applied without regard to technology and without regard to the question of whether we can afford the expensive technology. It is impossible to assert categorically that upon reaching a certain age people think that they have completed their life span. Furthermore, as technology progresses, the purchase price of advanced medical equipment falls. Later in the twenty-first century it may be possible to provide treatment, considered today to be costly and sophisticated, to a larger number of people at a lower cost. Callahan's claims are dependent on time and place. Even according to his own reasoning, we should not accept his assumptions as axioms that are always valid, or as arguments that should be applicable even in the next decade. His views were developed in a certain historical context, and at best they might be correct for the period in which they were written.[45]

Callahan further claims that we need to set priorities in light of certain financial limitations. Society must determine its most urgent needs and set boundaries on the economic possibilities that progress has made possible. If, for example, a society decided it could not afford artificial hearts for patients over the age of ninety, the decision would be an outcome of priorities stating that the health care system's primary purpose is to enable the young to grow old.[46] Another example provided by Callahan is that of bypass operations for patients aged eighty and over. In his opinion, such an operation poses a new problem, both ethically and financially. Callahan asks: Even if we agree that each person should have access to a decent level of health care, does this mean that the government must provide, at tax payers' expense, every technological development that science may bring, at any cost? Callahan answers this question, which to him seems purely rhetorical, in the negative.[47]

Callahan does not merely say that if we have two patients in exactly the same medical condition, one of eighty and the other of thirty, and only one scarce resource (such as a bed in an ICU), then we should give priority to the young over the old. This is a plausible suggestion. Other things being equal, we should give precedence to the person who has the prospect of living longer. Callahan's line of reasoning is far more general, arbitrary, and sweeping, speaking of age as a crude single criterion upon which we decide on priorities in allocation of resources in health care, no matter what is the medical condition of the patients under consideration. There are eighty-year-old patients whose physical and mental functioning is excellent and to whom a bypass operation could give them life. They need only a valve replacement to renew their vigor. On the other hand, there are forty-year-olds whose physical condition is so run down that neither a bypass operation nor a heart transplant would be sufficient to restore their health. The age criterion alone should not be the main consideration in decisions about transplanting or repairing a heart. The criteria of the patient's condition, the chances for the operation's success, and the chance to live as normal a life as possible after the treatment are more important.

A series of studies regarding patients in intensive care shows that the severity of the illness, not the patient's age, is the main criterion for predicting the chances of recovery. Other studies that analyze age as a factor in forecasting chances of recovery or death have found that the predictive power of this variable is minimal.[48] I agree that in cases where age is the single differentiating factor, unique or costly treatment should be provided to the patient with the longer life expectancy. The problem is that Callahan does not make any reference to such issues: For him the age criterion seems to play the role of trump card.[49]

Moreover, Callahan's writings imply that technological progress, as such, troubles him. In What Kind of Life, Callahan claims that there is a major contradiction between the public's desire to keep prices under control and the desire to improve public access to technologically advanced treatments. There are contradictions in our knowledge and behavior. We cannot have things both ways: progressing in medicine and at the same time restraining our budget. According to Callahan, advanced technologies should have a low priority in the comprehensive medical insurance plan in a reality in which resources are scarce. Callahan rebukes those who believe in a right to die with dignity when he points out that people speak of the right to die with dignity, while simultaneously enlarging budgets that seek cures for death-causing ailments.[50] Finally, Callahan's claim that, by virtue of technology, physicians are allowed to assume a godlike role, shifts the focus from the commitment of doctors to do everything possible to save lives to the commitment to preserve the dignity of patients. It might have been possible to agree with the essence of Callahan's words had he phrased them more carefully. In certain cases, such as those of Sue Rodriguez[51] or Benjamin Eyal,[52] the preservation of human dignity permits physician-assisted suicide. We must not see life as a cause that must be sanctified at all costs, regardless of the desires of the person who is living that particular life. However, Callahan's position is too inclusive, too paternalistic, and too utilitarian. In fact, Callahan's position demonstrates a lack of the requisite sensitivity to human life.

According to Callahan, ideas concerning prolonging life, stopping the process of aging, and conquering death are neither possible nor defensible. These are false causes, which divert medicine from its true purpose of defeating illness, rehabilitating patients, and improving human health. We ought to recognize our limitations: Instead of attempting to stop the aging process and thinking that old age can be changed into a permanent midlife stage, we must recognize that old age is an inevitable stage in life. Callahan claims that even if we had unlimited resources at our disposal, it would still be wiser to set boundaries.[53] Because old age and death are inevitable, there should not be an unlimited demand to fight them and to harness national resources for this mission.

Callahan adopts a collective posture whereby the place of the elderly in society is a group issue, not a personal one.[54] He justifies his position by asserting, in his comments on a draft of this chapter, that "policy must do that." Individualism should make way for the social, group idea, along with the recognition that we live in a reality of limited resources. The concept of autonomy, which lies at the heart of liberal ideology, does not receive due reference in Callahan's books. Moreover, the matter of reward is totally neglected. Callahan refrains from pondering the moral question of neglecting those who have contributed to society for many years. His calculation is utilitarian. His goal is to maximize benefits by reallocating resources to the younger population. My deontological criticism of Callahan's view focuses on his referring to sacrificing the older population as a means to achieving greater social happiness and prosperity, rather than as an end in itself. He is prepared to sacrifice the older population for the younger. This approach to cost efficiency largely excludes moral considerations. It is an efficient method insofar as it reduces funds spent on medical care, but it is not a just method. Older people need and deserve more care, not abandonment.[55]

Callahan explains, in his discussion of this chapter, that his train of thought is totally different from the thinking presented here. Callahan does not see his policy as one that sacrifices or abandons the older population. Rather, the elderly have already "won the game" by reaching an old age. The young have an obligation to allow the old a decent life; but at the same time, the old have an obligation not to pose excessive obligations on the health care system. Callahan draws an analogy between elderly people and marathon runners. Older people have finished the marathon and, in this respect, they are far better off in comparison with those who had to retire from the marathon at an early stage. We should allocate our resources in a way that would enable other people to start the race. According to Callahan, the fact of chief importance is that eighty-year-olds have reached this ripe old age. Other people should be helped to reach the same age.[56] The crude result of Callahan's policy is the sacrifice of some individuals for the common good, in accordance with the single criterion of age. In his view, people must accept some form of rationing, and once this rationing is accepted, some people will not get what they need.[57]

On the contrary, patients should be considered as individuals, regardless of their age. It is unjust to sacrifice individuals in the name of a predicted general benefit simply because they are old. Individuals must be considered as an end in themselves and should be accorded equal care to satisfy their needs and interests. Age should not serve as the sole utilitarian index when society makes decisions about life and death.[58] Other important considerations exist, such as the patient's quality of life, his or her wishes, efficacy of care, chances of recovery, and perhaps economic considerations such as the cost of treatment. Using age as the main variable of reference in medical decisions constitutes a utilitarian policy that ultimately is amoral.[59]

The problem with Callahan's position is that we are not merely logical and calculating creatures. We are also beings who act on sensations, instincts, and feelings, which do not always agree with cold rationalism. Often people knowingly act on the basis of irrational arguments. Many people take the liberty of expressing emotional experience socially, knowing that these emotional experiences contradict logical thought, and still these people prefer to give themselves that freedom. People enter into holy matrimony because they are in love, sometimes despite recognizing that they have very little in common.[60] Some people believe that there is no point in arguing with love. People wish to help their fellow humans not for utilitarian reasons but because they want to treat people as valuable ends, as human beings who are worthy of respect and deserving of human concern. John Stuart Mill's well-known example of a man who wishes to cross a bridge without knowing that it is unsafe is pertinent. Mill states: "If either a public officer or anyone else saw a person attempting to cross a bridge which had been ascertained to be unsafe, and there were no time to warn him of his danger, they might seize him and turn him back, without any real infringement of his liberty; for liberty consists of doing what one desires, and he does not desire to fall into the river."[61]

The idea here is that when all people treat their fellow human beings with respect and concern, society as a whole is better off. But under no circumstances should society be put before the individual, nor, in the name of an amorphous body called "society," should the basic rights of any particular sector be denied. Callahan's way of thinking might be appropriate in a world based on narrow financial considerations, utilitarian considerations, and rational computerized brains. However, this way of thinking seems too cold, detached, and impersonal.

Morals and emotions as well as pure reasoning may lead us to think that society must care for the elderly. One should consider their contribution to society in the past and remember that today's midlife generation is tomorrow's elderly community. To suggest that the state should help only those who can still help the state amounts to gross utilitarianism. According to Callahan, as long as citizens can contribute, participate in social activities, pay taxes, serve in the army when summoned, and fulfill civic responsibilities, the state must provide them with medical aid. But when citizens reach old age, the cost of maintaining their lives grows, and since they would have died in the pretechnological era anyway, Callahan asks us to think in a way that is devoid of context. He asks us to make believe that we do not have the medical means to save old people, so society should let them die. Precisely when the elderly need help most, the state's decision-makers are supposed to give up on them and apologetically deny them access to costly treatments that could preserve their lives.

In contrast to Callahan's view, the liberal state must not desert its citizens at the time and place where they need help more than ever. This follows the tradition of liberal thought, which should serve as a guide. The liberal state is founded on the principles of respect for others and not harming others. These principles must not be deserted when society deals with the elderly.

In utilitarian terms, there are important tasks to which the state allocates considerable resources, yet no one challenges the priority assigned to each task. The state of Israel allocates considerable resources to the cause of bringing home its prisoners of war. It is difficult to measure and calculate the efforts dedicated to the location of the navigator Ron Arad, who disappeared during the Lebanon War (1982–1985). Still, justly, no one has claimed that it would be better to put an end to the efforts to find him and to consider more worthy causes for those resources. Liberal countries devote considerable resources to ensure a fair trial for those suspected of felonies, and no one questions the set of priorities applied in this case. I have heard of no Callahan utilitarian equivalent in the area of law, wondering about decisions made by a jury and claiming that the maintenance of juries is too costly for the taxpayer. The cost per year of the O.J. Simpson trial alone was estimated at $9 million, most of the expenses covering the upkeep of the jurors and their replacements.[62] Even so, no voices were heard claiming that it would be better to find a different trial method because of financial considerations. The liberal state takes these stands because the right to a fair trial is seen as a basic one that must be preserved despite the cost.[63] At the root of this policy are the principles of not harming others and respecting others. The liberal state concerns itself with issues such as caring for POWs and maintaining a fair judicial system because any other form of behavior would mean neglecting these principles. The state's obligation to ensure citizens' right to live in dignity is no less important than its commitment to its POWs and the promise of the right to a fair trial. Rights do not expire when citizens reach a certain age.

Patients in Post-Coma Unawareness

Reading Callahan's writings, one cannot avoid suspecting that he selects the elderly community as a means of saving resources because of their weak position in society. The elderly no longer contribute to society, are not efficient, are often neglected, and sometimes constitute a burden on their families. It is easy to justify budget cuts pertaining to this segment of society. This same train of cold assertion guides Callahan's consideration of PCU patients. In the context of his discussion of the term *futile treatment*, Callahan writes that the phrase should be explained in two ways: Nothing positive will result from the treatment, and because of limited resources, the treatment is economically unjustifiable. Therefore, continues Callahan, we must reach a general social agreement concerning PCU patients and the right of doctors to deny treatment for such patients.[64] A social agreement should also be reached on the kinds of medical treatment that are to be considered useless for patients who are going to die of chronic disease or slow degeneration. Callahan suggests one end for all patients in a state of unconsciousness, no matter how long they have been in this state or what their chances are for some improvement in their condition. Hundreds and thousands of patients would be put to death if society accepted Callahan's claim that society must not keep them alive because of financial considerations. Some of these patients, who have a chance of returning to some viable form of life, would lose that chance altogether.[65] These patients, who need more devoted care than patients in other categories, would be deserted completely if society followed Callahan's reasoning, because in his opinion treating them is useless. Callahan believes this even though in quite a few cases there is a chance for rehabilitation (see chapter 2).

A possible solution to maintaining patients in PCU would be to enable individuals to purchase complementary insurance specifically geared to covering this expense. In any event, it should not be a policy to take the lives of others because their treatment is too costly.

There is a utilitarian approach that excludes treating certain diseases because of their cost. The Oregon plan is a result of such thinking.

The Exclusion of Certain Diseases:
An Examination of the Oregon Plan

As a matter of general principle, the purpose of a publicly funded service is not to generate revenue, but to meet a societal need and to respond to a societal right. Health is a major determining factor in people's ability to take advantage of the opportunities that are available in society. A just and equitable society, therefore, must try to minimize health-based differences to create a level playing field for all its citizens. Consequently, a just and equitable society has an obligation to meet the health care needs of its members so as to minimize health-based interpersonal differences. A publicly funded health care system is society's attempt to meet this obligation. It follows that a publicly funded health care system must start from the premise that health care is a right and not a commodity.[66]

In 1987, Oregon decided that it would no longer pay for organ transplants for Medicaid patients.[67] *Time* magazine reported that doctors admitted that applicants for new high-tech operations have to pass a "green screen" or "wallet biopsy," meaning that those who could afford to pay would be given first opportunity for the operations.[68] Between 1989 and 1991, the Oregon State Senate passed six laws that together changed the health care system in the state. These laws, which have come to be known as the Oregon plan, were meant to enable the Medicaid insurance plan to include tens and even hundreds of thousands more people from the lower classes who had been previously uninsured. A council of experts was formed to implement this goal, and the council's task was to grade the health services according to their importance, while conferring with health consumers representing the community.

Senate Bill 27 (1989) extended Medicaid coverage to every Oregonian with income below the federal poverty level and guaranteed them a basic benefit package based on a prioritized list of health services.[69] Senate Bill 935 (1989) required employers to cover all "permanent" employees and their dependents or pay into a special state insurance fund that would offer coverage to those employees. In turn, Senate Bill 534 (1989) founded the Oregon Medical Insurance Pool, which offers health insurance to people who cannot buy conventional coverage because of preexisting medical problems.[70]

In May 1990, the Oregon Health Services Commission declared that it had compiled a list of sixteen hundred medical procedures and treatments graded by computer on the basis of a formula that balanced the cost of treatment, the effect of the treatment on the quality of the patients' lives, and the number of people who would prosper from the provision of the treatment.[71] At the beginning, the scheme attracted a lot of criticism; it was argued that many of the rankings were clinically counterintuitive, assigning higher priorities to some services that were clearly less important than other, lower-ranked services.[72] Eventually, the list consisted of more than seven hundred medical conditions, each matched with a corresponding treatment, which were called condition-treatment pairs (CT pairs).[73] The state legislation then drew a line at item 587; treatments below the line would not be covered. Treatments that would prevent death and lead to full recovery were ranked first. Maternity care was ranked second. Treatments that prevented death without full recovery were ranked third. Treatments that resulted in minimal or no improvement in the quality of life were ranked last.[74] Rationing for the poor dictated that expensive medical operations be excluded because of their excessively high cost and the small number of patients in need of them. Thus, for instance, PCU patients were not included in the scheme. Those responsible for the plan estimated that it would provide medical treatment for double the number of previous recipients.[75] Interestingly, as of March 1998 assisted suicide was included on the list of services covered by Medicaid under the rubric of "comfort care."[76]

The legislative process continued, and during 1991 four further bills were passed. Senate Bill 1076 (1991) made affordable insurance available for small businesses. Senate Bill 1077 (1991) established a Health Resources Commission to examine the impact of capital expenditures on medical technologies. Senate Bill 1076 (1991) required the Health Services Commission to integrate mental health and chemical dependency services into future priority lists for the Legislature's consideration in funding. And Senate Bill 44 (1991) began the process of offering the standard benefit package to seniors and persons with disabilities on Medicaid, following legislative approval. In addition, three further bills— Senate Bill 5530 (1993), Senate Bill 152 (1995), and Senate Bill 1079 (1995)—outlined various mechanisms to implement the plan, to reform the insurance market, and to restructure the government bodies dealing with health care policy.[77]

In 1992, the Bush administration refused to authorize the Oregon plan on the grounds that it ran afoul of the American with Disabilities Act (1990). More specifically, the argument was that AIDS patients would be denied treatment. Once Oregon had made a few changes, President

Clinton approved the plan (in March 1993) and allowed the request for a waiver from normal Medicaid regulations, providing Medicaid to hundreds of thousands of people who previously had been denied any medical insurance. The Secretary of Health and Human Services, Donna E. Shalala, approved the plan to proceed for a five-year "experimental" period (1994–1999). In the first stage, the total number of Medicaid recipients was expanded from 240,000 to 360,000.[78] In July 1995, there were 402,000 people receiving benefits under the plan, among them 134,000 who were newly eligible.[79] Employers were mandated to provide health insurance for employees or be subject to a new payroll tax. Employers who "play" were said to offer health plans substantially similar to those on the Medicaid priority list and to bear at least 75 percent of the cost for employees and 50 percent of the cost for their dependents. Among the substantial conditions of federal approval, Secretary Shalala submitted that the Oregon Health Plan would not be permitted to consider "functional limitations" (such as inability to walk) or impairments that persisted after treatment as a measure of a treatment's "effectiveness." The state was also required not to rescind its guarantee of funding up to the level of 568 services without prior approval from HHS.[80]

The requirement that employers insure all their workers or contribute to a fund to cover them failed to gain support very early. Spending for the plan climbed to $2.1 billion in the 1997–1999 state budget period from $1.7 billion in the 1995–1997 period. Higher cigarette taxes did not offset the increase, requiring more money from the state's general fund. The state abandoned its promise of universal care. In addition, doctors routinely found ways to get around the rationing, and the practice of managed care involving doctors, clinics, and hospitals working together to control patient care broke down, especially in the rural areas.[81]

The plan's supporters characterize the Oregon plan as an organized effort intended to balance limited government resources with the high costs involved in providing technologically advanced medicine. P. R. Sipes-Metzler describes the plan as a thoughtful and deliberate blending of fact with public value for the purpose of responsible health policy.[82] Kristie Perry Dolan argues that the plan succeeded on many fronts: Emergency-room visits had decreased 5.3 percent by the end of 1994; charity care in hospitals plunged 30 percent, and hospital debt dropped 11 percent.[83] Some would question whether the decrease in emergency-room visits was a positive consequence. The emergency rooms were relatively quieter because hospitals were no longer strained by having to provide free emergency care. In no event should charity take the place of government to care for the citizens. Nevertheless, in a satisfaction survey the state conducted, Medicaid clients said the new plan was better than the plan it replaced.[84]

One of the criticisms of the Oregon plan focuses on its discrimination against the poor. The poor are covered by Medicaid, while those who can afford it buy full medical insurance, including the full medical treatment package. Unlike the basic Medicaid system, the Oregon plan offers care for people based solely upon their income and not according to their age, infirmities, and income. Arguments were also made that the plan discriminates against the disabled.[85] Critics maintained that the plan's promise to ration care was not only unfair, but also unnecessary. Eliminating administrative waste, squeezing drug companies and providers, and spending more represented, they argued, proven alternatives.[86] Furthermore, the methodology of Oregon's rationing plan was scrutinized. The attempt to conflate thousands of complex diagnoses and treatment scenarios into 709 homogeneous categories appeared to defy human and organizational ability. Oregon's approach of covering all services above a certain line and no services below that line regardless of an individual patient's medical condition or treatment prognosis meant that patients who stood to benefit greatly were denied care, while others who might benefit only slightly received it.[87] Finally, recent studies show that the plan did not generate substantial savings by rationing Medicaid services. Plans for setting priorities and drawing a "line" were never implemented. In striking contrast to the initial claim that prioritization would finance Medicaid expansion, the plan's administrators estimated that the list saved the state only 2 percent on total costs for the program over its first five years of operation.[88]

The supporters of the plan claim in response that most of Oregon's poor were much better off after the introduction of the plan than they were before.[89] However, like all utilitarian approaches, the Oregon plan focuses on numbers, and any particular individual does not always find a place in the general scheme. The focus on the forest causes many trees to be uprooted in the name of maximization of utility.[90] Attention should be focused on individuals' needs, as liberalism does, rather than ignoring the individual in the name of a majority.[91] To illustrate, one of the patients who suffered the consequences of the Oregon legislature's decision to stop paying for transplants was Coby Howard, a seven-year-old boy with acute lymphocytic leukemia. His plight and his family's efforts to raise money from public contributions received intense press coverage. When Coby died, the family was within $20,000 of the $100,000 needed for his treatment. The case was a classic example of the tension between an individual and society.[92]

A 1999 study showed that the administrators of the Oregon plan learned their lessons from the painful story of little Coby Howard. In the years after his death, coverage of transplants actually became more generous in comparison with coverage under the previous Medicaid system. The state voluntarily expanded coverage of transplants for a number of conditions, including bone marrow, heart, and lung transplants.[93]

Thomas Bodenheimer notes as a justification of the plan that physicians occasionally "game" the system, choosing a diagnosis above the line even though the patient has an illness that falls below the line.[94] However, physicians should not "game" the system. This is one of the problems of drawing an arbitrary line that does not consider specific needs of real patients. Physician discretion should be an integral part of the system, allowing physicians to use their judgment to meet the needs of their patients, for their benefit. Openness and honesty are required, not "gaming" and looking for loopholes.

The goal of eliminating discrimination between those who can afford complementary policies and those who receive only Medicaid insurance is distant yet viable.[95] The uninsured population in Oregon has dropped from 17 percent in 1989 to 11 percent.[96] The percentage of children without insurance has fallen from 21 percent to 8 percent.[97] The national average has remained about 16 percent.[98] Notwithstanding, the major ray of light in the Oregon plan is the way in which the list of treatments and diseases was formulated. The list was compiled on the basis of feedback from experts and other citizens of Oregon who democratically and freely stated their opinion and influenced the decision-making. The public process included community meetings, hearings, and telephone surveys. This is a desirable decision-making model toward which all may strive: It enlarges the circle of decision-makers regarding health issues that concern us all, and it involves citizens of all social classes in discussions concerning their future. Participation is at the heart of democracy, and active democratic participation should definitely be encouraged.[99] There is great importance in the provision of relevant information that furthers decision-making, so that the representatives of the public become aware of the ramifications of their decisions.

Conclusion

This appendix does not attempt to show that the state should assume the task of supporting all life as such. Patients suffering from irreversible brain-stem injury need not be sustained. Patients who specifically ask to die because a critical disease has deprived them of their desire to live should not be kept alive against their will. It is appropriate to recognize the autonomy of patients in determining their destiny, and the state should not implement inclusive paternalism against the better judgment of its citizens. Nor should the state invest scarce resources in supporting life in cases in which medical experience shows only slight chances of improvement, and the disease is defined as irreversible and incurable. For example, it is pointless to invest in costly chemotherapy for a cancer patient in the last stages of the illness, when it is known that such patients do not gain from these treatments and that their condition does not improve.

An important question is whether physicians have an obligation to be loyal to a single patient, even if this loyalty results in the allocation of large resources to that particular person; or whether physicians should be aware that they act within a social framework, that they must be loyal to society at large, and therefore must function in accordance with more general considerations that limit their responsibility to individual patients. Between personal accountability and inclusive social accountability there is constant tension. Avraham Steinberg is correct in stating that the physician carries the duty of properly considering the diagnostic tests, of responsibly and wisely choosing the treatment methods, and of acting in the best interest of the patient.[100] The classic codes of medicine, beginning with the Hippocratic Oath, place patients at the center of the doctor-patient relationship and demand the best for them. With this in mind, it is possible to foster the good of the patient on the basis of the medical norms that are accepted by society as a whole. The ideal situation would be for the clinical agent to represent the patient in good faith, without regard to possible problems of resource allocation, and the general policymakers should decide the possible frameworks for care on the basis of what society considers acceptable.

Moreover, physicians have an obligation to update their knowledge in the areas of diagnosis and treatment, including gaining insights on financial topics. In this manner, they can make a contribution to the welfare of the patients and to society at large. In addition, conversation time with patients should be mandated in health care packages. The situation today leaves physicians no time to hold proper conversations with their patients, to listen to them, to pay attention to their feelings, and to offer them encouragement.[101] A meaningful change in this impersonal situation can occur only through an allocation for patient-doctor conversations in the health care package.

The guiding concept of responsibility for all concerned parties is emphasized: decision makers at the state level, the medical system, and the individual. In most cases patients have the autonomy to decide on issues that concern their lives. Even patients incapable of decision-making have a guardian who decides for them in most cases. The physician is not the only one to decide for the patients. The assumption is that in most cases we deal with rational people who are capable of making decisions, choosing among options, and assessing efficiencies and costs. This approach emphasizes the autonomy of patients and encourages authorities to allow for the development of their abilities and to recognize their contribution to their own individual progress. Consulting others is effective as long as doctors and others whose views we respect do not become manipulative and allow patients to be exposed to different, sometimes conflicting opinions.[102]

Just as patients are expected to be responsible for making decisions about medical treatment, so are they expected to make decisions about the medical insurance that best suits them. Patients are the ones to decide which standards of medical care they may expect to receive on the basis of the insurance they have chosen. Such an approach respects the autonomy of patients, enables them to take part in the decision-making concerning their health, and allows for an open dialogue between the system and individual patients. This approach encourages competition among various insurance bodies, competition that in the long run will be in the best interest of the citizens. The aim is to expand the circle of people involved in the decision-making process, discussing citizens' expectations from the state, its policies, and assessments openly. Citizens cannot realistically expect to be eligible for complete treatment paid for by a nameless "someone." That someone is the citizen. The costs should be divided among the citizens, each deciding for him- or herself the scope of medical coverage each is interested in, and how much he or she is willing to pay. The state should guarantee a certain level of medical treatment to all its citizens, but it cannot be expected to provide the optimum. The optimum can be provided only for those who can pay for it. Nonetheless, the state may not exclude certain populations in advance, such as the poor, the elderly, PCU patients, or patients with locked-in syndrome. Of course, it is impossible to attain a system of absolute equality, and financial ability does in fact differentiate among people, but society must also strive to insure that everyone will receive the minimum required for continuation of a decent life.[103]

Some categories of treatment are too costly for most individuals in society. The sums of money involved in organ transplants are enormous, hundreds of thousands of dollars, and in these cases the state should help by devising special insurance schemes in which the state will assist those who commit themselves to having a transplant. The commitment could take two forms: special insurance for organ transplantation, and an explicit willingness to donate organs if certain conditions are fulfilled. Society must not reach a situation in which only the richest obtain these expensive operations. Charity and public fund-raising are options, but such donations must not be made obligatory; certainly they should not be considered an adequate substitute for state aid.[104] Special public committees comprised of people from diverse disciplines should make decisions concerning the allocation of costly treatments. It is preferable that these committees include doctors as well as various public representatives: ethicists, economists, sociologists, lawyers, social workers, and clergy. Together they will decide on proper priorities regarding the medical needs of each particular patient.

Notes

INTRODUCTION

1. Joseph Raz, *The Morality of Freedom* (Oxford, U.K.: Clarendon Press, 1986), 204. See also Lawrence P. Ulrich, *The Patient Self-Determination Act* (Washington, D.C.: Georgetown University Press, 1999), 149–151; Richard Dagger, *Civic Virtues* (New York: Oxford University Press, 1997), 11–40, 175–181; James F. Childress, *Practical Reasoning in Bioethics* (Bloomington and Indianapolis: Indiana University Press, 1997), 59–68; R. Cohen-Almagor, *The Boundaries of Liberty and Tolerance* (Gainesville: University Press of Florida, 1994), ch. 1; Tom L. Beauchamp and James F. Childress, *Principles of Biomedical Ethics* (New York: Oxford University Press, 1994), 120–132.
2. Immanuel Kant, *Foundations of the Metaphysics of Morals*, section 2, trans. Lewis White Beck (Indianapolis: Bobbs-Merrill Educational Publishers, 1969), 52–53.
3. The postulate "You ought never to tell lies" is an example of the categorical imperative. There is no way of evading the command or the moral requirement of practical reason that it expresses, for no end is mentioned, and there is therefore no end that can be given up. For further discussion, see J. Kemp, *The Philosophy of Kant* (Oxford, U.K.: Oxford University Press, 1979), 58.
4. On some issues the liberal state adopts a paternal approach that overrides individual decision-making. Thus, for instance, to protect our security the liberal state requires us to fasten seat belts when we travel by car and to wear crash helmets when we ride motorcycles. For further discussion, see John Stuart Mill, *Principles of Political Economy* (London: Longmans, Green, Reader and Dyer, 1869), book 5, "On the Influence of Government," 479–591.
5. John Rawls, "Liberty, Equality, and Law," in Sterling M. McMurrin (ed.), *Tanner Lectures on Human Values* (Cambridge, U.K.: Cambridge University Press, 1987), 1–87, section 3; "Justice as Fairness: Political Not Metaphysical," *Philosophy and Public Affairs* 14 (3) (1985): 223–251. See also Rawls, *Political Liberalism* (New York: Columbia University Press, 1993), "Fundamental Ideas," 3–46. Recently Rawls has broadened the scope of his theory

to argue for mutual respect among peoples. See his *The Law of Peoples* (Cambridge, Mass.: Harvard University Press, 1999), 62.

6. Cf. R. M. Dworkin, "Hard Cases," *Harvard Law Review* 88 (6) (1975): 1069–1071; *Taking Rights Seriously* (London: Duckworth, 1977), 150–183, 266–278; "Liberalism," in *A Matter of Principle* (Oxford, U.K.: Clarendon, 1985), 181–204. For further discussion, see A. E. Buchanan, "Assessing the Communitarian Critique of Liberalism," *Ethics* 99 (1989): 879.

7. Cf. James Griffin, *Well Being* (Oxford, U.K.: Clarendon Press, 1986), ch. 9.

8. Another tragic condition concerns patients in locked-in syndrome (LIS). The term *locked-in syndrome* was introduced by F. Plum and J. B. Posner in 1966 to describe a neurological condition associated with infraction of the ventral pons. Locked-in syndrome is a specific neurobehavioral problem caused by a lesion in the base of the pons and is characterized by complete immobility and severely limited ability to communicate. The patient remains conscious, alert, and cognitively aware of the environment but is unable to speak or communicate other than through vertical eye movements or blinking. Such patients are diagnosed with quadriplegia, lower cranial nerve paralysis, and mutism. There are various subclassifications of locked-in syndrome that relate to the extent of motor and verbal impairment ranging from complete to partial. Although minimal late neurologic recovery occurs in chronic locked-in syndrome patients, survival may, nonetheless, be prolonged with adequate supportive care. This example of consciousness without behavioral expression illustrates the need for a nonverificationist theory of the mind. See G. A. Kirkpatrick, "In re Rodas," *Issues in Law and Medicine* 2 (6) (May 1987): 471–480; Abraham Ohry, "The Locked-In Syndrome and Related States," *Paraplegia* 28 (1990): 73–75; M. Kurthen et al., "The Locked-In Syndrome and the Behaviorist Epistemology of Other Minds," *Theoretical Medicine* 12 (1) (March 1991): 69–79; American Congress of Rehabilitation Medicine, "Recommendations for Use of Uniform Nomenclature Pertinent to Patients with Severe Alterations in Consciousness," *Archives of Physical Medicine and Rehabilitation* 76 (2) (February 1995): 205–209; M. Onofrj et al., "Event Related Potentials Recorded in Patients with Locked-In Syndrome," *Journal of Neurology, Neurosurgery and Psychiatry* 63 (6) (December 1997): 759–764.

9. Raanan Gillon, "Why Keep People Alive? A Secular Medical Ethics Analysis," in *End-of-Life Medical Decisionmaking: Sanctity of Life and Death with Dignity,* International Conference, Tel Aviv University Faculty of Law (28–30 December 1998). See also R. Gillon, "Persistent Vegetative State, Withdrawal of Artificial Nutrition and Hydration, and the Patient's 'Best Interests,'" *Journal of Medical Ethics* 24 (April 1998): 75–76.

10. Responses to confirmatory tests to examine whether the brain stem is injured include fixed pupils with no response to light; corneal reflex absent; vestibulo-ocular reflexes absent; no motor responses elicited within the cranial nerve distribution; no gag reflex or response to bronchial stimulation by a suction catheter passed down the trachea; no respiratory movements when the patient is disconnected from the mechanical ventilator for long enough to ensure that the arterial CO_2 rises above the threshold for stimulating respiration. Cf. E. McClatchey, "Some Aspects of Euthanasia from the Point of View of a Family Doctor," in Amnon Carmi (ed.), *Euthanasia* (Berlin: Springer-Verlag, 1984), 106. See also Coordinating Council on Life-Sustaining Medical Treatment Decision Making by the Courts, *Guidelines for State Court Decision Making in Authorizing or Withholding Life-Sustaining Medical Treatment* (Williamsburg, Va.: National Center for State Courts,

1991); Christopher Kennard and Robin Illingworth, "Persistent Vegetative State," *Journal of Neurology, Neurosurgery and Psychiatry* 59 (October 1995): 347–348; Review by a working group convened by the Royal College of Physicians and endorsed by the Conference of Medical Royal Colleges and their faculties in the United Kingdom, "The Permanent Vegetative State," *Journal of the Royal College of Physicians of London* 30 (2) (March–April 1996): 119–121; Andreas Kampfl et al., "Prediction of Recovery from Post-traumatic Vegetative State with Cerebral Magnetic-resonance Imaging," *Lancet* 351 (13 June 1998): 1763–1767.

11. Joel Feinberg, "Voluntary Euthanasia and the Inalienable Right to Life," in Sterling M. McMurrin (ed.), *The Tanner Lectures on Human Values* (Salt Lake City: University of Utah Press, 1980), 254.

12. For a contrasting view, see Ronald Dworkin, *Life's Dominion* (New York: Knopf, 1993).

13. *Health Law Reporter* 3 (1994), 1673.

14. *State of Washington v. Glucksberg; Vacco v. Quill*, nos. 95–1858, 96–110 (10 December 1996). Brief for Ronald Dworkin, Thomas Nagel, Robert Nozick, John Rawls, Thomas Scanlon, and Judith Jarvis Thomson as amici curiae in support of respondents, see "Assisted Suicide: The Philosophers' Brief," *New York Review of Books*, 27 March 1997, 44. For a critique of the brief, see Richard Church, "The Rhetoric of Neutrality and the Philosophers' Brief: A Critique of the *Amicus* Brief of Six Moral Philosophers in *Washington v. Glucksberg* and *Vacco v. Quill*," *Law and Contemporary Problems* 61 (4) (autumn 1998): 233–247.

15. See John Hardwig, "Is There a Duty to Die?," *Hastings Center Report* 27 (2) (1997): 34–42.

16. Opening Procedure (Tel Aviv) 1141/90 *Eyal v. Dr. Wilensky and Others*, 1991.

CHAPTER 1   LANGUAGE AND REALITY AT THE END OF LIFE

1. Cf. U. Lowental, "Euthanasia: A Serene Voyage to Death," in Amnon Carmi (ed.), *Euthanasia* (Berlin: Springer-Verlag, 1984), 180–184. For discussion on the origin and rationale of the concept of dignity, see Kurt Bayertz, "Human Dignity: Philosophical Origin and Scientific Erosion of an Idea," in K. Bayertz (ed.), *Sanctity of Life and Human Dignity* (Dordrecht, The Netherlands: Kluwer, 1996), 73–90; David J. Velleman, "A Right of Self-Termination," *Ethics* 109 (3) (April 1999): 611–617.

2. Lawrence P. Ulrich, *The Patient Self-Determination Act* (Washington, D.C.: Georgetown University Press, 1999), 88.

3. Leon R. Kass, "Death with Dignity and the Sanctity of Life," in Barry S. Kogan (ed.), *A Time to Be Born and a Time to Die* (New York: Aldine DeGruyter, 1991), 133. Kass argues that one has no more right to dignity than one has to beauty or courage or wisdom. Although it is puzzling to speak of a right to beauty or courage or wisdom, I think all have a right to dignity. It is part of the fundamental principle of respect for others that underlies liberal democracies.

4. Haim Cohn holds that human dignity is the source from which human rights are derived and that it is, along with human rights, the foundation of freedom, justice and peace. Cf. Haim H. Cohn, "On the Meaning of Human Dignity," *Israel Yearbook of Human Rights* 13 (1983): 226.

5. An eloquent characterization of this transformation is presented in Margaret Edson's 1999 Pulitzer-winning play, *Wit.*

6. See John Harris, *The Value of Life* (London: Routledge and Kegan Paul, 1985);

Helga Kuhse, *The Sanctity of Life Doctrine in Medicine: A Critique* (Oxford, U.K.: Clarendon Press, 1987); and "Quality of Life and the Death of 'Baby M,'" *Bioethics* 6 (3) (1992): 233–250.

7. On the concept of paternalism, see James F. Childress, *Priorities in Biomedical Ethics* (Philadelphia: Westminster Press, 1981), 20–30; see also Childress, *Practical Reasoning in Bioethics* (Bloomington and Indianapolis: Indiana University Press, 1997), 44–46.

8. The New York Task Force on Life and the Law used the term "permanent unconsciousness." New York State Task Force on Life and the Law, *When Others Must Choose: Deciding for Patients Without Capacity* (Albany, N.Y.: Health Research Inc., March 1992).

9. Cf. Z. Groswasser and L. Sazbon, "Outcome in 134 Patients with Prolonged Posttraumatic Unawareness," *Journal of Neurosurgery* 72 (1990): 81; Concezione Tommasino, "Coma and Vegetative State Are Not Interchangeable Terms," *Anesthesiology* 83 (4) (October 1995): 888.

10. B. Jennet and F. Plum, "Persistent Vegetative State after Brain Damage: A Syndrome in Search of a Name," *Lancet* 1 (1972): 734–737.

11. Ibid., 735.

12. Bryan Jennett, "Clinical and Pathological Features of Vegetative Survival," in Harvey S. Levin and Arthur L. Benton (eds.), *Catastrophic Brain Injury* (New York: Oxford University Press, 1996), 5.

13. Ronald Dworkin has no qualms about referring to some patients as vegetables. See, for instance, *Life's Dominion* (New York: Knopf, 1993), 180, 230–232. See also Chris Borthwick, "The Proof of the Vegetable: A Commentary on Medical Futility," *Journal of Medical Ethics* 21 (1995): 206–208.

14. For further criticism of the word *terminal*, see Daniel Callahan and Margot White, "The Legalization of Physician-Assisted Suicide: Creating a Regulatory Potemkin Village," *University of Richmond Law Review* 30 (1) (January 1996): 45–52.

15. *Garry Lee v. State of Oregon*, Civil No. 94–6467–HO, United States District Court (3 August 1995), 13. On the Internet at www.islandnet.com/~deathnet/ergo_Hogan2.html.

16. Susan B. Rubin, *When Doctors Say No: The Battleground of Medical Futility* (Bloomington and Indianapolis: Indiana University Press, 1998), 42; Lance K. Stell, "Real Futility: Historical Beginnings and Continuing Debate About Futile Treatment," *North Carolina Medical Journal* 56 (9) (1995): 434.

17. Lawrence J. Schneiderman and Nancy S. Jecker, *Wrong Medicine* (Baltimore and London: Johns Hopkins University Press, 1995), 11; see also Schneiderman and Jecker, "Is the Treatment Beneficial, Experimental, or Futile?," *Cambridge Quarterly of Healthcare Ethics* 5 (2) (spring 1996): 249.

18. See Joanne Lynn and James F. Childress, "Must Patients Always Be Given Food and Water?," in J. Lynn (ed.), *By No Extraordinary Means* (Bloomington: Indiana University Press, 1986), 51.

19. John D. Lantos, "Futility Assessments and the Doctor-Patient Relationship," *Journal of the American Geriatrics Society* 42 (August 1994): 869.

20. Paul R. Helft et al., "The Rise and Fall of the Futility Movement," *New England Journal of Medicine* 343 (4) (27 July 2000): 293–296.

21. Moshe Sonnenblick et al., "Dissociation between the Wishes of Terminally Ill Parents and Decisions by Their Offspring," *Journal of the American Geriatric Society* 41 (6) (1993): 599–604.

22. See memorandum by Dr. David Lamb, House of Lords, *Select Committee on Medical Ethics*, session 1993–94, vol. 3, Minutes of Oral Evidence (London: HMSO, 1994), 133; Ulrich, *Patient Self-Determination Act*, 190.

23. Schneiderman and Jecker, *Wrong Medicine,* 97; L. J. Schneiderman et al.,

"Medical Futility: Its Meaning and Ethical Implications," *Annual International Medicine* 112 (1990): 949–954; L. J. Schneiderman et al., "Beyond Futility to an Ethic of Care," *American Journal of Medicine* 86 (1994): 110–114.

24. Robert D. Truog et al., "The Problem with Futility," *New England Journal of Medicine* 326 (23) (1992): 1561. For further criticism of Schneiderman et al., see Glenn G. Griener, "The Physician's Authority to Withhold Futile Treatment," *Journal of Medicine and Philosophy* 20 (1995): 216–218; C. Christopher Hook, "Medical Futility," in John F. Kilner et al. (eds.), *Dignity and Dying* (Grand Rapids, Mich.: William B. Eerdmans, 1996), 89–91.

25. John D. Lantos et al., "The Illusion of Futility in Clinical Practice," *American Journal of Medicine* 87 (July 1989): 81–83.

26. Council on Ethical and Judicial Affairs, American Medical Association, "Medical Futility in End-of-Life Care," *Journal of the American Medical Association* 281 (10) (10 March 1999): 938–940.

27. Rubin, *When Doctors Say No*, 115–117.

28. Childress, *Practical Reasoning*, 163. For a contrasting view, see Nancy S. Jecker, "Is Refusal of Futile Treatment Unjustified Paternalism?," *Journal of Clinical Ethics* 6 (2) (1995): 133–137.

29. Rubin, *When Doctors Say No*, 20.

30. South Australian Voluntary Euthanasia Society, "DID YOU KNOW? The Principle of Double Effect—SAVES," Fact Sheet No. 23 (October 1997).

31. Joseph Boyle wrote extensively on this topic. See, e.g., Joseph M. Boyle Jr., "Toward Understanding the Principle of Double Effect," *Ethics* 90 (July 1980): 527–538; and "Who Is Entitled to Double Effect?" *Journal of Medicine and Philosophy* 16 (1991): 475–494. See also the testimony of Dr. Walter R. Hunter before the Committee on the Judiciary (24 June 1999), on the Internet at www.house.gov/judiciary/hunt0624.htm; F. M. Kamm, "Physician-Assisted Suicide, the Doctrine of Double Effect, and the Ground of Value," *Ethics* 109 (3) (1999): 586–591; Charles F. McKhann, *A Time to Die: The Place for Physician Assistance* (New Haven, Conn.: Yale University Press, 1999), 102–106.

32. Cf. "When Doctors Might Kill Their Patients," *British Medical Journal* 318 (29 May 1999): 1431–1432. Further information on this and related issues is available from: Hon. Secretary, SAVES, PO Box 2151, Kent Town, SA 5071, Australia, fax 61–8 8265 2287; on the Internet at http://www.nejm.org/public/1998/0338/0019/1389/1.htm.

33. Timothy E. Quill et al., "The Rule of Double Effect—A Critique of Its Role in End-of-Life Decision Making," *New England Journal of Medicine* 337 (11 December 1997): 1768–1771. See also the correspondence on the rule of double effect in *New England Journal of Medicine* 338(19) (7 May 1998): 1389–1390.

34. Report of the Ad Hoc Committee of the Harvard Medical School to Examine the Definition of Brain Death, "A Definition of Irreversible Coma," *Journal of the American Medical Association* (August 1968): 337–340.

35. Stuart J. Youngner et al., "'Brain Death' and Organ Retrieval. A Cross-Sectional Survey of Knowledge and Concepts among Health Professionals," *Journal of the American Medical Association* 261 (15) (April 1989): 2205–2210.

36. Daniel Wikler and Alan J. Weisbard, "Appropriate Confusion over 'Brain Death,'" *Journal of the American Medical Association* 261 (15) (April 1989): 2246.

37. Robert D. Truog, "Organ Transplantation Without Brain Death," in R. Cohen-Almagor (ed.), *Medical Ethics at the Dawn of the 21st Century* (New York: New York Academy of Sciences, 2000), 229–239.

38. Robert D. Truog, "Is It Time to Abandon Brain Death?," *Hastings Center Report* 27 (1) (January–February 1997): 30.

39. Donnie J. Self and Evi Davenport, "Measurement of Moral Development in Medicine," *Cambridge Quarterly of Healthcare Ethics* 5 (2) (spring 1996): 269–277; Donnie J. Self et al., "Evaluation of Teaching Medical Ethics by an Assessment of Moral Reasoning," *Medical Education* 26 (1992): 178–184; S. Holm et al., "Changes in Moral Reasoning and the Teaching of Medical Ethics," *Medical Education* 29 (1995): 420–423.

40. Henry S. Perkins et al., "Challenges in Teaching Ethics in Medical Schools," *American Journal of the Medical Sciences* 319(5) (May 2000): 273–278.

41. Donnie J. Self et al., "Teaching Medical Ethics to First-Year Students by Using Film Discussion to Develop Moral Reasoning," *Academic Medicine* 68 (1993): 383–385.

42. Lantos argues that in the literature, the open-ended format and the relative intellectual marginality of the discipline allow questions to be raised about doctors and medicine, healing and illness, suffering and dying, that cannot be raised in any other discourse. The literature is thus avant-garde in raising these issues and beginning to question the patently messianic vision of medicine as a sort of secular salvation. See John Lantos, "Open Heart (Shiva M'Hodu)," in Cohen-Almagor (ed.), *Medical Ethics*, 41–51.

43. In the Yale Curriculum on Ethical and Humanistic Medicine, students and residents watch each other role-play clinical tasks such as obtaining informed consent, delivering bad news, and discussing do-not-resuscitate orders. Students compare the techniques they observe and perform, then discuss a list of practical suggestions specific to each interaction skill. Ellen Fox et al., "Medical Ethics Education: Past, Present, and Future," *Academic Medicine* 70 (9) (September 1995): 763. See also James W. Tysinger et al., "Teaching Ethics Using Small-Group, Problem-Based Learning," *Journal of Medical Ethics* 23 (5) (October 1997): 315–318; Edmund D. Pellegrino et al., "Teaching Clinical Ethics," *Journal of Clinical Ethics* 1 (3) (fall 1990): 175–180; Philip Hebert et al., "Evaluating Ethical Sensitivity in Medical Students: Using Vignettes as an Instrument," *Journal of Medical Ethics* 16 (3) (September 1990): 141–145.

44. Tony Hope and K.W.M. Fulford, "The Oxford Practice Skills Project: Teaching Ethics, Law and Communication Skills to Clinical Medical Students," *Journal of Medical Ethics* 20 (1994): 229–234; Françoise Baylis and Jocelyn Downie, "Ethics Education for Canadian Medical Students," *Academic Medicine* 66 (7) (July 1991): 413–414; Alister Browne et al., "Results of a Survey on Undergraduate Ethics Education in Canadian Medical Schools," Division of Biomedical Ethics, University of British Columbia (working paper).

45. Michael Parle et al., "The Development of a Training Model to Improve Health Professionals' Skills, Self-Efficacy and Outcome Expectancies When Communicating With Cancer Patients," *Social Science and Medicine* 44 (2) (1997): 231–240; K. Szauter et al., "Teaching Professionalism in Medical Grand Rounds," *Academic Medicine* 74 (5) (May 1999): 581–582; Kathryn M. Markakis et al., "The Path to Professionalism: Cultivating Humanistic Values and Attitudes in Residency Training," *Academic Medicine* 75 (2) (February 2000): 141–149.

46. See, e.g., Donnie J. Self et al., "The Effect of Teaching Medical Ethics on Medical Students' Moral Reasoning," *Academic Medicine* 64 (1989): 755–759.

47. Daniel P. Sulmasy et al., "Medical House Officers' Knowledge, Attitudes and Confidence Regarding Medical Ethics," *Archives of Internal Medicine* 150 (December 1990): 2509–2513; Sulmasy et al., "A Randomized Trial of Ethics Education for Medical House Officers," *Journal of Medical Ethics* 19 (3)

(September 1993): 157–163; Sulmasy and Eric S. Marx, "Ethics Education for Medical House Officers: Long-Term Improvements in Knowledge and Confidence," *Journal of Medical Ethics* 23 (1997): 88–92.

48. Neil S. Wenger et al., "Teaching Medical Ethics to Orthopaedic Surgery Residents," *Journal of Bone and Joint Surgery* 80A (8) (August 1998): 1125–1131.

49. Stephen Wear, *Informed Consent, Patient Autonomy and Clinician Beneficence within Health Care* (Washington, D.C.: Georgetown University Press, 1998), 61.

50. W. B. Carter et al., "Outcome-Based Doctor-Patient Interaction Analysis," *Medical Care* 20 (1982): 550–566; J. A. Hall et al., "Meta-Analysis of Correlates of Provider Behavior in Medical Encounters," *Medical Care* 26 (1988): 657–675; P. D. Cleary and B. J. McNeil, "Patient Satisfaction as an Indicator of Quality of Care," *Inquiry* 25 (1988): 25–36; D. L. Roter et al., "Communication Patterns of Primary Care Physicians," *Journal of the American Medical Association* 277 (1997): 350–356.

51. See Jennifer Garcia et al., "A Program to Elucidate Differences in Medical Students' Communication Skills," *Academic Medicine* 72 (5) (May 1997): 427–428; Jonathan Betz Brown et al., "Effect of Clinician Communication Skills Training on Patient Satisfaction," *Annals of Internal Medicine* 131 (1999): 826. See also Delia O'Hara, "Terminal Diagnosis: Tendering the Truth," *American Medical News* (3 July 2000).On the Internet at www.ama-assn.org/sci-pubs/amnews/pick_00/hlsa0703.htm.

52. Brown et al., "Effect of Clinician Communication," 828–829.

53. Irene S. Switankowsky, *A New Paradigm for Informed Consent* (Lanham, Md.: University Press of America, 1998), 105. See also Eric J. Cassell, *Talking with Patients* (Cambridge, Mass.: MIT Press, 1985), vols. 1, 2.

54. Jay Katz, *The Silent World of Doctor and Patient* (New York: Free Press, 1984), 4–5, 207–229.

55. Ulrich, *Patient Self-Determination Act*, 9.

56. W. Levinson, "In Context: Physician-Patient Communication and Managed Care," *Journal of Medical Practice Management* 14 (5) (March–April 1999): 226–230.

57. Wear, *Informed Consent*, 179.

CHAPTER 2   POST-COMA UNAWARENESS PATIENTS

1. Ronald E. Cranford and David Randolph Smith, "Consciousness: The Most Critical Moral (Constitutional) Standard for Human Personhood," *American Journal of Law and Medicine* 13 (2–3) (1987): 233–234.

2. Paolo Cattorini and Massimo Reichlin, "Persistent Vegetative State: A Presumption to Treat," *Theoretical Medicine* 18 (1997): 270.

3. Council on Scientific Affairs and Council on Ethical and Judicial Affairs, "Persistent Vegetative State and the Decision to Withdraw or Withhold Life Support," *Journal of the American Medical Association* 263 (3) (19 January 1990): 428.

4. Royal College of Physicians, *The Permanent Vegetative State* (London, April 1996), 3.

5. British Medical Association, *Guidelines on Treatment Decisions for Patients in Persistent Vegetative State* (London: BMA, June 1996), repeating the 1993 guidelines. See also Derick T. Wade and Claire Johnston, "The Permanent Vegetative State: Practical Guidance on Diagnosis and Management," *British Medical Journal* 319 (25 September 1999): 841–844.

6. Klaus Berek et al., "Euthanasia, Physician-Assisted Suicide, and Persistent Vegetative State," *Lancet* 348 (24 August 1996): 549.

7. Andrew Grubb et al., *Doctors' Views on the Management of Patients in Persistent Vegetative State (PVS): a UK Study* (London: Centre of Medical Law and Ethics, King's College, 1997), 14.

8. Multi-Society Task Force on PVS, "Medical Aspects of the Persistent Vegetative State," *New England Journal of Medicine* 330 (21) (26 May 1994): 1499–1508.

9. Sheila A. M. McLean, "Legal and Ethical Aspects of the Vegetative State," *Journal of Clinical Pathology* 52 (1999): 490–493. Sandra Horton writes that "the difference between coma and vegetative state is that coma appears to have gradations, whereas PVS is a 'permanent' state of unawareness." See Horton, "Persistent Vegetative State: What Decides the Cut-off Point?," *Intensive and Critical Care Nursing* 12 (February 1996): 41.

10. Cf. statements of Safar and Meisel in "Philosophical, Ethical and Legal Aspects of Resuscitation Medicine. III. Discussion," *Critical Care Medicine* 16 (10) (1988): 1069, 1074.

11. Cf. Hastings Center, *Guidelines on the Termination of Life-Sustaining Treatment and the Care of the Dying* (Bloomington: Indiana University Press, 1987), 112; Task Force on Ethics of the Society of Critical Care Medicine, "Consensus Report on the Ethics of Forgoing Life-Sustaining Treatments in the Critically Ill," *Critical Care Medicine* 18 (1990): 1435–1439; Robert D. Truog et al., "The Problem with Futility," *New England Journal of Medicine* 326 (23) (1992): 1563. For a critical review of this approach, see S. J. Youngner, "Futility in Context," *Journal of the American Medical Association* 264 (10) (1990): 1295–1296.

12. J. C. Hackler and F. C. Hiller, "Family Consent to Orders Not to Resuscitate, Reconsidering Hospital Policy," *Journal of the American Medical Association* 264 (10) (1990): 1281–1283; Gaetano F. Molinari, "Persistent Vegetative State, Do Not Resuscitate . . . and Still More Words Doctors Use," *Journal of the Neurological Sciences* 102 (1991): 125–127.

13. Gastone G. Celesia, "Persistent Vegetative State: Clinical and Ethical Issues," *Theoretical Medicine* 18 (1997): 222–233.

14. Charles L. Sprung and Leonid A. Eidelman, "Judicial Intervention in Medical Decision-making: A Failure of the Medical System?," *Critical Care Medicine* 24 (5) (1996): 730. Sprung and Eidelman note that one study showed that outpatients refused life-sustaining treatments in the case of persistent vegetative state in 85 percent of their responses. I assume that most of them are not aware of the possibility, meager as it is, of returning to some form of life.

15. Cranford and Smith, "Consciousness," 242. See also L. J. Nelson and R. E. Cranford, "Michael Martin and Robert Wendland: Beyond the Vegetative State," *Journal of Contemporary Health Law and Policy* 15 (1999): 427–453; G. A. den Hartogh, "Self-Determination and Compassion in the Dutch Euthanasia-Debate," *Rekenschap* 39 (2) (1992): 115.

16. Intractable coma is defined as an obstinate, difficult-to-control state of profound unconsciousness from which one cannot be roused. See *Stedman's Medical Dictionary*, 4th unabridged lawyers' ed. (Washington, D.C.: Jefferson Law Book Co., 1976).

17. In another essay Cranford drew a distinction between the vegetative and the minimally conscious state. However, it seems that Cranford believes that the distinction makes sense analytically and medically, in terms of prognosis, but he does not really think that it makes any difference at the practical level. See Ronald E. Cranford, "The Vegetative and Minimally Conscious States: Ethical Implications," *Geriatrics* 53 (supp. 1) (1998): S70–S73.

18. Chris Borthwick, "The Permanent Vegetative State: Ethical Crux, Medical Fiction?," *Issues in Law and Medicine* 12 (2) (1996): 178.

19. Keith Andrews, "Vegetative State—Background and Ethics," *Journal of the Royal Society of Medicine* 90 (November 1997): 594. On the problem of credible diagnosis, see the story of M.A., a twenty-four-year-old man who was involved in a car accident, as described by Davina Richardson, "To Treat or Not to Treat—PVS or Is He?," *Physiotherapy Research International* 2 (2) (1997): 1–6; and Julius Sim, "Ethical Issues in the Management of Persistent Vegetative State," *Physiotherapy Research International* 2 (2) (1997): 7–11.

20. "Position of the American Academy of Neurology on Certain Aspects of the Care and Management of the Persistent Vegetative State Patient," *Neurology* 39 (1989): 125–126. See also E. A. Freeman, "Protocols for the Vegetative State," *Brain Injury* 11 (11) (1997): 837–849.

21. "Persistent Vegetative State: Report of the American Neurological Association Committee on Ethical Affairs," *Annals of Neurology* 33 (4) (April 1993): 386–390.

22. Quite astonishingly, although Bryan Jennett recognizes the importance of these factors, he nevertheless makes an unqualified plea for letting "a vegetative patient" die by withdrawing tube-feeding. See "Letting Vegetative Patients Die," in John Keown (ed.), *Euthanasia Examined* (Cambridge, U.K.: Cambridge University Press, 1995), 170.

23. Council on Scientific Affairs and Council on Ethical and Judicial Affairs, "Persistent Vegetative State," 427. See also K. Higashi et al., "Five-Year Follow Up of Patients with Persistent Vegetative State," *Journal of Neurological Neurosurgical Psychiatry* 44 (1981): 552–554.

24. D. E. Levy et al., "Prognosis in Nontraumatic Coma," *Annals of Internal Medicine* 94 (1981): 293–301. See also Kenichiro Higashi, "Epidemiology of Catastrophic Brain Injury," in Harvey S. Levin and Arthur L. Benton (eds.), *Catastrophic Brain Injury* (New York: Oxford University Press, 1996), 26.

25. Gastone G. Celesia, "Persistent Vegetative State: Clinical and Ethical Issues," *Theoretical Medicine* 18 (1997): 224.

26. For further discussion, see Gaetano F. Molinari, "Brain Death, Irreversible Coma, and Words Doctors Use," *Neurology* 21 (4) (1982): 400–402; and Bryan Young et al., "Brain Death and the Persistent Vegetative State: Similarities and Contrasts," *Canadian Journal of Neurological Sciences* 16 (4) (November 1989): 388–393.

27. See S. L. Wilson et al., "Constructing Arousal Profiles for Vegetative State Patients—a Preliminary Report," *Brain Injury* 10 (2) (1996): 112.

28. M. Keatings, "The Biology of the Persistent Vegetative State, Legal and Ethical Implications for Transplantation: Viewpoints from Nursing," *Transplantation Proceedings* 2 (3) (1990): 998.

29. See S. J. Youngner et al., "'Brain Death' and Organ Retrieval: A Cross-Sectional Survey of Knowledge and Concepts Among Health Professionals," *Journal of the American Medical Association* 261 (15) (1989): 2205–2210. For further discussion, see D. Wikler and A. J. Weisbard, "Appropriate Confusion over 'Brain Death,'" *Journal of the American Medical Association* 261 (15) (1989): 2246; and Gaetano F. Molinari, "Persistent Vegetative State, Do Not Resuscitate . . . and Still More Words Doctors Use," *Journal of the Neurological Sciences* 102 (1991): 125–127.

30. "Position of the American Academy," 125.

31. Cranford and Smith, "Consciousness," 239.

32. Author discussion with Professor Tweeddale, Vancouver (1 September 1995).

33. Tweeddale, personal letter (3 January 1997).

34. Joseph S. Alport, "Persistent Vegetative State," *Archives of International Medicine* 151 (May 1991): 855–856. For further discussion, see Celesia,

"Persistent Vegetative State," 232; Chris Borthwick, "The Proof of the Vegetable: A Commentary on Medical Futility," *Journal of Medical Ethics* 21 (1995): 206–208.

35. Kirk Payne et al., "Physicians' Attitudes about the Care of Patients in the Persistent Vegetative State: A National Survey," *Annals of Internal Medicine* 125 (1996): 106. Another survey of American neurologists found that a significant number of physicians were "uncertain" about whether PCU patients could experience pain (31 percent) and suffering (26 percent): Ibid., 108.

36. Stephen Ashwal et al., "The Persistent Vegetative State in Children: Report of the Child Neurology Society Ethics Committee," *Annals of Neurology* 32 (1992): 575.

37. Council on Scientific Affairs and Council on Ethical and Judicial Affairs, "Persistent Vegetative State," 426–430.

38. Author discussions with Dr. Sazbon (19 October 1993 and 7 November 1993).

39. Multi-Society Task Force, "Medical Aspects of the Persistent Vegetative State," in *New England Journal of Medicine* 330 (22) (2 June 1994): 1572.

40. Borthwick, "The Permanent Vegetative State," 179.

41. U. T. Heindl and M. C. Laub, "Outcome of Persistent Vegetative State Following Hypoxic or Traumatic Brain Injury in Children and Adolescents," *Neuropediatrics* 27 (1996): 94–100.

42. Ashwal et al., "Persistent Vegetative State in Children," 570–576.

43. G. A. Rosenberg et al., "Recovery of Cognition after Prolonged Vegetative State," *Annals of Neurology* 2 (1977): 167–168.

44. P. G. May and R. Kaelbling, "Coma of a Year's Duration with Favourable Outcome," *Diseases of the Nervous System* (December 1968): 837–840.

45. Nancy L. Childs and Walt N. Mercer, "Brief Report: Late Improvement in Consciousness after Post-traumatic Vegetative State," *New England Journal of Medicine* 334 (4 January 1996): 24–25. See also the correspondence on "Late Improvement After Post-traumatic Vegetative State," in *New England Journal of Medicine* 334 (2 May 1996): 1201–1202.

46. H. S. Levin et al., "Vegetative State after Closed Head Injury: A Traumatic Data Bank," *Archives of Neurology* 48 (1991): 580–585.

47. K. Higashi et al., "Five-Year Follow Up," 552–554.

48. K. Higashi et al., "Epidemiological Studies on Patients with a Persistent Vegetative State," *Journal of Neurology, Neurosurgery and Psychiatry* 40 (1977): 876–885. See also K. Higashi et al., "Five-Year Follow Up," 552–554; W. Arts et al., "Unexpected Improvement after Prolonged Posttraumatic Vegetative State," *Journal of Neurology, Neurosurgery and Psychiatry* 48 (1985): 1300–1303; Council on Scientific Affairs and Council on Ethical and Judicial Affairs, "Persistent Vegetative State," 427–428; B. Steinbock, "Recovery from Persistent Vegetative State?: The Case of Carrie Coons," *Hastings Center Report* 19 (4) (1989): 14.

49. S. Sato et al., "Epidemiological Survey of Vegetative State Patients in Tohoku District, Japan: Special Reference to the Follow-up Study After One Year," *Neurologia Medico-Chirurgicala (Tokyo)* 19 (1979): 327–333 (in Japanese). See also Andreas Kampfl et al., "Prediction of Recovery from Post-traumatic Vegetative State with Cerebral Magnetic-resonance Imaging," *Lancet* 351 (13 June 1998): 1763–1767.

50. Adam Zeman, "Persistent Vegetative State," *Lancet* 350 (13 September 1997): 797. See also T. C. Britton, "Persistent Vegetative State, " *Lancet* 350 (1 November 1997): 1324; Jack Colover, "Persistent Vegetative State," *Lancet* 350 (1 November 1997): 1324.

51. Kirk Payne et al., "Physicians' Attitudes about the Care of Patients in the Persistent Vegetative State: A National Survey," *Annals of Internal Medicine* 125 (1996): 104.

52. Author discussions with Dr. Sazbon (19 October 1993 and 7 November 1993).
53. Letter from Dr. Keith Andrews, in House of Lords, *Select Committee on Medical Ethics*, session 1993–94, vol. 3, Minutes of Oral Evidence (London: HMSO, 1994), 222; Andrews, "Vegetative State," 594.
54. Andrews, "Vegetative State," 594. Author discussion with Dr. Andrews (23 September 1997).
55. Zeev Groswasser and Leon Sazbon, "Outcome in 134 Patients with Prolonged Posttraumatic Unawareness," *Journal of Neurosurgery* 72 (1990): 81–84.
56. Leon Sazbon et al., "Course and Outcome of Patients in Vegetative State of Nontraumatic Aetiology," *Journal of Neurology, Neurosurgery and Psychiatry* 56 (1993): 407–409.
57. Ibid.
58. The hospital was founded during the 1960s through the generosity of Paula Bart, who wanted to establish a place to take care of those who reached the final stage of their lives, whose families did not or could not assist them, to enable them to die with dignity. Lichtenstaedter is run by a public fellowship. Expenses are usually paid either by various health insurance companies or by the Ministry of Health, together with the help of the families. The Lichtenstaedter fellowship mobilizes funds from private sources for the purpose of development. In the United States, an estimate of cost of care of a PCU patient in a nursing facility varies from $126,000 to $180,000 per annum. It is estimated that between $1 billion and $7 billion may be spent annually on providing medical care for PCU patients in the United States. See Borthwick, "Permanent Vegetative State," 170–171; Payne et al., "Physicians' Attitudes," 104; Higashi, "Epidemiology," 28.
59. There are recorded cases of patients who regained their consciousness after longer periods of time. One eighteen-year-old woman, who was in PCU for two and a half years following a traffic accident, progressed to a state within the following three years of being able to comprehend and communicate, and to take a considerable interest in her environment, and she was able to reestablish interpersonal relationships. An even longer period of six years in a vegetative state was described concerning a twenty-five-year-old woman who was involved in a traffic accident. After fourteen months of rehabilitation she was able to feed and groom herself, and could dress and move around with some assistance, while her speech and cognitive function improved considerably. See Keith Andrews, "Managing the Persistent Vegetative State," *British Medical Journal* 305 (29 August 1992): 486–487; W.F.M. Arts et al., "Unexpected Improvement," 1300–1303; J. Tanheco and P. E. Kaplan, "Physical and Surgical Rehabilitation of Patient after Six Year Coma," *Archives of Physical and Medical Rehabilitation* 63 (1982): 36–38. More recently, Andrews reported about a man who first showed signs of recovery more than five years after the injury. Andrews emphasized that this was the exception that should not make the rule. Keith Andrews was cited in Clare Dyer, "Hillsborough Survivor Emerges from Permanent Vegetative State," *British Medical Journal* 314 (1997): 996, and in R. Hoffenberg et al., "Should Organs from Patients in Permanent Vegetative State Be Used for Transplantation?," *Lancet* 350 (1 November 1997): 1320. The *Los Angeles Times* reported the story of Happi White Bull, who lapsed into a coma in June 1983, at the age of twenty-seven, and regained consciousness after sixteen years in December 1999. Pauline Arrillaga, "Christmas Miracle Allows Family to Reclaim Its Past," *Los Angeles Times* (12 March 2000), B1, B3.
60. Payne et al., "Physicians' Attitudes," 106–109.

61. I am well aware of the possible criticism that in a reality of limited resources it is impossible to provide expensive medical treatment that has little probability of saving or restoring life. For a detailed discussion about the economic considerations involved in this issue, see appendix.

62. For discussion of locked-in syndrome, see R. T. Katz et al., "Long-Term Survival, Prognosis, and Life-Care Planning for 29 Patients with Chronic Locked-In Syndrome," *Archives of Physical Medicine and Rehabilitation* 73 (5) (May 1992): 403–408; T. Rechlin, "A Communication System in Cases of 'Locked-In' Syndrome," *International Journal of Rehabilitation Research* 16 (4) (December 1993): 340–342; R. R. Ockey et al., "Use of Sinemet in Locked-In Syndrome: A Report of Two Cases," *Archives of Physical Medicine and Rehabilitation* 76 (9) (September 1995): 868–870; J. S. Scott et al., "Autonomic Dysfunction Associated with Locked-In Syndrome in a Child," *American Journal of Physical and Medical Rehabilitation* 76 (3) (May–June 1997): 200–203; R. Firsching, "Moral Dilemmas of Tetraplegia: The 'Locked-in' Syndrome, the Persistent Vegetative State and Brain Death," *Spinal Cord* 36 (1998): 741–743. The locked-in syndrome is described in the introduction of this book.

63. Clare Dyer, "'Vegetative' Patient Wakes up after Seven Years," *Guardian*, 16 March 1996; Keith Andrews et al., "Misdiagnosis of the Vegetative State: Retrospective Study in a Rehabilitation Unit," *British Medical Journal* 313 (1996): 13–16; discussion with Dr. Andrews and his staff (23 September 1997). See also Derick T. Wade, "Misdiagnosing the Persistent Vegetative State," *British Medical Journal* 313 (1996): 942–943.

64. D. D. Tresch et al., "Clinical Characteristics of Patients in Persistent Vegetative State," *Archives of Internal Medicine* 151 (1991): 930–932.

65. N. L. Childs et al., "Accuracy of Diagnosis of Persistent Vegetative State," *Neurology* 43 (1993): 1465–1467.

66. Letter by A. Treloar, *Lancet* 351 (17 January 1998): 212. See also Derick T. Wade, "Ethical Issues in Diagnosis and Management of Patients in the Permanent Vegetative State," *British Medical Journal* 322 (10 February 2001): 352–354.

67. People who object to sustaining PCU patients argue that the saved financial resources can be used to save other patients' lives, both in larger numbers and to provide for higher quality. This claim is disputable, because health care funding is typically not a closed system, meaning that money saved in one part of the system does not necessarily go to another part of the system (it might instead return to the taxpayers, grant higher profits for doctors, sponsor incidental departmental expenses, etc.).

CHAPTER 3 SANCTITY AND QUALITY OF LIFE IN MEDICAL ETHICS

1. The first draft of this chapter was co-authored with attorney Merav Shmueli.

2. For further discussion, see James Lindemann Nelson, "Taking Families Seriously," *Hastings Center Report* 22 (4) (July–August 1992): 6–12; *Annals of Internal Medicine* 126 (15 January 1997): 97–106.

3. See, for example, Plato, "Criton," *The Trial and the Death of Socrates* (Tel Aviv: Shocken, 1979), 57, 64 (Hebrew); Aristotle, *Nicomachean Ethics*, 1100a 5–10.

4. E. W. Keyserlingk, *Sanctity of Life or Quality of Life* (Ottawa: A Study Written for the Law Reform Commission in Canada, 1980), 18; James F. Keenan, "The Concept of Sanctity of Life and Its Use in Contemporary Bioethical Discussion," in Kurt Bayertz (ed.), *Sanctity of Life and Human Dignity* (Dordrecht, The Netherlands: Kluwer, 1996): 1–18.

5. This principle has few exceptions. See the following discussion on the Jewish stance.

6. For a critical view of the death-with-dignity concept, see Paul Ramsey, "The Indignity of 'Death with Dignity,'" *Hastings Center Studies* 2 (2) (May 1974): 47–62.

7. Some Catholics would hold that they maintain sanctity of life while allowing shortening. Cohen argues that nothing in the central Christian tradition requires extending life as long as possible. Though there is a presumption that we have a duty to nurture and preserve life, this may be overcome when treatment is useless or overwhelmingly burdensome. Cynthia B. Cohen, "Christian Perspectives on Assisted Suicide and Euthanasia," in Margaret P. Battin et al. (eds.), *Physician Assisted Suicide* (New York and London: Routledge, 1998), 336.

8. Matthew P. Previn, "Assisted Suicide and Religion: Conflicting Conceptions of the Sanctity of Human Life," *Georgetown Law Journal* 84 (February 1996): 595. For deliberation on the collapse of the Catholic prohibition of suicide, see Fr. Robert Barry, "The Development of the Roman Catholic Teachings on Suicide," *Notre Dame Journal of Law, Ethics and Public Policy* 9 (1995): 482–491.

9. Robin Gill, "The Challenge of Euthanasia," in R. Gill (ed.), *Euthanasia and the Churches* (London and New York: Cassell, 1998), 18. For selected denominational perspectives on euthanasia, see Courtney S. Campbell, "Sovereignty, Stewardship, and the Self: Religious Perspectives on Euthanasia," in Robert I. Misbin (ed.), *Euthanasia: The Good of the Patient, the Good of Society* (Frederick, Md.: University Publishing Group, 1992): 178–181.

10. Keyserlingk, *Sanctity of Life*, 11; John J. Paris and Michael P. Moreland, "A Catholic Perspective on Physician-Assisted Suicide," in Battin et al., *Physician Assisted Suicide*, 326; Patricia A. Talone, *Feeding the Dying* (New York: Peter Lang, 1996): 56–57; Encyclical Letter, *Evangelium Vitae*, addressed by John Paul II to the Bishops and Others, para. 39.

11. Patricia L. Rizzo, "Euthanasia, Compassion in Dying v. State of Washington and Quill v. Vacco," *DePaul Journal of Health Care Law* 1 (winter 1996): 244. See also "Introduction," Encyclical Letter, *Evangelium Vitae*.

12. *Evangelium Vitae*, para. 57. Albin Eser, "Sanctity and Quality of Life in a Historical-Comparative View," in S. E. Wallace and A. Eser (eds.), *Suicide and Euthanasia* (Knoxville: University of Tennessee Press, 1981), 103, 105.

13. Eser, "Sanctity and Quality of Life," 103, 105.

14. Keyserlingk, *Sanctity of Life*, 11. See also Christian Medical and Dental Society Ethical Statement: Physician-Assisted Suicide, Approved by the 1992 House of Delegates, Passed unanimously (1 May 1992), St. Louis, Missouri, reported in *Issues in Law and Medicine* 8 (spring 1993): 553. According to Islamic law, God is the author of life and owns us. Since we do not own our lives, we cannot take them. Max Charlesworth, *Bioethics in a Liberal Society* (Cambridge, U.K.: Cambridge University Press, 1993), 42–43.

15. See Paul Ramsey, *Basic Christian Ethics* (New York: Charles Scribner's Sons, 1950), 249–284; Encyclical Letter, *Evangelium Vitae*, para. 34.

16. Encyclical Letter, *Evangelium Vitae*, para. 48.

17. Nathan Rotenstreich, "On the Sanctity of Life," in Yeshayahu Gafni and Aviezer Ravitzki (eds.), *The Sanctity of Life and the Defying of the Spirit* (Jerusalem: The Zalman Shazar Center for the Study of Jewish History, 1993), 27, 34 (Hebrew).

18. David Novak, *Jewish Social Ethics* (New York: Oxford University Press, 1992), 79; Novak, *Jewish-Christian Dialogue* (New York: Oxford University Press, 1989), 141; Talone, *Feeding the Dying*, 50; David E. Holwerda (ed.), *Exploring*

the Heritage of John Calvin (Grand Rapids, Mich.: Baker Book House, 1976), 209–235.

19. This is Professor John Finnis's view, espoused in Ronald Dworkin's seminar on "Abortion, Dementia and Euthanasia," Oxford University, February 1991.

20. Civil Appeal 506/88 *Scheffer v. The State of Israel*, P.D. 48 (1) 87: 116 (Hebrew).

21. Let it be noted that this principle has few exceptions. For example, three things that we must not commit even under the threat of death are idol worship, incest, and bloodshed (Sanhedrin, 74). These exceptions have specific halachic rationalizations, but the principle still is prohibition against the taking of human life.

22. Avraham Steinberg, "Euthanasia in Light of the *Halacha*," in Avraham Steinberg (ed.), *The Book of Assia* (Jerusalem: Reuven Mass, 1983), vol. 3, 424, 429–430 (Hebrew).

23. *Babylonian Talmud*, Sanhedrin 37a.

24. Cf. David J. Bleich, "Life as an Intrinsic Rather Than Instrumental Good: The 'Spiritual' Case Against Euthanasia," *Issues in Law and Medicine* 9 (2) (fall 1993): 140.

25. Shlomo Yosef Zoin (ed.), *The Talmudic Encyclopedia* (Jerusalem: The Talmudic Encyclopedia Publishing House, 1953), vol. 5, 395 (Hebrew).

26. Mishna, Shabbat, 151, 72.

27. Mishna, Smahot, 81.

28. Haim David Halevi, "Disconnecting a Patient Who Has No Chance of Surviving from an Artificial Resuscitation Machine," *Tchumin* (Alon Shevut, Israel, 1981), vol. 2, 297, 298 (Hebrew).

29. Cf. H. H. Cohn, "On the Dichotomy of Divinity and Humanity in Jewish Law," in A. Carmi (ed.), *Euthanasia* (Berlin: Springer-Verlag, 1984), 31–67.

30. Steinberg, "Euthanasia in Light of the *Halacha*," 435.

31. Ibid., 440.

32. Halevi, "Disconnecting a Patient," 298–299.

33. Maimonides, *The Laws of Murder and Preservation of Life*, II, 7.

34. Yeshayahu Leibowitz, "Medicine and Values of Life," in *Faith, History, Values* (Jerusalem: Acadmon, 1982), 243–255 (Hebrew).

35. Yeshayahu Leibowitz, "On Euthanasia," in Ruth Gavizon and Hagai Shniedor (eds.), *Human and Civil Rights in Israel—A Reader* (Jerusalem: The Civil Rights Movement, 1991), vol. 1, 179 (Hebrew).

36. Sanhedrin, 45, 1.

37. Fred Rosner, *Modern Medicine and Jewish Law* (New York: Yeshiva University Press, 1972), 120; A. Carmi, "Live Like a King: Die Like a King," in Carmi, *Euthanasia*, 3–28.

38. Civil Appeal 506/88 *Scheffer v. The State of Israel*, P.D. 48 (1) 87, 142.

39. Exodus 17 (14–16); Deuteronomy 25 (17–19).

40. *Cruzan v. Director Mo. Health Dept.* 497 U.S. 261 (1990), 111 L. Ed. 2d 224, 110 S. Ct. 2841; *Cruzan v. Harmon*, 760 S.W. 2d 408 (Mo. Banc 1988).

41. *Cruzan v. Harmon*, 432.

42. Halevi, "Disconnecting a Patient," 305. It should be noted that this view is exceptional among halachic thinkers.

43. Noam Zohar, "A Person as a Possession of God," in Daniel Statman and Avi Sagie (eds.), *Between Religion and Morality* (Ramat Gan: Bar Ilan University Press, 1993), 149–150 (Hebrew).

44. Ibid., 150–152. See also Zohar, "Jewish Deliberations on Suicide," in Battin et al., *Physician Assisted Suicide*, 362–372.

45. Keyserlingk, *Sanctity of Life*, 15–17.

46. See, for example, Daniel Callahan and Margot White, "The Legislation of Physician-Assisted Suicide: Creating a Regulatory Potemkin Village," *University of Richmond Law Review* 30 (1) (January 1996): 1–81.

47. *Cruzan v. Director Mo. Health Dept.* 497 U.S. 261 (1990), 111 L. Ed. 2d 224, 244.

48. Keyserlingk, *Sanctity of Life*, 19–21; John A. Robertson, "*Cruzan* and the Constitutional Status of Nontreatment Decisions for Incompetent Patients," *Georgia Law Review* 25 (5) (summer 1991): 1139–1202.

49. Talone, *Feeding the Dying*, 59.

50. For further discussion, see Ronald Dworkin, *Life's Dominion* (New York: Knopf, 1993), 84–89.

51. Roy W. Perrett, "Valuing Lives," *Bioethics* 6 (3) (1992): 185.

52. Ibid., 187.

53. Helga Kuhse, *The Sanctity of Life Doctrine in Medicine* (Oxford, U.K.: Clarendon Press, 1987), 211–213; Helga Kuhse and Peter Singer, *Should the Baby Live? The Problem of Handicapped Infants* (Oxford, U.K.: Oxford University Press, 1985), 123. For further discussion, see John Harris, *The Value of Life* (London: Routledge and Keagan Paul, 1985); Paula Boddington and Tessa Podpadec, "Measuring Quality of Life in Theory and in Practice: A Dialogue Between Philosophical and Psychological Approaches," *Bioethics* 6 (3) (1992): 201–217; E. Haavi Morreim, "The Impossibility and the Necessity of Quality of Life Research," *Bioethics* 6 (3) (1992): 218–232; Klemens Kappel and Peter Sandoe, "Qalys, Age and Fairness," *Bioethics* 6 (4) (1992): 297–316; Lakshmipathi Chelluri et al., "Intensive Care For Critically Ill Elderly: Mortality, Costs, and Quality of Life," *Archives of Internal Medicine* 155 (22 May 1995): 1013–1022.

54. The vitalist scholars do not accept this view. For them the mere biological existence of human life is important.

55. Peter Singer, *Practical Ethics* (Cambridge, U.K.: Cambridge University Press, 1993), 2nd ed., 83.

56. Helga Kuhse, "Quality of Life and the Death of 'Baby M,'" *Bioethics* 6 (3) (1992): 250.

57. Peter Singer repeats these statements in his article "All Animals Are Equal," in Peter Singer (ed.), *Applied Ethics* (Oxford, U.K.: Oxford University Press, 1986), 222; and in *Practical Ethics*, 88.

58. According to Kuhse and Singer, infants are not persons. They only have a potential to become persons. Thus Singer argues that if a train instantly killed an infant, the death would not have been contrary to the interests of the infant, because the infant would never have had the concept of existing over time. To have a right to life, according to Singer, one must have, or at least at one time have had, the concept of having a continued existence. Singer, *Practical Ethics*, 98.

59. Ibid., 89–90.

60. Ibid., 105–107.

61. Ibid., 107. For further discussion, see David Wiggins, *Sameness and Substance* (Oxford, U.K.: Basil Blackwell, 1980), 169–175.

62. Kuhse, *Sanctity of Life Doctrine*, 211–213.

63. For a different perspective defending a more comprehensive framework of rights for animals, see Tom Regan, *The Case for Animal Rights* (London and New York: Routledge, 1988), 2nd ed. See also Robert Nozick, *Anarchy, State, and Utopia* (New York: Basic Books, 1974), 35–45.

64. R. S. Downie and Elizabeth Telfer, *Caring and Curing* (London and New York: Methuen, 1980), 39–40. For further discussion on the concept of the person, see Ludger Honnefflder, "The Concept of a Person in Moral Philosophy," in Bayertz, *Sanctity of Life*, 139–160.

65. Downie and Telfer, *Caring and Curing*, 46.
66. Joseph Fletcher, "Indicators of Humanhood: A Tentative Profile of Man," *Hastings Center Report* 2 (1972): 1–4.
67. Cf. Alan D. Shewmon, "Active Voluntary Euthanasia: A Needless Pandora's Box," *Issues in Law and Medicine* 3 (3) (winter 1987): 237.
68. Kuhse and Singer, *Should the Baby Live?*, 120; and Kuhse, *Sanctity of Life Doctrine*, 211–213.
69. See David Heyd, *Genethics* (Berkley: University of California Press, 1992), in which he contends that coming to life is neither a harm nor a gift. The quality of life of the prospective subject cannot play any role in the decision whether to bring him or her to life. Heyd maintains that the existence of people with "restricted lives" can no more be considered "intrinsically undesirable" than the existence of happy people can be considered intrinsically desirable (109–110).
70. We distinguish between gross and soft paternalism. Gross paternalism does not involve the person in question to any extent in the decision-making regarding treatment. Soft paternalism takes some consideration of the patient's view in the decision-making, but the doctors have the final say with regard to the question of what would serve the patient's best interests.
71. Cf. Warren T. Reich (ed.), *Encyclopedia of Bioethics* (New York: The Free Press, 1978), vol. 4, 1749, 1784.
72. This responsibility has been recognized and repeated in U.S. court decisions. See for example *Superintendent of Belchertown v. Saikewicz* Mass 370 N.E. 2d. 417 (1977), at 426; *In re Conroy*, 486 A.2d 1209, 1223 (N.J. 1985). For general discussion, see James Jr. Bopp, "Is Assisted Suicide Constitutionally Protected?," *Issues in Law and Medicine* 3 (2) (fall 1987): 132–133; Sanford H. Kadish, "Letting Patients Die: Legal and Moral Reflections," *California Law Review* 80 (1992): 863.
73. Kuhse and Singer, *Should the Baby Live?*, v.
74. Ibid., ch. 6.
75. In his comments on this chapter, Peter Singer wrote that he and Kuhse explicitly say that parents should be the ones who choose whether their disabled infant lives or dies. If they choose that the infant should live, "then we think it should get more resources to help it live a good life than most societies presently give to disabled children and adults." Personal communication (14 February 2000).
76. Kuhse and Singer, *Should the Baby Live?*, ch. 5.
77. Ibid., 99.
78. Ibid., 107.
79. Ibid., 108.
80. Singer writes: "When the death of a defective infant will lead to the birth of another infant with better prospects of a happy life, [Could we know this for certain when we kill the infant?—RCA] the total amount of happiness will be greater if the defective infant is killed. The loss of happy life for the first infant is outweighed by the gain of a happier life for the second. Therefore, if killing the haemophiliac infant has no adverse effect on others, it would, according to the total view, be right to kill him." *Practical Ethics*, p. 134. Singer's utilitarian ethics holds that humanity should strive for the greatest possible happiness for the greatest number of people. He is trying to lay down rules for human behavior that are divorced from emotion and intuition. Yet when his mother fell ill with Alzheimer's disease, Singer hired a team of home health care aides to look after her. When asked how he reconciled this with his writing that we ought to do what is morally right without regard to proximity or family relationships, Singer an-

swered: "I think this has made me see how the issues of someone with these kinds of problems are really very difficult. . . . Perhaps it is more difficult than I thought before, because it is different when it's your mother." Cf. Michael Specter, "The Dangerous Philosopher," *New Yorker* (6 September 1999), 55. See also Peter Berkowitz, "Other People's Mothers," *New Republic* (10 January 2000): 27–37.

81. Kuhse and Singer, *Should the Baby Live?*, 110–111. See the same method exhibited in their discussion, 131–136.

82. See Kuhse and Singer, *Should the Baby Live?*, 123.

83. Ibid., 160. See also Kuhse, *Sanctity of Life Doctrine*, 218.

84. Ibid., 204–218; Kuhse and Singer, *Should the Baby Live?*, 160–161.

85. *Should the Baby Live?*, 122–123. Singer explains that infants lack rationality, autonomy, and self-consciousness. Therefore killing them cannot be equated with killing older human beings. Instead, the principles that govern the wrongs of killing nonhuman animals that are sentient, but not rational or self-conscious, apply to them. *Practical Ethics*, 182–183.

86. Ibid., 118. For further critique of Singer's views, see Jan C. Joerden, "Peter Singer's Theories and Their Reception in Germany," in R. Cohen-Almagor (ed.), *Medical Ethics at the Dawn of the 21st Century* (New York: New York Academy of Sciences, 2000), 150–156.

87. Opening Procedure (Tel Aviv) 1141/90 *Eyal v. Dr. Wilensky and Others*, 1991 (3) 187, 199.

88. See Dworkin, *Life's Dominion*, 222–229.

89. *Cruzan v. Director Mo. Health Dept.* 497 U.S. 261 (1990), 251.

90. See Victor Frankel, *Man's Search for Meaning* (Tel Aviv: Dvir, 1981), 95–106 (Hebrew).

91. Andrew Devine, age thirty, was injured in the 1989 Hillsborough disaster when one of the gates of the soccer stadium collapsed. He was diagnosed as a "vegetable" with no chance of recovery. His family insisted on keeping him alive. In March 1997, after eight years, he began to react and to communicate. See Mody Krietman, "Diagnosed as 'a Total Vegetable' and Awoke after Eight Years," *Yedioth Ahronoth* (Israeli daily), 27 March 1997, 17. A similar case occurred a year earlier. See Clare Dyer, "'Vegetative' Patient Wakes Up after Seven Years," *Guardian*, 16 March 1996.

92. *Superintendent of Belchertown v. Saikewicz* Mass 370 N.E. 2d. 417 (1977), 432.

93. See Koby Nissim, "Asking to Die," *Al Ha'mishmar* (Israeli daily), 20 August 1993. In this interview a man described how during his period of hospitalization, even though he suffered great pain, he still "felt wonderful" looking out the window and enjoying the beauty of nature.

94. Norman St. John Stevas, *Life, Death and the Law* (London: Eyre and Spottiswoode, 1961), 272. See also Paul Badham, "Should Christians Accept the Validity of Voluntary Euthanasia?," in Gill, *Euthanasia and the Churches*, 49–50.

95. Previn, "Assisted Suicide and Religion," 596. On the other hand, Cardinal Roger Mahony of Los Angeles endorsed a belief "in acting to relieve needless suffering." See Richard M. Doerflinger, "The Good Samaritan and the 'Good Death': Catholic Reflections on Euthanasia," *Issues in Law and Medicine* 11 (fall 1995): 158. For further discussion, see Talone, *Feeding the Dying*, 83–103, 107–108.

96. Miguel de Unamuno, "The Tragic Sense of Life," in *Men and Notions*, trans. A. Kerrigan, Bollingen Series 85, No. 4 (Princeton, N.J.: Princeton University Press, 1972), 224.

97. Edmund D. Pellegrino, "Doctors Must Not Kill," in Misbin, *Euthanasia: The Good*, 31.

98. Civil Appeal 506/88 *Scheffer v. The State of Israel*, P.D. 48 (1) 87, 100. We should note that in this case, the patient was a minor, and it is therefore impossible to determine what her will would have been and what she might consider dignity if she were an adult. This discussion focuses on adults who were born healthy, and according to the circumstances of their lives prior to the illness, we can appraise their will.

99. Justice Stevens in his dissenting opinion stated that the interests of Nancy Cruzan include how those whose opinions mattered to her will think of her after her death. *Cruzan v. Director Mo. Health Dept*, 497 U.S. 261 (1990), 283.

100. For further discussion, see Frederick H. Lowy, "The Ethical Professor of Medicine: Challenges for the 21st Century," and John Lantos, "Open Heart (Shiva M'Hodu)," both in Cohen-Almagor, *Medical Ethics at the Dawn of the 21st Century.*

101. Diana Crane, *The Sanctity of Social Life: Physicians' Treatment of Critically Ill Patients* (New Brunswick, N.J.: Transaction Books, 1977), 199; G. A. Meeburg, "Quality of Life: A Concept Analysis," *Journal of Nursing* 18 (1993): 32–38.

102. *In re Phillip*, 92 Cal. App. 3d 796 (1979).

103. In contrast to the *Phillip* ruling, in *Custody of a Minor* 379 NE2d 1053, 97 ALR3d 401 (1978, Mass.) the court decided that the state could intervene when the child's parents declined to administer the only type of medical treatment that evidence before the court indicated could save their child's life. And in *In re Rotkowitz* 175 Misc 948, 25 NYS2d 624 (1941) the court ordered an operation on a child's foot to arrest and correct a progressive deformity resulting from an attack of poliomyelitis, despite the fact that the father objected. For further discussion, see John C. Williams, "Power of Court or Other Public Agency to Order Medical Treatment for Child Over Parental Objections Not Based on Religious Grounds," *American Law Reports* 97 (1980): 421–426.

104. See Rebecca S. Dresser and John A. Robertson, "Quality of Life and Non-Treatment Decisions for Incompetent Patients: A Critique of the Orthodox Approach," *Law, Medicine and Health Care* 17 (3) (fall 1989): 234–244.

CHAPTER 4 PASSIVE AND ACTIVE EUTHANASIA

1. For further discussion, see Natalie Abrams, "Active and Passive Euthanasia," *Philosophy* 53 (1978): 257–263; Philip Montague, "The Morality of Active and Passive Euthanasia," *Ethics in Science and Medicine* 5 (1978): 39–45; Bruce Jennings, "Active Euthanasia and Forgoing Life-Sustaining Treatment: Can We Hold the Line?" *Journal of Pain and Symptom Management* 6 (5) (July 1991): 312–316.

2. For further discussion, see James Rachels, "Killing and Letting People Die of Starvation," *Philosophy* 54 (208) (April 1979): 159–171.

3. Daniel Callahan, *The Troubled Dream of Life* (New York: Simon and Schuster, 1993), 76. See also Paul Ramsey, *The Patient as Person* (New Haven, Conn.: Yale University Press, 1970).

4. James Rachels, "Active and Passive Euthanasia," *New England Journal of Medicine* 292 (2) (9 January 1975): 79. A similar claim is made by Michael Tooley, "An Irrelevant Consideration: Killing Versus Letting Die," in Bonnie Steinbock (ed.), *Killing and Letting Die* (Englewood Cliffs, N.J.: Prentice Hall, 1980), 56–62. For further discussion, see Sophie Botros, "Acts, Omissions and Keeping Patients Alive in a Persistent Vegetative State," *Philosophy* 70 (supp. 38) (15 July 1995): 102–106; Charles F. McKhann, *A Time to Die: The*

Place for Physician Assistance (New Haven, Conn.: Yale University Press, 1999): 100–102.

5. The same claim of self-righteousness is voiced against religious authorities that base their objection to active euthanasia on the grounds that it contradicts God's will. God and nature are applied to express the same rationale. See the discussion in chapter 3.

6. In his comments on an earlier draft of this chapter, Beauchamp argued that it is a wrong strategy to take when Callahan argues that "when we let a patient die, the illness is the agent that causes the death." This takes argument, not mere assertion, and Callahan needs to have a theory of causation to make the argument. In Beauchamp's view, the agent may be the doctor or may be the illness, or may be both. It depends on the context and on the theory of causation needed for that context. Callahan also illicitly links causation to killing, which Beauchamp would avoid or, Beauchamp maintains, "at least be very clear about what the link is."

7. Callahan, *Troubled Dream of Life*, 76–82, 103. Callahan writes "euthanasia" when he means "active euthanasia." He does not oppose passive euthanasia.

8. Daniel Callahan and Margot White, "The Legalization of Physician-Assisted Suicide: Creating a Regulatory Potemkin Village," *University of Richmond Law Review* 30 (1) (January 1996): 1–81.

9. See, for instance, Memorandum by the British Medical Association, in House of Lords, *Select Committee on Medical Ethics*, session 1993–94, Minutes of Oral Evidence (London: HMSO, 1994); Edmund D. Pellegrino, "Doctors Must Not Kill," in Robert I. Misbin (ed.), *Euthanasia: The Good of the Patient, the Good of Society* (Frederick, Md.: University Publishing Group, 1992), 27–41.

10. Most Dutch doctors are willing to perform euthanasia under certain conditions. Some of them prefer assisted suicide to active euthanasia because then they are sure that this is what the patient wants. The patients themselves are taking the lethal drugs. Fieldwork in the Netherlands (July–August 1999).

11. Some doctors believe that forgoing life-sustaining systems is more acceptable than withdrawing from them. See The Society of Critical Care Medicine Ethics Committee, "Attitudes of Critical Care Medicine Professionals Concerning Forgoing Life-Sustaining Treatments," *Critical Care Medicine* 20 (3) (1992): 321.

12. Warren T. Reich (ed.), *Encyclopedia of Bioethics* (New York: Free Press, 1978), vol. 4, 1731.

13. Ibid.

14. This example was inspired by discussions and communications with Isaiah Berlin.

15. For discussion of the hospice facility, see Joan K. Harrold and Joanne Lynn (eds.), *A Good Dying: Shaping Health Care for the Last Months of Life* (New York: Haworth Press, 1998); Anne Munley, *The Hospice Alternative* (New York: Basic Books, 1983); on the Internet at http://www.hospiceforhemlock.com/; http://www.oregonhospice.org/.

16. In a public opinion poll that was conducted in the United States in 1990, 33 percent of the interviewees said that being a heavy burden on the family constitutes a moral right to end one's life. See "Fear of Dying," *The Gallup Poll* (Wilmington, Del.: Scholarly Resources Inc., 1991), 4.

17. *Sue Rodriguez v. The Attorney General of Canada*, File No. 23476 (September 1993). For further discussion, see Eike-Henner Kluge, "Doctors, Death and Sue Rodriguez," *Canadian Medical Association Journal* 148 (6) (1993): 1015–1017.

18. In February 1993 the Second Chamber of the Dutch Parliament accepted these provisions. See Margaret P. Battin, *The Least Worst Death* (New York: Oxford University Press, 1994), 130–131. See also Sjef Gevers, "Physician Assisted Suicide: New Developments in the Netherlands," *Bioethics* 9 (3/4) (1995): 309–312, and RDMA, *Euthanasia in the Netherlands*, 4th ed. (Utrecht, The Netherlands: RDMA, December 1995).

19. See "The Netherlands: Bill on Euthanasia and Assisting Suicide in the Netherlands," *European Journal of Health Law* 5 (1998): 299–324; Tony Sheldon, "Netherlands Gives More Protection to Doctors in Euthanasia Cases," *British Medical Journal* 321 (9 December 2000): 1433; Rory Watson, "MEPs Try to Mobilise Public Opinion against Extension of Euthanasia," *British Medical Journal* 322 (17 March 2001): 638.

20. Initiative for Death with Dignity, Washington Initiative No. 119 (1991); The California Death with Dignity Act, California Proposition No. 161 (1992).

21. Defendants' Reply Memorandum in Support of Motion for Summary Judgement, *Garry Lee v. State of Oregon*, Civil No. 94–6467–HO, U.S. District Court (3 August 1995), 9.

22. The voter turnout was 57 percent. A breakdown of the results showed that the vote was 55 percent for and 45 percent against in the affluent areas. It lost in most rural counties with smaller populations. Mark O'Keefe, "Assisted-Suicide Measure Survives," *The Oregonian* (Portland), 10 November 1994, A1.

23. *Lee v. Oregon*, 869 F.Supp. 1491 (D. Oregon 1994).

24. *Lee v. Oregon*, 891 F.Supp. 1429 (D. Oregon 1995). For criticism of this court ruling, see Charles H. Baron et al., "A Model State Act to Authorize and Regulate Physician-Assisted Suicide," *Harvard Journal of Legislation* 33 (1) (1996): 14–16.

25. *Lee v. Oregon*, 107 F.3d 1382, 1392 (9th Cir. 1997).

26. Assisted suicide is a crime by statute in the following states: Alaska, Arizona, Arkansas, California, Colorado, Connecticut, Delaware, Florida, Georgia, Hawaii, Illinois, Indiana, Iowa, Kansas, Kentucky, Louisiana, Maine, Minnesota, Mississippi, Missouri, Montana, Nebraska, New Hampshire, New Jersey, New Mexico, New York, North Dakota, Oklahoma, Pennsylvania, Rhode Island, South Dakota, Tennessee, Texas, Washington, and Wisconsin. Common law forbids assisted suicide in: Alabama, Idaho, Massachusetts, Nevada, Vermont, and West Virginia. States in which physician-assisted suicide is considered a criminal act through statutes and common law are: Maryland, Michigan, and South Carolina. States without common laws or statute laws on assisted suicide are North Carolina, Utah, and Wyoming. In addition, Virginia has neither clear case law nor any statute on assisted suicide but does have a state statute that imposes civil sanctions on persons assisting in a suicide, and the Ohio Supreme Court ruled in October 1996 that assisted suicide is not a crime. Source: National Conference of State Legislatures (November 1997), reported by the Associated Press, Status of Assisted Suicide by State (5 January 1998), and by American Medical News (May 2000). For discussion on the legislative attempts to legalize PAS in ten states during 1997, see Russell Korobkin, "Physician-Assisted Suicide Legislation: Issues and Preliminary Responses," *Notre Dame Journal of Law, Ethics and Public Policy* 12 (2) (1998): 449–472.

27. *Compassion in Dying v. State of Washington* 850 F. Supp. 1454 (W. D. Wash. 1994). For further discussion, see Ronald Dworkin, *Freedom's Law* (Cambridge, Mass. Harvard University Press, 1996), 143–146.

28. *Compassion in Dying v. State of Washington*, 49 F. 3d 586 (9th Cir. 1995), 592.

29. *Compassion in Dying v. State of Washington*, 79 F. 3d 790 (9th Cir. 1996).
30. *Compassion in Dying v. State of Washington*, 96 C.D.O.S. 1507, 2.
31. Ibid.
32. *Washington v. Glucksberg*, 117 S. Ct. 2258 (1997).
33. Ibid., 2275.
34. *Schloendorff v. Society of New York Hosp.*, 211 N.Y. 125, 129 (1914); *In re Storar*, 52 NY2d 363, 420 NE2d 64, cert denied, 454 U.S. 858, 70 L.Ed 2d 153, 102 S.Ct. 309 (1981); *In re Eichner* 52 N.Y. 2d 363, 438 N.Y.S. 2d 266, 420 N.E. 2d 64 (1981); *Rivers v. Katz*, 67 N.Y. 2d 485 (1986).
35. *Quill v. Vacco*, U.S. Court of Appeals for the Second Circuit (2 April 1996), No. 95–7028, 12.
36. *Vacco v. Quill* 117 S.Ct. 2293 (1997), 2295, 2301. For analysis of *Washington v. Glucksberg*, *Compassion in Dying v. State of Washington*, and *Vacco v. Quill*, see Yale Kamisar, "On the Meaning and Impact of the Physician-Assisted Suicide Cases," *Minnesota Law Review* 82 (1998): 895–922; Cass R. Sunstein, *One Case at a Time* (Cambridge, Mass.: Harvard University Press, 1999), 75–116. For an overview of the legalization efforts of physician-assisted suicide in the United States, see Carol A. Pratt, "Efforts to Legalize Physician-Assisted Suicide in New York, Washington and Oregon: A Contrast Between Judicial and Initiative Approaches—Who Should Decide?," *Oregon Law Review* 77 (winter 1998): 1027–1123.
37. Mich. Comp. Laws Ann. 752.1027 (West Supp. 1995). See Janet M. Branigan, "Michigan Struggle with Assisted Suicide and Related Issues as Illuminated by Current Case Law: An Overview of *People v. Kevorkian*," *University of Detroit Mercy Law Review* 72 (1995), 959–960.
38. *State of Michigan v. Kevorkian*, Michigan Cir. Ct. (Oakland City), verdict 8, March 1996. Kevorkian outlines his rationale for assisted suicide in *Prescription: Medicide* (New York: Prometheus Books, 1991). For further discussion of developments in American law, see David Orentlicher, "The Legalization of Physician Assisted Suicide: A Very Modest Revolution," *Boston College Law Review* 28 (3) (May 1997): 443–475.
39. Rights of the Terminally Ill Act 1995 (NT), Section 4.
40. Ibid., Section 7.
41. Ibid., Section 8.
42. Ibid., Section 7.
43. Ibid., Section 7.
44. Ibid., Section 9.
45. Ibid., Section 9.
46. Ibid., Section 10.
47. Ibid., Section 7. For further discussion, see Simon Chesterman, "Last Rights: Euthanasia, the Sanctity of Life, and the Law in the Netherlands and the Northern Territory of Australia," *International and Comparative Law Quarterly* 47 (April 1998): 386–387; Andrew L. Plattner, "Australia's Northern Territory: The First Jurisdiction to Legislate Voluntary Euthanasia, and the First to Repeal It," *DePaul Journal of Health Care Law* 1 (spring 1997): 647–648.
48. Philip Nitschke, "Do No Harm," *Family Circle*, 1 April 1998, 126; Gay Alcorn, "First Death under NT mercy law," *The Age* (Melbourne), 27 September 1996. On Dr. Nitschke and his campaign for euthanasia in Darwin and Australia, see "Australia Has Its own 'Kevorkian,'" *Associated Press,* 11 January 1998; film *The Road to Nowhere*, Four Corners, ABC (broadcast in Australia on 8 July 1996). See also South Australian Voluntary Euthanasia Society (SAVES): http://www.on.net/clients/saves/ and http://www.protection.net.au/deliverance/index.htm.

49. See the film *Where Angels Fear to Tread*, produced by the Australian Film Finance Corporation Ltd. and Annamax Media Pty. Ltd. (broadcast on the Science Channel No. 8 in Israel on 4 November 1998).

50. Helga Kuhse, "From Intention to Consent," in Margaret P. Battin et al. (eds.), *Physician Assisted Suicide* (New York and London: Routledge, 1998), 252.

51. Darren Gray, "Doctor: I Helped 15 Patients Die," *The Age* (Melbourne), 27 November 1998. Chris Ryan, "Right-to-die Bill Pleases Doctor," *The Age* (Melbourne), 11 July 1997. Further information is available from: Hon. Secretary, SAVES, P.O. Box 2151, Kent Town, SA 5071, Australia; fax + 61 8 8265 2287. For further discussion of end-of-life practice in Australia see H. Kuhse et al., "End-of-Life Decisions in Australian Medical Practice," *Medical Journal of Australia* 166 (1997): 191–196.

52. "Experts want Switzerland as first nation with legal euthanasia," right_to_die@efn.org, e-mail sent 30 April 1999.

53. Derek Humphry and Ann Wicket, *The Right to Die* (New York: Harper and Row, 1986), 221–222; on the Internet at http://www.finalexit.org/world.fed.html.

54. "Experts want Switzerland"; "Swiss assisted suicide policy draws attention at euthanasia meeting," APF news story, 15 October 1998. I am grateful to Sylvia Gerhard for relating the information.

55. The Swiss Academy of Medical Sciences takes the view that helping a patient to commit suicide is beyond the scope of medical practice. This makes it difficult to use the law, given that the doctor is the person most qualified to give help to a terminally ill person who wants assistance in suicide. South Australian Voluntary Euthanasia Society, "DID YOU KNOW? Assisted Suicide in Switzerland," SAVES Fact Sheet No. 20, issued February 1997.

56. Article 115 of the Swiss Penal Code deals with inciting and assisting suicide. It holds: "Anyone with a selfish motive who incites a person to commit suicide or who helps that person to commit suicide, if the suicide is consummated or attempted, will be punished by a maximum of five years reclusion or imprisonment." If there is no selfish motive, assisted suicide is legal. I am grateful to EXIT A.D.M.D. Suisse Romande for sending me the information; e-mail: exit@freemail.ch. See also http://www.exit-geneve.ch.

57. "The Practice of Assisted Suicide in Switzerland," a report by Meinrad Schaer, M.D., president of EXIT, Society for Human Dying, Switzerland; http://www.finalexit.org/swissframe.html. See also Jérome Sobel, "Assisted Suicide," EXIT A.D.M.D. I am grateful to Sandrine Rohmer for supplying this information.

58. Fact sheet based on a paper by Professor Meinrad Schaer (16 December 1996), published by the South Australian Voluntary Euthanasia Society. The data were verified by Derek Humphry (personal correspondence on 4 January 1999), who said that there has never been a prosecution for abuse of the law. Further information is available at: Exit A.D.M.D. Suisse Romande, C.P. 100, 1222 Vesenaz, Geneva, Switzerland. Telephone: 41–22–735–7760; fax: 41–22–735–7765; EXIT/Vereinigung fr humanes Sterben (German-speaking) Feldeggstraase 3, P.O. Box 309, CH-8034 Zurich, Switzerland. Telephone: 41–1–383 33 53; fax: 41–1–383 33 78.

59. Luc Deliens et al., "End-of-Life Decisions in Medical Practice in Flanders, Belgium: A Nationwide Survey," *Lancet* 356 (25 November 2000): 1806–1811.

60. *R. v. Adams*, *Criminal Law Review* (1957): 365–377.

61. See "GMC Tempers Justice with Mercy in Cox Case," *British Medical Journal* 305 (November 1992): 1311.

62. *Bolam v. Friern Hospital Management Committee* (1957), 2 All ER 118.

63. *F v. West Bershire Health Authority* (1989) 2 All ER 545, 546. See also *In Re J* (1990) 3 All ER 930.

64. *In Re J*, 938.

65. *Airedale NHS v. Bland* (1993) 1 All ER 821.

66. Ibid.

67. Ibid., 894. For further discussion, see *Law Hospital NHS Trust v. Lord Advocate and Others*, Court of Session: Inner House (First Division) (22 March 1996), Inner House Cases; Joan Loughrey, "Medical Decision Making and the Human Rights Act 1998," *Proceedings of the 13th World Congress on Medical Law* (Helsinki, 6–10 August 2000), vol. 2: 687–695.

68. Gary Edwards and Josephine Mazzuca, "Three Quarters of Canadians Support Doctor-Assisted Suicide," Gallup News Service, 24 March 1999. See also Frederick H. Lowy et al., *Canadian Physicians and Euthanasia* (Ottawa: Canadian Medical Association, 1993), 3.

69. *Nancy B. v. Hotel-Dieu de Québec et al.* (1992), 86 DLR (4th) 385 (Que Sup Ct). For criticism of this ruling, see Arthur Fish and Peter A. Singer, "Nancy B.: The Criminal Code and Decisions to Forgo Life-sustaining Treatment," *Canadian Medical Association Journal* 147 (September 1992); 637–642; Bernard M. Dickens, "Medically Assisted Death: *Nancy B. v. Hotel-Dieu de Québec*," *McGill Law Journal* 38 (4) (October 1993): 1053–1070.

70. For general discussions concerning the progressive neuromuscular disease amyotrophic lateral sclerosis (ALS) and assisted suicide, see the 1 October 1998 issue of the *New England Journal of Medicine*; on the Internet at http//:www.nejm.org.

71. (Tel Aviv) 1141/90 *Benjamin Eyal v. Dr. Nachman Willensky and Others* 51 (3): 187, 192.

72. R.S.C. 1985, c. C-46.

73. For a critical discussion, see Lorraine Eisenstat Weinrib, "The Body and the Body Politic: Assisted Suicide under the Canadian Charter of Rights and Freedoms," *McGill Law Journal* 39 (1994): 619–644; Jerome E. Bickenbach, "Disability and Life-Ending Decisions," in Battin et al., *Physician Assisted Suicide*, 123–132.

74. Personal discussion at the Canadian Supreme Court, Ottawa (28 September 1998). In 1997, Robert Latimer was convicted of second-degree murder for the mercy killing of his severely disabled daughter. In January 2001, the Supreme Court of Canada upheld Latimer's life sentence. See http://www.abilityinfo.com/latimer.html.

75. For further discussion of the role of the media in covering such matters, see E. Haavi Morreim, "Bioethics and the Press," *Journal of Medicine and Philosophy* 24 (2) (April 1999): 103–107; Albert Rosenfeld, "The Journalist's Role in Bioethics," *Journal of Medicine and Philosophy* 24 (2) (April 1999): 108–129; Martyn Evans, "Bioethics and the Newspapers," *Journal of Medicine and Philosophy* 24 (2) (April 1999): 164–180.

76. Province of British Columbia, Ministry of Attorney General, B.C. Coroners Service, "Judgement of Inquiry into the death of Susan Jane Rodriguez" (12 February 1994). I thank Chief Coroner J. V. Cain for sending me the report.

77. Discussion with Margo Somerville (18 September 1998). See also Margaret A. Somerville, "Euthanasia in the Media: Journalists' Values, Media Ethics and 'Public Square' Messages," *Humane Health Care International* 13 (1) (spring 1997): 17–20; Margaret A. Somerville, "'Death Talk' in Canada: The *Rodriguez* Case," *McGill Law Journal* 39 (1994): 602–617.

78. Somerville, "Euthanasia in the Media," 20.

79. Ronald Dworkin, *Life's Dominion* (New York: Knopf, 1993): 201–213.

CHAPTER 5   WHAT INTERESTS DO WE HAVE?

1. A Do Not Resuscitate (DNR) order is a directive by a physician to withhold cardiopulmonary resuscitation in the event that a patient experiences cardiac or respiratory arrest.
2. Ronald Dworkin, *Life's Dominion* (New York: Knopf, 1993), 201–213.
3. Bernard Williams, "Persons, Character and Morality," in Williams, *Moral Luck* (Cambridge, U.K.: Cambridge University Press, 1981), 1–19.
4. Dworkin, *Life's Dominion*, 71–84. For a different view, see David Heyd's critique of *Life's Dominion* in *European Journal of Philosophy* 3 (1995): 105–109. A further distinction can be made between objective and subjective values: Objective values are values we all share and support, such as knowledge, love, and friendship; subjective values are connected to certain "significant others" with whom people identify: country, ethnic affiliation, etc.
5. Dworkin, *Life's Dominion*, 236.
6. Ibid., 210.
7. Ibid., 215.
8. Cf. *Airedale NHS v. Bland* (1993) 1 All ER 821, 870.
9. For instance, Dworkin, *Life's Dominion*, 180, 230–232.
10. Ibid., 232.
11. Alzheimer's disease is the prototypical dementia, the most common neurological disease of adult life, affecting four million people in the United States alone. See Arthur R. Derse, "Making Decisions About Life-Sustaining Medical Treatment in Patients with Dementia: The Problem of Patient Decision-Making Capacity," *Theoretical Medicine and Bioethics* 20 (1) (January 1999): 59.
12. Dworkin, *Life's Dominion*, 226–233. For further discussion that supports Dworkin's view on Margo's precedent autonomy, see Michael J. Newton, "Precedent Autonomy: Life-Sustaining Intervention and the Demented Patient," *Cambridge Quarterly of Healthcare Ethics* 8 (1999): 189–199. For critique of Dworkin's position, see Agnieszka Jaworska, "Respecting the Margins of Agency: Alzheimer's Patients and the Capacity to Value," *Philosophy and Public Affairs* 28 (2) (1999): 105–138.
13. Dworkin, *Life's Dominion*, ch. 8. For further discussion, see John Harris, "Euthanasia and the Value of Life," in John Keown (ed.), *Euthanasia Examined* (Cambridge, U.K.: Cambridge University Press, 1995), 12–19; John Finnis, "The Fragile Case for Euthanasia: A Reply to John Harris," Ibid., 50–53.
14. Following Dworkin, let us suppose that a person reaches an irreversible stage where she is able to enjoy only a small number of things, like the taste of ice cream and the smell of lilies, and nothing else. From her previous directives it is understood that when she was competent she thought that this sparse kind of pleasure was not worth living for. However, current evidence indicates that upon reaching the stage of permanent dementia, this patient, who now leads a nonautonomous life, nevertheless hangs on to life and finds pleasure in those things that had no importance for her in the past. It seems that her world is filled with joy when she eats ice cream or smells fresh lilies, and she now gives no indication that she wants to depart from life. In such a case, the patient's present priorities should play the role of trump card to win over past considerations.
15. An advance directive (AD) is a document that allows patients to describe the life-sustaining treatments they want and to designate whom they want to make these decisions for them. In the United States, more than forty states have enacted legislation supporting the use of ADs. For further discussion, see Joseph J. Fins, "The Patient Self-Determination Act and Patient-Physician

Collaboration in New York State," *New York State Journal of Medicine* 92 (November 1992): 489–493; Nitsa Kohut and Peter A. Singer, "Advance Directives in Family Practice," *Canadian Family Physician* 39 (May 1993): 1087–1093; Maarthen Reinders and Peter A. Singer, "Which Advance Directive Do Patients Prefer?," *Journal of General Internal Medicine* 9 (January 1994): 49–51; Dallas M. High, "Families' Roles in Advance Directives," *Hastings Center Report*, special supplement (November–December 1994): S16–S18; Stuart Hornett, "Advance Directives: A Legal and Ethical Analysis," in Keown, *Euthanasia Examined*, 297–314; Hans-Martin Sass et al. (eds.), *Advance Directives and Surrogate Decision Making in Health Care* (Baltimore: Johns Hopkins University Press, 1998); Lawrence P. Ulrich, *The Patient Self-Determination Act* (Washington, D.C.: Georgetown University Press, 1999), 219–251; David Degarzia, "Advance Directives, Dementia, and 'The Someone Else' Problem," *Bioethics* 13 (5) (1999): 373–391; D. William Molloy et al., "Systematic Implementation of an Advance Directive Program in Nursing Homes," *Journal of the American Medical Association* 283 (11) (15 March 2000); and Joan M. Teno, "Advanced Directives for Nursing Home Residents," *Journal of the American Medical Association* 283 (11) (15 March 2000), on the Internet at http://jama.ama-assn.org/issues/v283n11/toc.html; Paul Biegler et al., "Determining the Validity of Advance Directives," *Medical Journal of Australia* 172 (2000): 545–548.

16. See *In the Matter of Roche*, 296 N.J.Super. 583, 687 A.2d 349 (3 September 1996).

17. Keith Andrews, "Euthanasia in Chronic Severe Disablement," *British Medical Bulletin* 52 (2) (1996): 287. Author discussion with Dr. Andrews (23 September 1997).

18. Andrews, "Euthanasia," 287.

19. Ibid.

20. We should be aware of the possibility of abuse. The emphasis is on the competency of the patient. Dementia is a condition of progressive deterioration, and we should not honor living wills signed at the early stage of the dementia, when their content might be influenced by partisan interests of family members who would manipulate the patient into signing a document that he or she does not really endorse.

21. John A. Robertson, "Second Thoughts on Living Wills," *Hastings Center Report* 21 (6) (November–December 1991): 7. On the status of living wills in the United States, Great Britain, Canada, Australia, New Zealand, and Denmark, see Alexander Morgan Capron, "Advance Directives," in Helga Kuhse and Peter Singer (eds.), *A Companion to Bioethics* (Oxford, U.K.: Blackwell, 1998), 262–270.

22. Robertson, "Second Thoughts," 6–9. Childress stresses the necessity to continue to appraise a person's degree of autonomy over time to determine whether he or she is autonomously revoking previous consents or dissents. He maintains that for patients who have never been autonomous or for previously autonomous patients whose prior preferences and values cannot be reliably traced, it is more defensible to rely on a best-interests standard, based on nonmaleficence and beneficence, rather than on a substituted-judgment standard, based on autonomy. Childress categorically asserts that the standard of substituted judgment should be rejected in such situations as an illegitimate fiction. Cf. James F. Childress, "The Place of Autonomy in Bioethics," *Hastings Center Report* 20 (1) (January–February 1990): 12–17. Kadish argues that an advance competent choice has force, but not the conclusive moral force of a contemporary choice and not so much force as to preclude consideration of the possibly conflicting experiential interests of

the patient. Sanford H. Kadish, "Letting Patients Die: Legal and Moral Reflections," *California Law Review* 80 (1992): 857–888.

23. Robertson, "Second Thoughts," 8.

24. Dworkin, *Life's Dominion*, ch. 8.

25. Ibid., 231. For further discussion on dementia, see Piero Antuono and Jan Beyer, "The Burden of Dementia: A Medical and Research Perspective," *Theoretical Medicine and Bioethics* 20 (1) (January 1999): 3–13.

26. Edmund D. Pellegrino, "Doctors Must Not Kill," in Robert I. Misbin (ed.), *Euthanasia: The Good of the Patient, the Good of Society* (Frederick, Md.: University Publishing Group, 1992), 30. See also Herbert Hendin, *Seduced by Death* (New York: W. W. Norton, 1997), 25.

27. Author discussions with Dr. Susak (19 October and 7 November 1993).

28. Fieldwork in Lichtenstaedter Hospital, November–December 1993.

29. Personal communication (8 October 1999).

30. Personal letter from Dr. Keith Andrews (12 November 1999).

31. Series of interviews held in Canada during August–September 1995. At the 10th World Congress on Medical Law (Jerusalem, 28 August–1 September 1994), Dr. Holloway said that according to the Attorney of Queensland, only a handful of cases of patients had ever requested withdrawal of machines. A pending question that deserves separate (preferably comparative) analysis concerns the number of patients wishing to die.

32. Personal communication (8 October 1999).

33. Paul van der Maas et al., "Euthanasia, Physician-Assisted Suicide, and Other Medical Practices Involving the End of Life in the Netherlands, 1990–1995," *New England Journal of Medicine* 335 (22) (28 November 1996): 1700; Gerrit K. Kimsma and Evert van Leeuwen, "Euthanasia and Assisted Suicide in the Netherlands and the USA: Comparing Practices, Justifications and Key Concepts in Bioethics and Law," in David C. Thomasma et al. (eds.), *Asking to Die* (Dordrecht, The Netherlands: Kluwer, 1998), 46–50.

34. We might disregard some relevant data required for making a decision, either because we do not acknowledge its relevance, or because its meaning is incomprehensible. Sometimes we may find it preferable to ignore some facts because they conflict with beliefs that we are not willing to yield. Nevertheless, we are still said to be autonomous. We are not coerced into choosing one alternative over another. Our ability (or lack of it) as deciding agents might restrain us from taking the best alternative available. Yet from our point of view, we are taking the best one that we can possibly conceive of, given our inherent deficiencies. Choosing the best option or thinking correctly is not a requirement for autonomy so long as the person exercises careful judgment in assessing the alternatives. The emphasis is not on deciding the "best" options, or on holding the "true" opinions, but on the way in which we come to make the decisions and to hold our opinions. See R. Cohen-Almagor, *The Boundaries of Liberty and Tolerance* (Gainesville: University Press of Florida, 1994), 11–15.

35. Robert G. Twycross, "Where There Is Hope, There Is Life: A View From the Hospice," in Keown, *Euthanasia Examined*, 141.

36. Ezekiel J. Emanuel et al., "Euthanasia and Physician-Assisted Suicide: Attitudes and Experiences of Oncology Patients, Oncologists, and the Public," *Lancet* 347 (29 June 1996): 1809.

37. *Cruzan v. Director Mo. Health Dept.*, 497 U.S. 261. (1990), 111 L.Ed 2d 224, 110 S.Ct. 2841, 245.

38. Ronald Dworkin, "The Right to Death," *New York Review of Books* 38 (3) (1991): 14, 16. For further critique, see Martha Minow, "The Role of Families in Medical Decisions," *Utah Law Review* 1 (1) (1991), 2–13, 16–17.

39. Dworkin, *Life's Dominion*, 199.
40. American courts respect living wills when they are signed. In *Saunders v. State* (129 Misc. 2d 45, 492 N.Y.S.2d 510, S.Ct. 1985), the court considered the issue of living wills, arguing that a living will constitutes an informed medical consent statement; it is highly persuasive evidence, a clear and convincing demonstration of a patient's wishes and should be given great weight by hospital authorities. In *In re Application of Kruczlnicki* (IAS No. 56/1–89–0077, N.Y. Sup. Ct. 1989), the court directed the removal of life support, based on the patient's living will. In *Doe v. Wilson* (No. 90–364–II, Tenn.Ch.Ct., 16 February 1991), the right to forgo life-sustaining care was upheld following a request of a sixty-two-year-old terminally ill patient, made in oral statements and a living will. In *State of Georgia v. McAfee* (259 Ga. 579, 385 S.E.2d 651, 1989), a competent patient suffering from quadriplegia testified that he wanted to die. The court asserted that the patient should be allowed to end his life, and that he has the right to be free from pain at the time the ventilator is shut off. A similar case is *McKay v. Bergstedt*, No. 21207, 106 Nev. 808, 801 P.2d 617 (30 November 1990). In *In re Jane Doe* (16 Phila. 229, 1987), the court ordered a ventilator to be disconnected following the directives of a sixty-four-year-old competent and terminally ill patient, who communicated her wish by writing letters on the bedsheets asking that the ventilator be shut off. Oral statements were also conceived as sufficient justification for removal of life-sustaining treatment. In *Satz v. Perlmutter*, withdrawal of a ventilator was authorized, honoring oral statements made by the patient (362 So.2d 160 Fla. Dis.Ct.App. 1978). See also *In the Matter of Deel*, No. 90–CV-80, 729 F.Supp. 231 (24 January 1990); *Elbaum v. Grace Plaza of Great Neck Inc.*, 148 A.D.2d 244, 544 N.Y.S.2d 840 (1989); *Gammon v. Albany Memorial Hospital*, N.Y. Sup. Ct. (3 April 1989), competent adults have the right to self-determination, including the right to refuse life-sustaining treatment; *In re Hallahan*, No. 16338/1989, N.Y.Sup. Ct. (28 August 1989); *Tune v. Walter Reed Army Medical Hospital*, 602 F. Supp. 1452 D. D.C (1985). For further deliberation, see John D. Dolley, "Death by Right: A Call for Change to Michigan's Health Care Decisions Law," *University of Detroit Mercy Law Review* 72 (1995): 927–939; and "Appendix," Ibid., 946–958.
41. *Cruzan by Cruzan v. Harmon*, 760 S.W.2d 408 (Mo. Banc. 1988), 411; *Cruzan v. Director Mo. Health Dept*, 497 U.S. 261. (1990), 234.
42. See, for instance, *Frontline* TV program, "The Death of Nancy Cruzan," PBS Video (24 March 1992).
43. In a public opinion poll that was conducted in the United States in 1990, 20 percent of the interviewees said that they have a living will, and 75 percent said that they would like to have one at some point in the future. See "Fear of Dying," *The Gallup Poll* (Wilmington, Del.: Scholarly Resources Inc., 1991), 5.
44. Ronald Dworkin, *Freedom's Law* (Cambridge, Mass.: Harvard University Press, 1996), 135.
45. Dworkin made this point in his seminar on "Abortion, Dementia, and Euthanasia," Oxford University, January–February 1991.
46. Cf. Daniel Callahan, *The Troubled Dream of Life* (New York: Simon and Schuster, 1993); *Setting Limits* (New York: Simon and Schuster, 1987), and "Response to Roger W. Hunt," *Journal of Medical Ethics* 19 (1993): 24–27.
47. Such, for instance, was the case in *Blackman et al. v. New York City Health and Hospitals Corp.*, 173 Misc.2d 562, 660 N.Y.S.2d 643 (12 May 1997). The court held that the hospital was required to honor the patient's request to remove oral endotracheal ventilator tube.

48. As discussed in chapter 3, this is the stance of the Catholic Church. See Encyclical Letter, *Evangelium Vitae*, addressed by John Paul II to the Bishops and Others, para. 23; on the Internet at http://www.vatican.va/holy_father/john_p . . . ii_enc_25031995_evangelium-vitae_. John Finnis expressed this view in Dworkin's seminar "Abortion, Dementia and Euthanasia," Oxford University, January–February 1991.

49. Cf. Dworkin, "The Right to Death," 15.

50. For further discussion, see Lawrence J. Schneiderman and Nancy S. Jecker, *Wrong Medicine* (Baltimore and London: Johns Hopkins University Press, 1995), 63–64; Editorial, "How Living Wills Can Help Doctors and Patients Talk about Dying," *British Medical Journal* 320 (17 June 2000): 1618–1619.

CHAPTER 6   THE ROLE OF THE PATIENTS' LOVED ONES

1. For a study describing the process of family members letting go, see Valerie Swigart et al., "Letting Go: Family Willingness to Forgo Life Support," *Heart and Lung* 25 (6) (1996): 483–494.

2. Civil Appeal 506/1988. *Yael Scheffer, through Talila Scheffer v. The State of Israel* (arguments published December 1993).

3. The factors of pain and suffering (physical, psychological, and spiritual) are of crucial importance. If it became impossible to control Grace's pain and suffering (quite a rare circumstance), then she probably would not be able to enjoy the company and affection of her family. Grace's family, in turn, may come to the conclusion that, on balance, it is in Grace's best interest to depart from life.

4. Evidence about the abuse of the elderly by their relatives is reported in Clive Seale and Julia Addington-Hall, "Dying at the Best Time," *Social Science and Medicine* 40 (5) (1995): 590.

5. The strain might bring people to "get rid of" their relatives. This was the case of Roswell Gilbert, who shot his wife, Emily, twice in the head and claimed that he had done this to end her suffering. Emily suffered from osteoporosis and Alzheimer's disease. She left no written document stating a will to die. She was always neat and well dressed, wearing makeup, jewelry, and coordinated outfits. Her doctor testified that Emily could have lived for another five to ten years. She was never bedridden or completely incapacitated. On the day of the shooting, when Emily interfered yet again in one of her husband's meetings, Roswell interpreted her saying "Please, somebody help me" as a plea for ending her life. *Roswell Gilbert v. State of Florida*, No. 85–1129, 487 So. 2d 1185 (30 April 1986). Another problematic case is *In the Matter of R.H.*, No. 93–P-1267, 35 Mass.App.Ct. 478, 622 N.E.2d 1071 (17 November 1993), in which the mother of a thirty-three-year-old mentally retarded patient was vehemently opposed to the initiation of dialysis treatment for her daughter, despite knowing that her decision might lead to her daughter's death. The court rejected the substituted judgment of the mother, saying that proper consideration of the patient's expressed preferences strongly suggested her desire to enjoy and prolong life.

6. It is possible that parents play a greater role in Israel than, for example, in the United States, where parents and children frequently may live thousands of miles apart.

7. Seale and Addington-Hall found that spouses were less likely than children or some other relatives—particularly sons-in-law and daughters-in-law—to have said that an earlier death would have been better. Spouses' feelings were influenced by their concern about the loss that the death represented for them, fearing the grief of bereavement and the experience of loneliness. See "Dying at the Best Time," 591, 594.

8. In *In re Department of Children and Family Services, on behalf of Kennedy*, No. 97–2562, 698 So.2d 1382 (18 September 1997), the court authorized the performance of a surgical procedure on developmentally disabled adult quadriplegic patient against the wishes of his mother, who opposed the procedure. The court noted that Kennedy's treating physician testified that if the requested surgery "is not performed, Kennedy will die," and that "the benefits of the procedure far outweigh the risks." Since the physician's opinion was unrefuted, the court saw no reason to accept the opposition of Kennedy's mother.

9. New York Publication Health Law, quoted in *Quill v. Vacco*, U.S. Court of Appeals for the Second Circuit (2 April 1996), No. 95–7028, 12.

10. *In re Eichner* 52 N.Y. 2d 363, 378–380; 438 N.Y.S. 2d 266, 420 N.E. 2d 64 (1981).

11. *In the Matter of Charlotte F. Tavel*, 661 A.2d 1061 (2 August 1995), 1069.

12. Cf. *In re O'Connor*, 72 N.Y.2d 517, 531 NE.2d 607 (1988), 617 (Hancock J.). See also *Doe v. Wilson*, No. 90–364–II, Tenn. Ch. Ct. (16 February 1991). Oral statements were also conceived sufficient to remove life-sustaining treatment. See *Satz v. Perlmutter*, 362 So.2d 160 Fla. Dis.Ct App. (1978); *Gray v. Romeo*, 697 F. Supp. 580 D.R.I. (1988), to be discussed later in the chapter; *Elbaum v. Grace Plaza of Great Neck Inc.*, 148 A.D.2d 244, 544 N.Y.S.2d 840 (1989); *Gammon v. Albany Memorial Hospital*, N.Y. Sup. Ct. (3 April 1989).

13. *Wickel v. Spellman*, 552 N.Y.S.2d 437 (12 March 1990). See also *Hayner v. Child's Nursing Home*, RJI No. 0188015609, N.Y. Sup. Ct. (1988).

14. *In re Storar*, 52 N.Y. 2d 363, 438 N. Y. S. 2d 266, 420 N. E. 2d 64, cert. Denied 454 U.S. 858, 102 s. Ct. 309, 70 L. Ed. 2d 153 (1981).

15. *In re Michael Martin*, Nos. 99699, 99700, 450 Mich. 204, 538 N.W.2d 399 (22 August 1995).

16. *Hayner v. Child's Nursing Home*, RJI No. 0188015609, N.Y.Sup. Ct. (1988). See also *In the Matter of the Application of Morrey Barsky, as Guardian of Virginia E. Kyle*, 165 Misc.2d 175, 627 N.Y.S.2d 903 (9 May 1995).

17. In a substituted-judgment hearing, a judge attempts to decide what decision regarding treatment the incompetent patient would make if he or she were competent. Factors to be considered include the patient's expressed preferences regarding treatment, the patient's religious convictions, the impact of the decision on the patient's family, the probability of adverse side effects, and the prognosis of the patient with and without treatment. See *Guardianship of Roe*, 383 Mass. 415, 444, 421 N.E.2d 40 (1981); *Guardianship of Brandon*, 424 Mass. 482, 677 N.E.2d 114 (13 March 1997).

18. *Nancy Cruzan v. Robert Harmon*, 760 S. W. 2d 408 (1988); *Nancy Cruzan v. Director, Missouri Department of Health*, 497 U. S. 261 (1990), 110 S. Ct. 2841. For further discussion, see Martha Minow, "The Role of Families in Medical Decisions," *Utah Law Review* 1 (1) (1991): 1–24; Tom L. Beauchamp and James F. Childress, *Principles of Biomedical Ethics* (New York: Oxford University Press, 1994), 4th ed., 170–188.

19. Jeremiah Suhl et al., "Myth of Substituted Judgment: Surrogate Decision Making Regarding Life Support Is Unreliable," *Archives of Internal Medicine* 154 (1994): 94. For further critique, see John Hardwig, "The Problem of Proxies with Interests of Their Own," in *Is There a Duty to Die?* (New York and London: Routledge, 2000), 45–60.

20. *In the Matter of Marie Moorhouse*, 250 N.J.Super. 307, 593 A.2d 1256 (5 August 1991). The court relied on *Rova Farms Resort v. Investors Ins. Co. of America*, 65 N.J. 474, 484, 323 A.2d 495 (1974); *State v. Johnson*, 42 N.J. 146, 162–163, 199 A.2d 809 (1964).

21. *In re Quinlan*, 70 N.J., 355 A.2d (1976), 664.
22. As a matter of fact, Karen Quinlan did not die immediately. She continued breathing without the help of the respirator for a further nine years.
23. *In re Conservatorship of Wanglie*, No. PX-91–283, Minn. Dist. Ct. (28 June 1991), reviewed in 16 [1] MPDLR 46.
24. *In the Matter of the Welfare of Bertha Colyer*, 660 P.2d 738 (Wash. 1983). See also *In re Lawrance*, 579 N.E. 2d 32 (Ind. 1991); *In re Estate of Greenspan*, No. 67903, 137 Ill.2d 1, 558 N.E.2d 1194, 146 Ill.Dec. 860 (9 July 1990). The "best interests" standard pertains to be an objective analysis under which the benefits and burdens to the patient in treatment are assessed by the guardian in conjunction with any statements made by the patient, if such statements are recorded. In making the best interests determination, the guardian must begin with a presumption that continued life is in the best interests of the ward. Whether that presumption may be overcome depends upon a good-faith assessment by the guardian of several objective factors including the degree of humiliation, dependence, and loss of dignity probably resulting from the condition and treatment; the life expectancy and prognosis for recovery with and without treatment; the various treatment options; and the risks, side effects, and benefits of each of those options. Cf. *In the Matter of the Guardianship of L.W.*, No. 89–1197, 167 Wis.2d 53, 482 N.W.2d 60 (1 April 1992), at 86. See also *In the Matter of Sue Ann Lawrence*, No. 29S04–9106–CV-00460, 579 N.E.2d 32 (16 September 1991).
25. No 95–2719, 210 Wis.2d 557, 563 N.W.2d 485 (12 June 1997).
26. The court relied on *In re Guardianship of L.W.*, 167 Wis.2d 53, 482 N.W.2d 60 (1992).
27. *In re Daniel Fiori*, 543 Pa. 592, 673 A.2d 905 (2 April 1996).
28. Ibid., 606. See also *In re Daniel Fiori*, 438 Pa.Super. 610, 652 A.2d 1350 (17 January 1995); *In re Guardianship of Crum*, No. 404369, 61 Ohio Misc.2d 596, 580 N.E.2d 876 (19 September 1991). It should be noted that not all courts accept this line of reasoning. In *Mack v. Mack*, 329 Md. 188, 618 A.2d 744 (2 February 1993), the court said that Maryland did not permit withholding of nutrition and hydration to patient (Ronald Mack) who was in PCU. The patient's wife asked to remove artificial feeding and the court held that when no clear and convincing evidence was produced to show that this would have been the patient's choice, life-sustaining treatment should be maintained. Judge Rodowsky wrote that "sustaining Ronald and other persons like him, whose desires concerning the withdrawal of artificial sustenance cannot clearly be determined, is a price paid for the benefit of living in a society that highly values human life" (760).
29. The President's Commission for the Study of Ethical Problems and Biomedical and Behavioral Research, *Deciding to Forgo Life-Sustaining Treatment* (1983), 28.
30. John Rawls, *A Theory of Justice* (Oxford, U.K.: Oxford University Press, 1973), 209.
31. Cf. *In re Guardianship of McInnis*, No. 145869, 61 Ohio Misc.2d 790, 584 N.E.2d 1389 (1 November 1991); *John F. Kennedy Memorial Hospital Inc. v. Bludworth*, 452 So 2d 921, (Fla 1984), 926; *In re Jobes*, 108 NJ 394, 529 A 2d 434, (NJ 1987): 444–447; *In re L.H.R.*, 321 SE 2d 716, (Ga 1984), 723.
32. *DeGrella v. Elston*, No. 92–SC-756–TG, 858 S.W.2d 698 (15 July 1993).
33. Ibid., 709. A somewhat similar case is *In re Guardianship of Browning*, No. 74174, 568 So. 2d 4 (13 September 1990), in which a guardian of an incompetent patient petitioned to terminate the patient's artificial life support. The Supreme Court of Florida held that a surrogate or proxy may exercise the constitutional right of privacy for one who has become incom-

petent and who, while competent, expressed his or her wishes orally or in writing.

34. *Airedale NHS v. Bland* (1993) 1 All ER 821, at 836. Keith Andrews testified that he has encountered quite a number of relatives of patients in the vegetative state who feel that it is appropriate that artificial nutrition and hydration be withdrawn. Their argument is nearly always that the patient died at the time of the brain damage and that all they have left is the body but that they are unable to mourn. Personal letter (12 November 1999).

35. Cf. *Sidaway v. Bethlem Royal Hospital Governors* (1985) 1 All ER 643, 665–666.

36. *Superintendent of Belchertown v. Saikewicz*, Mass. 370 N.E.2d 417 (1977).

37. *In re Quinlan* 70 N.J. 10, 355 A.2d 647 (1976); *Nancy Cruzan v. Robert Harmon*, 760 S.W.2d 408 (1988); *Nancy Cruzan v. Director, Missouri Department of Health*, 497 U.S. 261 (1990), 110 S. Ct. 2841. The *Gray* decision is discussed later.

38. In her criticism of the *Saikewicz* decision, Lynn D. Wardle writes that the so-called consent of many incompetent individuals is nothing more than a shabby legal fiction, like the fiction of "separate but equal," which was adopted by the U.S. Supreme Court in *Plessy v. Ferguson*, 163 U.S. 537 (1896), and which for decades was the justification for racial discrimination as officially accepted in the United States until it was overruled nearly sixty years later in *Brown v. Board of Education*, 347 U.S. 483, 495 (1954). Cf. Lynn D. Wardle, "Sanctioned Assisted Suicide: 'Separate But Equal' Treatment for the 'New Illegitimates,'" *Issues in Law and Medicine* 3 (3) (winter 1987): 262. For further discussion, see Ira Mark Ellman, "Can Others Exercise an Incapacitated Patient's Right to Die?," *Hastings Center Report* 20 (1) (January–February 1990): 47–50.

39. *Care and Protection of Beth*, 412 Mass. 188, 587 N.E.2d 1377 (11 March 1992).

40. Ibid., 1381.

41. Ibid., 1383. See also the judgment of Justice Abrams, and the dissent of Justice Nolan in *Guardianship of Jane Roe*, 411 Mass. 512, 583 N.E.2d 1263 (6 January 1992).

42. *Care and Protection of Beth*, 1381–1382.

43. *In the Matter of Spring*, Mass. App. 399 N.E.2d 493 (1979).

44. If the conditions were different, a preferable solution may have been to relieve the Spring family from its responsibilities to Earl Spring by providing him with private nursing care.

45. Cf. John Hardwig, "What About the Family?," *Hastings Center Report*, 20 (2) (March–April 1990): 5–10. For further discussion on the role of the family, see Joseph Richman, "Sanctioned Assisting Suicide: Impact on Family Relations," *Issues in Law and Medicine* 3 (1) (summer 1987): 53–63; Bruce Jennings, "Last Rights: Dying and the Limits of Self-Sovereignty," *In Depth* 2 (3) (fall 1992): 103–118; Beauchamp and Childress, *Principles of Biomedical Ethics*, 170–181.

46. *Gray by Gray v. Romeo*, 697 F. Supp. 580 (D.R.I. 1988).

47. Such a council is necessary to prevent clashes of opinion between the medical staff and the patient's family that might lead to lawsuits. See *Causey et al v. St. Francis Medical Center and Others*, No. 30732–CA, La.App. 2 Cir. 719 So.2d 1072 (26 August 1998). For further discussion on cases of conflict between the medical staff and the patient's agents, see Lawrence J. Schneiderman et al., "Who Decides Who Decides?," *Archives of Internal Medicine* 155 (24 April 1995): 793–796.

48. Civil Appeal 506/1988. *Yael Scheffer, through Talila Scheffer v. The State of Israel* (arguments published December 1993).

49. For further discussion, see *In re Jane Doe*, No. S92A0325, 262 Ga. 389, 418 S.E.2d 3 (6 July 1992). Jane's mother agreed to a DNR order; her father did not.

50. See, for instance, *Tune v. Walter Reed Army Medical Hospital*, 602 F. Supp. 1452 D. D.C (1985); *In re Gardner*, 534 A.2d 947 (Me. 1987) (Maine); *Elbaum v. Grace Plaza of Great Neck Inc.*, 148 A.D.2d 244, 544 N.Y.S.2d 840 (1989); *Gammon v. Albany Memorial Hospital*, N.Y. Sup. Ct. (3 April 1989); *In re Hallahan*, NO. 16338/1989, N.Y. Sup. Ct. (28 August 1989); *In re Swan*, 569 A.2d 1202 (15 February 1990). Under the Maryland Health Care Decisions Act, an effective advance directive must be made in the presence of the attending physician and must be documented as part of the patient's medical record. See *Wright et al v. Johns Hopkins Health Systems Corp. et al.*, 353 Md. 568, 728 A.2d 166 (20 April 1999), 127.

51. *In the Matter of Nickolas Christopher for an Order Authorizing the Involuntary Medical Treatment of Anna Kushnir*, 177 Misc.2d 352, 675 N.Y.S.2d 807 (21 May 1998).

52. Ibid., 809.

CHAPTER 7   AN OUTSIDER'S VIEW OF DUTCH EUTHANASIA POLICY AND PRACTICE

Interviews in the Netherlands (summer 1999)

John Griffiths, department of legal theory, faculty of law, University of Groningen (Groningen, 16 July 1999).

J. K. Gevers, professor of health law, University of Amsterdam (Amsterdam, 19 July 1999).

Evert van Leeuwen, chairperson, department of metamedicine, Free University of Amsterdam (Amsterdam, 19 July 1999; Haarlem, 28 July 1999).

Dick Willems, Institute for Research in Extramural Medicine, department of social medicine, Amsterdam (Amsterdam, 20 July 1999).

Bert Thijs, director, Medical Intensive Care Unit, VU Hospital, Amsterdam (Amsterdam, 20 July 1999).

A. van Dantzig, retired expert in psychiatry (Amsterdam, 20 July 1999).

H.J.J. Leenen, formerly professor of social medicine and health law, medical faculty and faculty of law, University of Amsterdam (Amsterdam, 21 July 1999).

Gerrit van der Wal, Institute for Research in Extramural Medicine, department of social medicine, Free University of Amsterdam (Amsterdam, 21 July 1999).

Jaap J. F. Visser, Ministry of Health, department of medical ethics, The Hague (Amsterdam, 21 July 1999).

Heleen Dupuis, department of metamedicine, University of Leiden (Leiden, 22 July 1999).

Margo Trappenburg, department of political science, University of Leiden (Leiden, 22 July 1999).

Henri Wijsbek, department of medical ethics, Erasmus University of Rotterdam (Rotterdam, 23 July 1999).

Arie J. G. van der Arend, health ethics and philosophy, Maastricht University (Maastricht, 26 July 1999).

George Beusmans, Maastricht Hospital (Maastricht, 26 July 1999).

G. F. Koerselman, Sint Lucas Andreas Hospital, Amsterdam (Amsterdam, 27 July 1999).

Henk Jochemsen, director, professor, Lindeboom Institute (Ede Wageningen, 27 July 1999).

Gerrit K. Kimsma, department of metamedicine, Free University of Amsterdam (Koog aan de Zaan, 28 July 1999).

James Kennedy, Department of History, Hope College, Michigan. Visiting research fellow at the Institute for Social Research, Amsterdam (Amsterdam, 29 July 1999).

Paul van der Maas, department of public health, faculty of medicine, Erasmus University, Rotterdam (Amsterdam, 29 July 1999).

Chris Rutenfrans, *Trouw* newspaper (Amsterdam, 30 July 1999).

Arko Oderwald, department of metamedicine, Free University of Amsterdam (Amsterdam, 30 July 1999, 8 August 1999).

Barbara de Boer and her three children (Amsterdam, 2 August 1999).

Egbert Schroten, director, Center for Bioethics and Health Law, Utrecht University (Utrecht, 5 August 1999).

Govert den Hartogh, faculty of philosophy, University of Amsterdam (Amsterdam, 10 August 1999).

Johannes J. M. van Delden, senior researcher, Center for Bioethics and Health Law, Utrecht University (Utrecht, 10 August 1999).

Rob Houtepen, health ethics and philosophy, Maastricht University (Maastricht, 11 August 1999).

Ron Berghmans, Institute for Bioethics, Maastricht University (Maastricht, 11 August 1999).

Ruud ter Meulen, director, Institute for Bioethics, and professor at the University of Maastricht (Maastricht, 11 August 1999).

1. Herbert Hendin, *Seduced by Death* (New York: W.W. Norton, 1997), 23.
2. The Medical Association Executive Board emphasized that there are only limited possibilities for verifying whether suffering is unbearable and without prospect of improvement. The board considered it in any case the doctor's task to investigate whether there are medical or social alternatives that can make the patient's suffering bearable. John Griffiths et al., *Euthanasia and Law in the Netherlands* (Amsterdam: Amsterdam University Press, 1998), 66.
3. John Keown, "The Law and Practice of Euthanasia in the Netherlands," *Law Quarterly Review* 108 (January 1992): 56.
4. The Royal Dutch Medical Association's refinements of the 1984 Guidelines (25 August 1995). Cf. Marlise Simons, "Dutch Doctors to Tighten Rules on Mercy Killings," *New York Times,* 11 September 1995, A3.
5. Supreme Court of the Netherlands, Criminal Chamber (21 June 1994), no. 96.972. For translation, see Griffiths et al., *Euthanasia and Law*, Appendix II (2), 329–340.
6. On the Internet at http://www.euthanasia.org/dutch.html#remm. See also Marcia Angell's editorial, "Euthanasia in the Netherlands—Good News or Bad?," *New England Journal of Medicine* 335 (22) (28 November 1996); Adriaan Jacobovits, "Euthanasia in the Netherlands," *Washington Post*, 23 January 1997, A16; General Health Council, "A Proposal of Advice Concerning Careful Requirements in the Performance of Euthanasia" (The Hague, 1987).
7. Cf. P. J. van der Maas et al., *Euthanasia and other Medical Decisions Concerning the End of Life*, Health Policy Monographs (Amsterdam: Elsevier, 1992).
8. For further discussion, see Johannes J. M. van Delden et al., "Deciding Not to Resuscitate in Dutch Hospitals," *Journal of Medical Ethics* 19 (1993): 200–205; Tony Sheldon, "Euthanasia Law Does Not End Debate in the Netherlands," *British Medical Journal* 307 (11 December 1993): 1511–1512; Henk Jochemsen, "Euthanasia in Holland: An Ethical Critique of the New Law," *Journal of Medical Ethics* 20 (1994): 212–217; Chris Ciesielski-Carlucci and Gerrit Kimsma, "The Impact of Reporting Cases of Euthanasia in Holland: A Patient and Family Perspective," *Bioethics* 8 (2) (1994): 151–158; J.K.M. Gevers, "Physician Assisted Suicide: New Developments in the Netherlands,"

Bioethics 9 (3/4) (1995): 309–312. A recent study conducted in Belgium repeats the Dutch death-certificate study on end-of-life decisions. See Luc Deliens et al., "End-of-Life Decisions in Medical Practice in Flanders, Belgium: A Nationwide Survey," *Lancet* 356 (25 November 2000), 1806–1811.

9. Van der Maas et al., *Euthanasia and other Medical Decisions*, 41.
10. Gerrit van der Wal and Paul J. van der Maas, "Empirical Research on Euthanasia and Other Medical End-of-Life Decisions and the Euthanasia Notification Procedure," in Thomasma et al., *Asking to Die*, (Dordrecht, Netherlands: Kluwer, 1998) 171. See also Bill Mettyear, "Advocating Legalising Voluntary Euthanasia" (South Australian Voluntary Euthanasia Society, February 1997), on the Internet at http://www.on.net/clients/saves/.
11. Van der Maas et al., *Euthanasia and other Medical Decisions*, 58.
12. Ibid., 61.
13. Ibid., 62.
14. In another study among family doctors, one quarter of the physicians said that they did not ask for a second opinion before administering euthanasia or assisted suicide. Twelve percent of the GPs had no kind of consultation with any professional health worker. Cf. G. van der Wal et al., "Euthanasia and Assisted Suicide. II. Do Dutch Family Doctors Act Prudently?," *Family Practice* 9 (2) (1992): 140.
15. Van der Maas et al., *Euthanasia and other Medical Decisions*, 65.
16. Ibid., 66.
17. Henk A.M.J. ten Have, "Euthanasia: The Dutch Experience," *Annals de la Real Academia Nacional de Medicina*, Tomo CXII (Madrid, 1995), 429.
18. See 1996 Study Findings, "Euthanasia and Other Decisions Concerning the End of Life in the Netherlands," Foreign Information Department, Netherlands Ministry of Foreign Affairs.
19. Remmenlink Commission, *Rapport Medische Beslissingen Rond het Levenseinde* (The Hague: SDU, 1991), 37. See also ten Have, "Euthanasia: The Dutch Experience," 429. In his comments on the first draft of this study, Leenen wrote that the proposal of the Remmelink Commission was rejected by nearly all the Dutch commentators and also by the government. Letter (25 July 2000).
20. In his letter (5 June 1999), Dr. Chabot wrote: "After four years waiting for the final court judgment (1991–1995) and discussing the case with many people from abroad, I hope you will understand that I prefer to remain in the background now and not to make an appointment with you." He agreed, however, to answer via e-mail some specific questions relating to his conduct that brought about the charges against him.
21. My questionnaire comprised fifteen questions. The Dutch comprehensive study of 1995 consisted of 120 pages (!), and the interviews lasted for an average of 2.5 hours. The pace of questioning was, apparently, frantic. Cf. Paul J. van der Maas et al., "Euthanasia, Physician-Assisted Suicide, and Other Medical Practices Involving the End of Life in the Netherlands, 1990–1995," *New England Journal of Medicine* 335 (22) (28 November 1996): 1700.
22. Carlos F. Gomez, *Regulating Death* (New York: Free Press, 1991), 59–60.
23. In her remarks on the first draft of this chapter, Heleen Dupuis wrote: "We do not want to defend our views, nor do we want to persuade others to adopt them. We are just very weary when the hundred and umpteenth foreigner comes with questions we already have discussed the same number of times. Personally I am very tired by the endless interrogations, whereas I feel that euthanasia is a private matter, such as abortion, and even more so. I also feel that there is a certain exaggeration when it comes to the gravity of the problem." Personal communication (25 July 2000).

24. In his comments on the first draft of this study, Leenen wrote that he doesn't agree that there is a lack of criticism in the Netherlands: "We have for more than 25 years discussed euthanasia publicly and between all kinds of opinions in a good atmosphere. Nobody was excluded. I personally lectured in meetings of opponents who invited me. I don't know of a country where this is possible." Leenen maintained that gradually a kind of consensus has grown "within a majority" and the problem is that "people like Fenigsen" never took part in this debate and only ventilated their critique elsewhere. Letter (25 July 2000).

25. Gomez, *Regulating Death*. John Keown, "The Law and Practice of Euthanasia in the Netherlands," *Law Quarterly Review* 108 (January 1992): 51–78; Keown, "Euthanasia in the Netherlands: Sliding Down the Slippery Slope?," *Notre Dame Journal of Law, Ethics and Public Policy* 9 (1995): 407–448; Hendin, *Seduced by Death*.

26. This statement spurred van der Maas to react by saying: "I consider myself as an independent researcher, with a primary responsibility in collecting reliable data and basing impartial estimates and interpretations on that empirical information. I see no position for myself in a pro versus contra euthanasia debate and I think such kind of debate is entirely unproductive. As a researcher I think my responsibility is to find out what people do and how that might fit in high quality end of life medicine. During the last years part of our study has been replicated in Australia and Belgium and we have obtained funding from the European Union for an international collaborative study in order to establish empirical comparisons between countries." Personal communication (18 September 2000).

27. Keown, "Law and Practice," 68.

28. *Death on Request*, IKON, Interkerkelijke Omroep Nederland, Postbus 10009, 1201 D. A. Hilversum. I thank IKON for sending me a copy of this film. For deliberation and critique of the content of this film, see Hendin, *Seduced by Death*, 114–120.

29. G. van der Wal et al., "Euthanasia and Assisted Suicide. II. Do Dutch Family Doctors Act Prudently?," *Family Practice* 9 (2) (1992): 113, 115.

30. Bregje Dorien Onwuteaka-Philipsen, *Consultation of Another Physician in Cases of Euthanasia and Physician-assisted Suicide* (Doctoral thesis. Amsterdam: Vrije Universiteit, 1999), 29, 31.

31. Bregje D. Onwuteaka-Philipsen et al., "Consultants in Cases of Intended Euthanasia or Assisted Suicide in the Netherlands," *Medical Journal of Australia* 170 (1999): 360–363.

32. Onwuteaka-Philipsen et al., "Consultants," 360–363.

33. Henri Wijsbek reiterated this point of lenient courts saying he did not know of any prosecutions for lack of consultation, and that consultation should be "observed and complied closely." Leenen, on the other hand, wrote that it is incorrect to say that the courts are very lenient toward lack of consultation. Letter (25 July 2000). However, it is clear from the *Chabot* case that the courts do not regard consultation (except in cases of nonsomatic suffering) as an absolute requirement.

34. Jacqueline M. Cuperus-Bosma et al., "Physician-Assisted Death: Policy-Making by the Assembly of Prosecutors General in the Netherlands," *European Journal of Health Law* 4 (1997): 232.

35. In his book, Griffiths writes that 12 percent of Dutch doctors are principally unwilling to perform euthanasia and that most of them would refer a patient requesting it to another doctor. See Griffiths et al., *Euthanasia and Law*, 253. According to van der Maas et al., 9 percent of all physicians would never perform euthanasia and assisted suicide but would refer patients seeking

it to another physician. Three percent would never perform the practices or refer patients. Cf. van der Maas et al., "Euthanasia, Physician-Assisted Suicide,1990–1995," 1702.

36. Bert Thijs, Rob Houtepen, Arie van der Arend, Jaap Visser, Ruud ter Meulen, and Henk Jochemsen.

37. Leenen maintained that consultation might be a problem in small villages. But in May 1999, following SCEA, the government initiated the organization of consultation teams all over the country. Consultants will travel to small villages to examine medical files and to see patients. Hospital specialists are required to examine the files. The scheme is not fully worked out yet, and time will tell to what extent it will succeed, but Leenen thinks the consultation mechnism has gradually improved.

38. Freud recognized that doctors' unconscious has an impact on their relations with patients. Countertransference has been defined in the psychoanalytic literature as reactions in the therapist engendered by the patient. Cf. Jay Katz, *The Silent World of Doctor and Patient* (New York: Free Press, 1984), 147.

39. I have asked Paul van der Maas what the difference is between requests for euthanasia "at a later time" and requests for euthanasia "at a particular time." In response, Agnes van der Heide wrote (on 27 March 2001) that the first category generally refers to requests from persons who ask their doctor whether she would be willing to give assistance in dying in hypothetical future circumstances, e.g., when this person suffers hopelessly and unbearably and asks for such assistance. The second category refers, in turn, to requests from persons who are already in such circumstances and who ask their doctor to give assistance in dying, that is, perform euthanasia or assist in suicide, at short notice.

40. Bert Keizer, *Dancing with Mister D* (London: Black Swan, 1997), 117.

41. Interviews with Evert van Leeuwen, John Griffiths, J. K. Gevers, Dick Willems, Gerrit van der Wal, Jaap Visser, H.J.J. Leenen, Henk Jochemsen, Gerrit Kimsma, Paul van der Maas, Govert den Hartogh, and Johannes van Delden.

42. Onwuteaka-Philipsen, *Consultation*, 91.

43. Personal communication (27 August 2000).

44. Ibid.

45. As a nurse, van der Arend is dissatisfied because nurses are not represented on the committees. He believes that it would be better to have a balance of ideas before the euthanasia decision is made, by including nurses and independent physicians, and by following the rules of careful procedure in detail.

46. Cf. Gevers, den Hartogh, van Delden, Visser, as well as Leenen and Jochemsen.

47. Van Leeuwen, Griffiths, Gevers, Thijs, Houtepen, Jochemsen, van der Arend, den Hartogh, van Delden, Visser, and van der Maas.

48. District Court, Leeuwarden, 8 April 1997. Griffiths et al. argue that the facts found by the district court, involving multiple and serious failures to conform to the requirements of careful practice, seem to call for a serious medical disciplinary measure, perhaps revocation of the license to practice medicine. See Griffiths et al., *Euthanasia and Law*, 293, n. 56.

49. John Griffiths, "Effective Regulation of Euthanasia and Other Medical Behavior that Shortens Life," draft paper (14 October 1998): 10, 11; Griffiths et al., *Euthanasia and Law*, 236–237.

50. In his comments on the first draft of this chapter, Griffiths denied saying that the criminal law is "ineffective." He wrote: "I do not regard it as perfect, the imperfections are a matter of concern, and something should be done about them. As a matter of fact, something is being done: unlike other

countries, the Dutch are continually working on the adequacy of control of this sort of intrinsically dangerous medical behavior." Personal communication (10 July 2000).

51. For further discussion, see Griffiths et al., *Euthanasia and Law*, ch. 6.
52. Cf. Jacqueline M. Cuperus-Bosma et al., "Assessment of Physician-Assisted Death by Members of the Public Prosecution in the Netherlands," *Journal of Medical Ethics* 25 (1999): 8–15.
53. Sjef Gevers, Rob Houtepen, Ruud ter Meulen, Margo Trappenburg, Ron Berghmans, Henk Leenen, and Egbert Schroten.
54. Van der Maas and his colleagues stated that after performing euthanasia and assisted suicide, three quarters of the general practitioners and about two thirds of the specialists reported "natural death" in the declaration of death. The most important reasons for falsely declaring natural death were: the "fuss" of a legal investigation (55 percent), fear of prosecution (25 percent), the desire to safeguard relatives from judicial inquiry (52 percent), and negative experiences in the past with describing the cause of death as nonnatural (12 percent). Van der Maas et al., *Euthanasia and Other Medical Decisions*, 46–48. See also van der Wal et al., "Evaluation of the Notification Procedure," *New England Journal of Medicine* 335 (22) (28 November 1996), 1707; Martien Tom Muller, *Death on Request* (Doctoral thesis. Amsterdam: Vrije Universiteit, 1996), 73.
55. Most notably of Trappenburg, Wijsbek, van Leeuwen, Gevers, Thijs, Willems, and Schroten.
56. Martien T. Muller et al., "Euthanasia and Assisted Suicide: Facts, Figures and Fancies with Special Regard to Old Age," *Drugs and Aging* 13 (3) (September 1998): 190.
57. Evert van Leeuwen and Gerrit Kimsma, "Problems Involved in the Moral Justification of Medical Assistance in Dying: Coming to Terms with Euthanasia and Physician Assisted Suicide," in R. Cohen-Almagor (ed.), *Medical Ethics at the Dawn of the 21st Century* (New York: New York Academy of Sciences, 2000), 157–173.
58. This is an agency, independent of the public prosecution. Its activities may lead to disciplinary law trials.
59. Personal communication (27 August 2000).
60. In the first draft of this chapter, van Delden explained that his hesitation to disclose numbers at that time derived from the fact that these numbers had not yet been made public. He emphasized that he had "no inclination to hide anything." Personal communication (4 August 2000).
61. In his comments the first draft of this study, van Dantzig wrote that this assertion is fundamentally incorrect: "The whole of Dutch society is based on the cohabitation of people who fundamentally disagree on everything. The sometimes very creative solutions (soft drugs may not be bought by coffee shops, but their sale is not punished within certain limits) have given rise to the word 'poldermodel,' which expressly means living by compromise, or as I have once put it, the fair division of discontent. I write to you because such a fundamental misunderstanding may harm the quality of your paper." Personal communication (14 July 2000).
62. J. S. Mill, *Utilitarianism, Liberty, and Representative Government* (London: J. M. Dent, 1948), Everyman's ed., 78–113.
63. In his comments on the first draft of this essay, Griffiths reacted to this statement by writing: "Nowhere do you suggest that anywhere else there is a *better* system. The Dutch know about the system's defects and are working to improve it. Can you tell me about another country where that is true? In short, I think you need to think again, and a lot more carefully, about what

you are writing about, before you can expect to be taken seriously." Personal communication (10 July 2000).

Griffiths, it seems, finds a lot of comfort in comparative studies to the point of blurring his own careful thinking about happenings in his country.

64. In his remarks on the first draft of this study, Griffiths wrote that this assertion is "of course pretty silly." He asked: "Do you know of a single legal policy that 'works' 100%? The fact that the Guidelines are not yet effective *enough* does not mean they are having no effect at all. I would argue that the situation in the Netherlands is *much better* than elsewhere, that the difference is that here *we know* the extent to which control is not yet adequate." Personal communication (10 July 2000).

65. For discussion of the range of what "unbearable suffering" means, see Gomez, *Regulating Death*, 99–104.

66. See Griffiths's analysis in "Assisted Suicide in the Netherlands: The *Chabot* Case," *Modern Law Review* 58 (March 1995): 239–248.

67. Muller, *Death on Request*, 52.

68. For further discussion, see Jacqueline M. Cuperus-Bosma et al., "Physician-Assisted Death: Policy-Making by the Assembly of Prosecutors General in the Netherlands," *European Journal of Health Law* 4 (1997): 225–238.

69. In his comments on the first draft, van Dantzig wrote: "Please remove this, this is far from true!" Personal communication (8 July 2000).

70. The number of citizens who approve of euthanasia at the patient's explicit request grew from 40 percent in 1966 to over 60 percent (in some polls almost 80 percent) in 1993. Likewise the number of opponents decreased steadily (21 percent in 1986, 17 percent in 1989, 12 percent in 1994). Cf. Joop van Holsteyn and Margo Trappenburg, "Citizens' Opinions on New Forms of Euthanasia. A Report from the Netherlands," *Patient Education and Counseling* 35 (1998) 64. A 1998 poll indicated that 92 percent of the population supports the practice of euthanasia. Cf. "Dutch Might Legalize Euthanasia," Associated Press, 12 July 1999.

71. In his comments on the first draft, Jochemsen asked me to add that he does realize that in the present situation a simple reiteration of the prohibition would not improve the practice straight away. This would require a whole package of measures. Personal communication (5 July 2000).

72. Arie van der Arend contested my argument that there is not enough reflective thinking about euthanasia, arguing that (a) I cannot expect extensive and balanced reflective thinking during interviews with people who were busy with totally different tasks at that moment; (b) my study does not cover the extensive Dutch literature on the subject; (c) I did not interview one of the best "reflective thinkers," Beemer; and (d) that such a value judgment could have been justified only after I had compared the Dutch practice to the situation in other countries. Personal communication (3 July 2000).

73. Hendin reached a similar conclusion. Cf. Hendin, *Seduced by Death*, 100.

74. Tony Sheldon, "Netherlands Gives More Protection to Doctors in Euthanasia Cases," *British Medical Journal* 321 (9 December 2000), 1433.

75. Ibid.

76. Cf. R. Cohen-Almagor, "The Patients' Right to Die in Dignity and the Role of Their Beloved People," *Annual Review of Law and Ethics* 4 (1996): 213–232; "Reflections on the Intriguing Issue of the Right to Die in Dignity," *Israel Law Review* 29 (4) (1995): 677–701; "Autonomy, Life as an Intrinsic Value, and Death with Dignity," *Science and Engineering Ethics* 1 (3) (1995): 261–272.

77. Cf. Hendin, *Seduced by Death*, 122.

CHAPTER 8   THE OREGON DEATH WITH DIGNITY ACT

1. This chapter was coauthored with attorney Monica G. Hartman.
2. See Patrick M. Curran, Jr., "Regulating Death: Oregon's Death with Dignity Act and the Legalization of Physician-Assisted Suicide," *Georgetown Law Journal* 86 (1998): 725–726.
3. Daniel Callahan and Margot White, "The Legalization of Physician-Assisted Suicide: Creating a Regulatory Potemkin Village," *University of Richmond Law Review* 30 (1) (January 1996): 42.
4. See Initiative for Death with Dignity, Washington Initiative No. 119 (1991).
5. The California Death with Dignity Act, California Proposition No. 161 (1992).
6. Tom Bates and Mark O'Keefe, "On Suicide Measure, Oregon Is a Maverick Again," *The Oregonian* (Portland), 13 November 1994, A1.
7. U.S. Bureau of the Census, *Statistical Abstract of the United States: 1997* (Washington, D.C.: U.S. Bureau of the Census; 1997), 117th ed.; P. V. Caralis et al., "The Influence of Ethnicity and Race on Attitudes toward Advance Directives, Life-Prolonging Treatments, and Euthanasia," *Journal of Clinical Ethics* 4 (2) (1993): 157–159.
8. Bates and O'Keefe, "On Suicide Measure," A1.
9. See Mark O'Keefe, "Founding Father: Derek Humphry Began the Assisted Suicide Movement, But His Views May Be Too Extreme for Measure 16 Strategists," *The Oregonian* (Portland), 2 November 1994, A1.
10. Ibid.
11. 13 Oregon Revised Statute § 2.01 (1998).
12. Measure 16 was approved by a vote of 618,751 to 586,702 (51 percent to 49 percent). The act is codified at Or. Rev. Stat. § 127.800 et seq. For articles describing and discussing the statute, see, e.g., Mark O'Keefe, "Assisted Suicide Measure Survives Heavy Opposition," *The Oregonian* (Portland), 10 November 1994, A1; Melinda A. Lee and Susan W. Tolle, "Oregon's Assisted Suicide Vote: The Silver Lining," *Annals of Internal Medicine* 124 (1996): 267; Kathy T. Graham, "Last Rights: Oregon's New Death with Dignity Act," *Willamette Law Review* 31 (1995): 601; David M. Smith and David Pollack, "A Psychiatric Defense of Aid in Dying," *Community Mental Health Journal* 34 (1998): 547.
13. See 13 Or. Rev. Stat. § 2.01 (1998).
14. 13 Or. Rev. Stat. § 1.01 (1998).
15. 13 Or. Rev. Stat. § 2.01 (1998).
16. *Lee v. Oregon*, 891 F. Supp. 1421 (D. Or. 1995).
17. See Kim Murphy, "Voters in Oregon Soundly Endorse Assisted Suicide," *L.A. Times*, 5 November 1997, A1.
18. On the Internet at http://www.ohd.hr.state.or.us/cdpe/chs/pas/pas.htm.
19. 13 Or. Rev. Stat. §§ 3.09, 3.11 (1998).
20. For comprehensive critical discussions, see Carlos F. Gomez, *Regulating Death* (New York: Free Press, 1991); Herbert Hendin, *Seduced by Death* (New York: W. W. Norton, 1997); Cohen-Almagor, *Euthansia in the Netherlands* (forthcoming).
21. 13 Or. Rev. Stat. § 2.01 (1998).
22. See Amy D. Sullivan et al., "Legalized Physician-Assisted Suicide in Oregon—The Second Year," *New England Journal of Medicine* 342 (8) (24 February 2000): 598–604 (hereafter *OHD Report 2*).
23. "Oregon Battles Over Suicide Law," *Newsday*, 5 December 1994, A17.
24. By contrast, both of the OMA's counterparts in Washington and California had voiced strong opposition to the assisted suicide initiatives in their respective states. In addition, the Oregon Hospice Association (OHA) refused to take a firm position on the act, and the act was supported by the state's

Democratic party and a moderate wing of the Oregon Republican party. See Curran, "Regulating Death," 727–728.

25. See Erin Hoover and Patrick O'Neill, "The AMA Is Wary of Legislation's Effect on Pain Management But Remains Opposed to Assisted Death," *The Oregonian* (Portland), 6 June 1998; Melinda A. Lee et al., "Legalizing Assisted Suicide—Views of Physicians in Oregon," *New England Journal of Medicine* 334 (5) (1 February 1996): 310, 312 (hereafter *OHSU Survey*). This is a higher percentage than the journal has found in studies of U.S. physicians nationwide, although results have varied, with anywhere from "20 to 70 percent of physicians favor[ing] the legalization of physician-assisted suicide" in various U.S. studies. Kathleen M. Foley, "Competent Care for the Dying Instead of Physician-Assisted Suicide," *New England Journal of Medicine* 336 (2 January 1997): 54.

26. Cf. Lee et al., *OHSU Survey*, 312. It is important to note that the OHSU survey did not include all eligible physicians in Oregon, but approximately 69–70 percent (only those who responded to the survey).

27. See Lee et al., *OHSU Survey*, 313. The study also showed that religious beliefs strongly influenced physicians' willingness to participate. In addition, physicians practicing in small towns or rural communities were less likely to be willing to participate. Ibid., 312.

28. Lee et al., *OHSU Survey*, 313.

29. See, e.g., George J. Annas, "Death By Prescription: The Oregon Initiative," *New England Journal of Medicine* 331 (1994): 1240, 1243 (arguing that the act will injure patients with terminal diseases); "The Oregon Death with Dignity Act [Letters]," *New England Journal of Medicine* 332 (1995): 1174–1175 (assorted responses to Annas's article); Timothy Egan, "Suicide Law Placing Oregon on Several Uncharted Paths," *New York Times*, 25 November 1994, A1 (quoting supporters and opponents of the act).

30. See Curran, "Regulating Death," 728.

31. *Lee v. Oregon*, 869 F.Supp. 1491 (D. Oregon 1994).

32. Ibid., 1496–1497.

33. *Lee v. Oregon*, 891 F.Supp. 1429 (D. Oregon 1995). For criticism of this court ruling, see Charles H. Baron et al., "A Model State Act to Authorize and Regulate Physician-Assisted Suicide," *Harvard Journal of Legislation* 33 (1) (1996): 14–16.

34. *Lee v. Oregon*, 891 F.Supp. 1429 (D. Oregon 1995).

35. *Lee v. Oregon*, 107 F.3d 1382, 1392 (9th Cir. 1997).

36. *Washington v. Glucksberg*, 117 S. Ct. 2258 (1997); *Vacco v. Quill*, 117 S. Ct. 2293 (1997). In *Washington v. Glucksberg*, the Court rejected the plaintiffs' claim that individuals have a liberty interest in assisted suicide protected by the Due Process clause. See *Glucksberg*, 117 S. Ct., 2269–2271. In *Vacco v. Quill*, the Court rejected the plaintiffs' claim that allowing terminally ill patients to be disconnected from life support is, in effect, giving them a right to die, and therefore laws that deny the same right to terminally ill patients who are not on life support violate the Equal Protection Clause. See *Vacco*, 117 S. Ct., 2305–2306. For an overview of the legalization efforts of physician-assisted suicide in the United States, see Carol A. Pratt, "Efforts to Legalize Physician-Assisted Suicide in New York, Washington and Oregon: A Contrast Between Judicial and Initiative Approaches—Who Should Decide?," *Oregon Law Review* 77 (1998): 1027–1080.

37. See David J. Garrow, "The Oregon Trail," *New York Times*, 6 November 1997, A2. For further discussion, see Tom L. Beauchamp, "The Autonomy Turn in Physician-Assisted Suicide," in R. Cohen-Almagor (ed.), *Medical Ethics at the Dawn of the 21st Century* (New York: New York Academy of Sciences, 2000), 111–126.

38. Yale Kamisar, "On the Meaning and Impact of the Physician-Assisted Suicide Cases," *Minnesota Law Review* 82 (1998): 897.

39. Carole Pateman, *Participation and Democratic Theory* (Cambridge, U.K.: Cambridge University Press, 1979); Richard Dagger, *Civic Virtues* (New York: Oxford University Press, 1997), ch. 9.

40. P.L. No. 105–12, 111 Stat. 23 (1997) (codified at 42 U.S.C. 14401 et seq.).

41. 42 U.S.C.A. 14401(b) (West 1998 Pamphlet).

42. See Timothy Egan, "Threat from Washington Has Chilling Effect on Oregon Law Allowing Assisted Suicide," *New York Times*, 19 November 1997, A18.

43. Ibid.

44. See, e.g., Rebecca Dresser, "Nervous Doctors," *New York Times*, 24 November 1997, A22.

45. "Reno: Justice Reviewing Advice on Oregon's Assisted-Suicide Law," Associated Press, 14 November 1997, available in 1997 WL 2562712.

46. Ibid. See also "Justice Dept. Bars Punishing Oregon Doctors Aiding Suicides," *New York Times*, 24 January 1998, A6.

47. See "Reno Won't Fight Oregon Suicide Law," *Associated Press Online*, 6 June 1998.

48. S 2151, 105th Cong. (1998); HR 4006, 105th Cong. (1998).

49. H.R. 2260, 106th Congress (1999). The actual text of H.R. 2260 (Title I) is, in relevant part:

> For purposes of this Act and any regulations to implement this Act, alleviating pain or discomfort in the usual course of professional practice is a legitimate medical purpose for the dispensing, distributing, or administering of a controlled substance that is consistent with public health and safety, even if the use of such a substance may increase the risk of death. Nothing in this section authorizes intentionally dispensing, distributing, or administering of a controlled substance for the purpose of causing death or assisting another person in causing death.
> (2) Notwithstanding any other provision of this Act, in determining whether a registration is consistent with the public interest under this Act, the Attorney General shall give no force and effect to State law authorizing or permitting assisted suicide or euthanasia.
> (3) Paragraph (2) applies only to conduct occurring after the date of enactment of this subsection.

50. H.R. 2260, 106th Congress (1999). The measure was written in response to Attorney General Janet Reno's announcement that federal drug agents will not try to prosecute or revoke the drug licenses of doctors who help patients suffering from a terminal disease die under Oregon's law. See Mark O'Keefe, "Congress Deals Blow to Assisted Suicide," *The Oregonian* (Portland), 14 September 1999; "Anti-Assisted Suicide Bill Approved," Associated Press, 14 September 1999. See also http://hotnews.oregonlive.com; http://www.euthanasia.com/found.html.

51. The legislation would make it impossible for Oregon physicians to prescribe federally controlled substances, but there are other lethal medications that are not covered by the federal law, and Oregon physicians would remain free to prescribe them.

52. Patrick McMahon and Wendy Koch, "Assisted Suicide: A Right or a Surrender?," *USA Today*, 22 November 1999, 21A.

53. Based on personal conversation with Congressional Aide Thomas R. Bullock, III, about the Pain Relief Promotion Act of 1999 and issues surrounding the legislative debate (7 December 1999).

54. See the brief of Henry J. Hyde, chairman of the Committee on the Judiciary. On the Internet at http://www.house.gov/judiciary/ib062399.htm. For further favorable views of the act, see the testimonies of Thomas J. Marzen and Physi-

cians for Compassionate Care before the Committee on the Judiciary (24 June 1999). On the Internet at http://www.house.gov/judiciary/marz0624.htm; http://www.house.gov/judiciary/hami0624.htm.

55. See David A. Pratt, "Too Many Physicians: Physician-Assisted Suicide After *Glucksberg/Quill*," *Albany Law Journal of Science and Technology* 9 (1999): 161, n. 149–154.

56. Brad Cain, "Oregon Medical Association Opposes Congressional PAS Bill," Associated Press, 3 August 1999.

57. Patrick McMahon and Wendy Koch, "Assisted Suicide: A Right or a Surrender?," *USA Today*, 22 November 1999, 21A.

58. See Thomas: Legislative Information on the Internet at http://thomas.loc.gov.

59. Ben Fox, "Assisted Suicide on Doctors' Agenda," Associated Press, 8 December 1999. Reported by Euthanasia Research and Guidance Organization (ERGO) staff; ergo@efn.org.

60. Press statement, "Congress Strikes at Civil Liberties," distributed on 26 October 2000 by ERGO: ergo@efn.org.

61. See Steve Woodward, "Oregon Will Cover Assisted Suicide," *The Oregonian* (Portland), 27 February 1998, A1.

62. Ibid.; Joseph P. Shapiro, "Assisted Suicide, Casting a Cold Eye on 'Death with Dignity': Oregon Studies Year 1 of a Benchmark Law," *U.S. News and World Report*, 1 March 1999, 56.

63. See Diane M. Gianelli, "Suicide Opponents Rip Oregon Medicaid's Pain Control Policy," *American Medical News* (28 September 1998), available in 1998 WL 20198702. The commission sought to reduce coverage of antidepressants because it claimed that physicians were prescribing them too frequently.

64. See "Bills Aim to Curb Assisted-Suicide Law," *The Columbian*, 22 January 1999, B6.

65. Ibid.

66. Ibid.

67. See Erin Hoover Barnett, "Bill Clarifying Assisted-Suicide Law Passes House by a Wide Margin," *The Oregonian* (Portland), 25 May 1999, E1.

68. See 13 Or. Rev. Stat. § 3.14 (1998).

69. "Capable" is defined as "having the ability to make and communicate health care decisions to a health care provider" (Ibid. § 1.01(6)). An adult is an individual who is at least eighteen years of age (Ibid. § 1.01(6)). The residency requirement was intended to prevent individuals from other states from rushing to Oregon to take advantage of the act (Ibid. § 3.10). See Annette E. Clark, "Autonomy and Death," *Tulane Law Review* 71 (1996): 45, n. 43.

70. 13 Or. Rev. Stat. § 2.01 (1998). Voluntary euthanasia occurs when an individual, usually a physician, administers a lethal drug at a patient's request, thus producing the patient's death. See David Orentlicher, "Physician Participation in Assisted Suicide," *Journal of the American Medical Association* 262 (1989): 1844.

71. 13 Or. Rev. Stat. § 4.01(1) (1998). Without this provision, physicians who assisted a suicide would be civilly and criminally liable under Or. Rev. Stat. § 163.125 (1995), which makes it a crime to intentionally cause or aid another in committing suicide.

72. 13 Or. Rev. Stat. § 3 (1998), "Safeguards."

73. The statute contains a form for the written request (see 13 Or. Rev. Stat. § 6.01 [1998]), and requires that two witnesses affirm that the patient is capable and is acting voluntarily in making the request. Ibid., § 2.02.

74. The "attending physician" is the doctor with primary responsibility for the care of the patient. Ibid., § 1.01.

75. The rationale might be to involve a close member of the family in the decision-making process, thinking that he or she would, in the majority of cases,

seek to protect the best interests of the patient. Hendin and colleagues criticized this, saying that the law should insist that neither of the two witnesses could be a beneficiary. Herbert Hendin et al., "Physician-Assisted Suicide: Reflections on Oregon's First Case," *Issues in Law and Medicine* 14 (winter 1998): 254.
76. 13 Or. Rev. Stat. § 2.01, 2.02.
77. 13 Or. Rev. Stat. § 3.07 (1998).
78. Ibid., § 3.01(2)(a)–(e).
79. 13 Or. Rev. Stat. § 3.08 (1998).
80. Section 7 of Rights of the Terminally Ill Act (1995) (NT); for further discussion, see Andrew L. Plattner, "Australia's Northern Territory: The First Jurisdiction to Legislate Voluntary Euthanasia, and the First to Repeal It," *DePaul Journal of Health Care Law* 1 (spring 1997): 647–648.
81. Darien S. Fenn and Linda Ganzini, "Attitudes of Oregon Psychologists toward Physician-Assisted Suicide and the Oregon Death with Dignity Act," *Psychology: Research and Practice* 30 (3) (1999): 235–244.
82. Personal communication (9 July 2000); Linda Ganzini et al., "Physicians' Experiences with the Oregon Death with Dignity Act," *New England Journal of Medicine* 342 (8) (24 February 2000): 561. For further discussion, see Howard Wineberg, "Oregon's Death With Dignity Act: Fourteen Months and Counting," *Archives of Internal Medicine* 160 (1) (10 January 2000); on the Internet at http://archinte.ama-assn.org/issues/v160n1/full/icm90010.html. The report of the first year's experience said, without explanation, that six of the twenty-three patients who received prescriptions for lethal medications died from underlying illness. The report of the second year said that five of the thirty-three patients who received such prescriptions died from underlying illnesses. See Arthur E. Chin et al., "Legalized Physician-Assisted Suicide in Oregon: The First Year's Experience," *New England Journal of Medicine* 340 (7) (18 February 1999): 577–583 (hereafter *OHD Report*), and Amy D. Sullivan et al., *OHD Report 2*: 598–600. Interestingly, when R. Cohen-Almagor specifically asked Katrina Hedberg about this issue, her answer was that "we don't have any information on people who have started the request process, but didn't complete it, either because they were not eligible, they changed their minds, or because they died during the waiting period. We have heard anecdotally that many people die during the fifteen-day waiting period, but we only get the forms for those who have completed the process." Personal communication (7 June 2000).
83. The consulting physician is the doctor qualified by specialty or experience to render a professional diagnosis and prognosis about the patient's condition. See 13 Or. Rev. Stat. § 1.01.
84. 13 Or. Rev. Stat. § 3.01(3).
85. Ibid., § 3.01(5). However, the physician may not require notification as a condition of assistance.
86. For further discussion, see Fenn and Ganzini, "Attitudes of Oregon Psychologists"; Franklin G. Miller et al., "Can Physician-Assisted Suicide Be Regulated Effectively?," *Journal of Law, Medicine and Ethics* 24 (1996): 226; Hendin et al., "Physician-Assisted Suicide," 250.
87. Bregje Onwuteaka-Philipsen, *Consultation of Another Physician in Cases of Euthanasia and Physician-Assisted Suicide* (Doctoral thesis. Amsterdam: Department of Social Medicine, Vrije Universiteit, 1999), 104–118. For further discussion, see chapter 7.
88. 13 Or. Rev. Stat. §§ 3.01(4), 3.03 (1998). No physician may write a prescription until the counselor determines that the patient is not suffering from any mental illness.

89. See Lee et al., *OHSU Survey*, 313.

90. Ganzini et al., "Physicians' Experiences," 559.

91. Chin et al., *OHD Report*, 577–583.

92. Ibid., 578.

93. Families were interviewed for the second-year OHD report.

94. The report has been criticized for providing "nothing approaching a full picture of the extent to which physicians (and others) both have and have not complied with the law. . . . A report, like Oregon's, that relies heavily on physician self-reporting will tend to show that the law is operating well and its provisions are regularly being followed. And that is what the Oregon report shows. . . . A report that makes no serious efforts to uncover the extent of covert assisted suicide does not inspire much faith that legalizing assisted suicide brings the practice into the open, as some proponents told us it would." Marc Spindelman, "Flaws Mar Oregon Report on Dying Law," *Detroit News*, 7 March 1999.

95. Chin, *OHD Report*, 582.

96. Ibid., 578, 579.

97. Ibid.

98. According to the 2000 annual report, sixteen patients had used the drugs and died. See http://www.ohd.hr.state.or.us/chs/pas/ar-tbl-3.htm.

99. Chin, *OHD Report*, 577, 579. See also James D. Moore, "One Year Down: Oregon's Assisted-Suicide Law," *Commonweal* 126 (5) (12 March 1999): 10.

100. Chin, *OHD Report*, 577–583.

101. See Sam Verhovek, "Oregon Reporting 15 Deaths in Year under Suicide Law; Officials See No Abuses," *New York Times*, 18 February 1999, A1; "Assisted Suicide, in Practice," *New York Times*, 27 February 1999. See also the *Los Angeles Times* about how the physician-assisted suicide law in Oregon works in practice, on the Internet at http://www.latimes.com/news/reports/suicide/lat_law991114.html; and "Mercy in Oregon," *Albany Times Union*, 22 February 1999.

102. John Hughes, "New Doctors' Group Criticizes Oregon Death with Dignity Report," Associated Press, 26 February 1999; Spindelman, "Flaws Mar Oregon Report."

103. Amy D. Sullivan, Katrina Hedberg and David W. Fleming, *OHD Report 2*: 598–600.

104. Amy D. Sullivan et al., "Legalized Physician-Assisted Suicide in Oregon, 1998–2000," *New England Journal of Medicine* 344 (22 February 2001): 8.

105. Ibid.; see also "Assisted Suicide-Box," Associated Press (21 February 2001).

106. "Assisted Suicide-Box"; Sullivan et al., "Legalized Physician-Assisted Suicide."

107. Erin Hoover Barnett and Don Colburn, *The Oregonian* (Portland), 22 February 2001; Sullivan et al., "Legalized Physician-Assisted Suicide."

108. Editorial, "Physician-assisted suicide: When pain trails other concerns," *American Medical News* (19 March 2001); Sullivan et al., "Legalized Physician-Assisted Suicide." See also Erin Hoover Barnett, "Oregon's Death With Dignity Act Influences End-of-Life Care Across the State As Doctors Wrestle with Prescribing Pain Treatment," *The Oregonian* (Portland), 18 February 2001.

109. See http://www.ohd.hr.state.or.us/chs/pas/arresult.htm; http://www.ohd.hr.state.or.us/chs/pas/ar-tbl-3.htm.

110. Erin Hoover Barnett and Don Colburn, *The Oregonian* (Portland), 22 February 2001.

111. *Ibid.*

112. Reported by ERGO, to the Right to Die list (2 March 2000); e-mail communication.

113. Ninety-three percent (twenty-five patients) died at home in 1999 and also in 2000. Eighty-one percent (fifteen patients) died at home in 1998. See Sullivan et al., *OHD Report 2*, 601.
114. Chin et al., *OHD Report*, 578.
115. See http://www.ohd.hr.state.or.us/chs/pas/ar-tbl-3.htm.
116. Sullivan et al., *OHD Report 2*, 599.
117. Johanna H. Groenewoud et al., "Clinical Problems with the Performance of Euthanasia and Physician-Assisted Suicide in the Netherlands," *New England Journal of Medicine* 342 (8) (24 February 2000): 551–556.
118. See Oregon State Ballot Measure 51: Repeal of 1994 Assisted Suicide Ballot Measure, published in *City Club of Portland Bulletin* 79 (20) (17 October 1997), on the Internet at http://www.pdxcityclub.org/ballot51.html; International Anti-Euthanasia Task Force, *Special Report: Oregon Takes a Closer Look at Assisted Suicide*, on the Internet at <http://www.iaetf.org>, citing Barbara Coombs Lee et al., "Physician Assisted Suicide," *Oregon Health Law Manual* 2; *Life and Death Decisions*, Oregon State Bar (1997): 8–12. See also Mark O'Keefe and Gail Kinsey Hill, "Suicide Methods Come into Question," *The Oregonian* (Portland), 15 August 1997.
119. See Lee et al., *OHSU Survey*, 313.
120. Legislative attempts to legalize PAS that were introduced during 1997 in Connecticut, Illinois, and Massachusetts stated that the physician may assist the patient in making use of the means to hasten death, so long as the actual use is a voluntary physical act of the patient. The Maine bill requires the responsible physician to be present when the patient self-administers the lethal medication. See Russell Korobkin, "Physician-Assisted Suicide Legislation: Issues and Preliminary Responses," *Notre Dame Journal of Law, Ethics and Public Policy* 12 (2) (1998): 464.
121. Patients ingesting lethal medications in 2000 represented an estimated 9/10,000 total Oregon deaths. By comparison, 1998 PAS patients represented 6/10,000 deaths; 1999 PAS patients, 9/10,000 deaths. See http://www.ohd.hr.state.or.us/chs/pas/arresult.htm.
122. See 13 Or. Rev. Stat. § 4.01 (1998)
123. *OHD Report 2*, 601. See also *OHD Report*, 582.
124. Sullivan et al., *OHD Report 2*, 599.
125. Ganzini et al., 559.
126. Richard S. Mangus et al., "Medical Students' Attitudes toward Physician-Assisted Suicide," *Medical Student Journal of the American Medical Association* (MSJAMA) 282 (1 December 1999): 2080–2081.
127. *OHSU Survey*, 312.
128. *OHSU Survey*, 312.
129. Section 7, Rights of the Terminally Ill Act (1995) (NT).
130. Sullivan et al., *OHD Report 2*, 601.
131. http://www.ohd.hr.state.or.us/chs/pas/ar-tbl-3.htm.
132. Ibid.
133. Paul van der Maas and Linda L. Emanuel, "Factual Findings," in L. L. Emanuel (ed.), *Regulating How We Die* (Cambridge, Mass.: Harvard University Press, 1998), 173.
134. *OHD Report*, 582. It should be noted that it was argued that more than one patient feared pain. See Joseph P. Shapiro, "Casting a Cold Eye on 'Death with Dignity' Oregon Studies Year 1 of a Benchmark Law," *U.S. News & World Report* (1 March 1999): 56.
135. Ezekiel J. Emanuel et al., "Euthanasia and Physician-assisted Suicide: Attitudes and Experiences of Oncology Patients, Oncologists, and the Public," *Lancet* 347 (29 June 1996): 1809.

136. Sullivan et al., *OHD Report 2*, 601.
137. Ganzini et al., "Physicians' Experiences with the Oregon Death with Dignity Act," 559.
138. Kathleen Foley, "Dismantling the Barriers: Providing Palliative and Pain Care," *Medical Student Journal of the American Medical Association* 283 (5 January 2000), 115; on the Internet at http://www.ama-assn.org/sci-pubs/ msjama/articles/vol_283/no_1/jms90045.html
139. S. Ward et al., "Patient-Related Barriers to Management of Cancer Pain," *Pain* 53 (1993): 319–324; Charles S. Cleeland et al., "Pain and Its Treatment in Outpatients with Metastatic Cancer," *New England Journal of Medicine* 330 (1994): 592–596; Cleeland, "Controlling Cancer Pain: Many Missed Opportunities," *Medical Student Journal of the American Medical Association* 283 (5 January 2000); on the Internet at http://www.ama-assn.org/sci-pubs/ msjama/articles/vol_283/no_1/cleeland.htm.
140. Catherine S. Magid, "Pain, Suffering, and Meaning," *Medical Student Journal of the American Medical Association* 283 (5 January 2000), 114; on the Internet at http://www.ama-assn.org/sci-pubs/msjama/articles/vol_283/no_1/ jms90044.htm.
141. To institute effective pain control, new programs for the training and certification of palliative care consultants need to be developed and implemented. See Franklin G. Miller et al., "Regulating Physician-Assisted Death," *New England Journal of Medicine* 331 (2) (14 July 1994): 119–123; Timothy E. Quill et al., "Palliative Options of Last Resort," *Journal of the American Medical Association* 278 (23) (17 December 1997): 2099–2104; P. D. Doyle et al. (eds.), *Textbook of Palliative Medicine* (New York: Oxford University Press, 1998); Anne Scott, "Autonomy, Power, and Control in Palliative Care," *Cambridge Quarterly of Healthcare Ethics* 8 (2) (1999): 139–147; Janet L. Abrahm, "The Role of the Clinician in Palliative Medicine," *Medical Student Journal of the American Medical Association* 283 (5 January 2000): 116; on the Internet at http://www.ama-assn.org/sci-pubs/msjama/articles/vol_283/no_1/ jms90047.htm.
142. *OHD Report*, 583; *OHD Report 2*, 603.
143. *OHD Report*, 583.
144. See Gerrit van der Wal et al., "Evaluation of the Notification Procedure for Physician-Assisted Death in the Netherlands," *New England Journal of Medicine* 335 (28 November 1996): 1706, 1710; John Griffiths et al., *Euthanasia and Law in the Netherlands* (Amsterdam: Amsterdam University Press, 1998), 259–298.
145. Van der Maas and colleagues decided not to include pharmacists in their comprehensive study about the Dutch practice of euthanasia. They explained: "While, in several instances, pharmacists are aware of the preparation or carrying out of euthanasia, they often are not. Therefore it did not appear necessary to interview pharmacists, either for reliable quantification or to obtain an insight into the background for this type of decisions, although they might be able to provide interesting additional information in a number of cases." Paul J. van der Maas et al., *Euthanasia and Other Medical Decisions Concerning the End of Life*, Health Policy Monographs (Amsterdam: Elsevier, 1992), 12.
146. One such case was reported in 1998 (Chin et al., *OHD Report*, 582). In 1999, twenty-four patients died within four hours, and three patients died after eleven hours or more (Sullivan et al., *OHD Report 2*, 599).
147. Chin et al., *OHD Report*, 579.
148. Sullivan et al., *OHD Report 2*, 602. See also the conclusions of Ganzini et al., "Physicians' Experiences," 563.

149. See http://www.ohd.hr.state.or.us/chs/pas/arresult.htm.
150. "Surveys: More Favor Assisted-Suicide Law," *The Oregonian* (Portland), 11 March 1997, D1; Roper Organization of New York City, "The 1988 Roper Poll on Attitudes toward Active Voluntary Euthanasia" (Los Angeles, Calif.: National Hemlock Society, 1988); Mark Gillespie, "Kevorkian to Face Murder Charges," Gallup News Service, 19 March 1999; Sheryl Gay Stolberg, "In Survey, Few Doctors Admit to Helping Terminal Patients Die," *New York Times*, 23 April 1998. See also Charles F. McKhann, *A Time to Die: The Place for Physician Assistance* (New Haven, Conn.: Yale University Press, 1999); http://www.nejm.org/public/1998/0338/0017/1193/1.htm; http://www.medscape.com.
151. Maine had a referendum on physician-assisted suicide in November 2000. The ballot measure to legalize PAS failed by a 51 percent to 49 percent decision. For further information, see Tim Christie, "Voters in Maine Reject Assisted-Suicide Law," *The Register-Guard* (Eugene, Ore.), 14 November 2000; Mainers for Death with Dignity; Maine Citizens Against the Dangers of Physician-Assisted Suicide, on the Internet at http://www.noassistedsuicide.com; text of ballot questions, on the Internet at http://www.state.me.us/sos/cec/refguide.htm.
152. Emanuel and his colleagues found that patients who had seriously considered and prepared for euthanasia or PAS were significantly more likely to be depressed. See Emanuel et al., "Euthanasia and Physician-Assisted Suicide," 1809.
153. Sullivan et al., *OHD Report 2*, 598–604. See also David Brown, "A Picture of Assisted Suicide: Most Who Use Oregon Law Are Educated, Insured; Some Change Their Minds," *Washington Post*, 24 February 2000, A03.

CONCLUSIONS

1. Notorious among them are the Hemlock Society in the United States and the corresponding association in Vancouver, British Columbia. Sue Rodriguez disassociated herself from the British Columbia association after she felt they used her and betrayed her trust. For further discussion, see Sue Woodman, *Last Rights* (New York: Plenum Trade, 1998), 17–24, 54–56, 119–137; Derek Humphry and Mary Clement, *Freedom to Die* (New York: St. Martin's Griffin, 2000); ERGO, on the Internet at http://www.FinalExit.org/world.fed.html.

   In November 1999, a weekend conference was held in Seattle dealing with methods of self-deliverance from a terminal illness using new equipment. Only those with hands-on experience with assisting death were invited, and the conference location was kept secret. Derek Humphry, whose Euthanasia Research and Guidance Organization sponsored the two-day meeting, explained that they did not want "observers, moralists, philosophers or protesters." See the *Seattle Times*, on the Internet at http://www.seattletimes.com/news/local/html98/suic_19991115.html.

   In the Netherlands, a Web site provides a how-to guide for suicide methods. Step-by-step instructions guide the reader through wrist-slashing, sleeping pills, jumping off buildings, and the "reasonably painless . . . death of carbon monoxide poisoning." The Pink Floyd song "Goodbye Cruel World" can be heard on the home page, along with verses from the William Butler Yeats poem "An Irish Airman Foresees His Death." "Suicide Web Site Sparks Controversy," *New York Times*, 31 January 2000. See also http://huizen.dds.nl/~thisbe/ and http://huizen.dds.nl/7/8thisbe/verder.
2. Opening Motion (Tel-Aviv) 1141/1990. *Benjamin Eyal v. Lichtenstaedter Hospital.* P.M. 1991 (3), 194.

3. Ibid., 187. For further discussion of similar cases, see 1030/95 *Israel Gilad v. Soroka Medical Center and Others*, Beer Sheva District Court (23 October 1995); Opening Motion 2339 + 2242/95 *A.A. and Y. S. v. Kupat Holim and State of Israel*, Tel Aviv District Court (11 January 1996); Opening Motion 2242/95 *Eitay Arad v. Kupat Holim and State of Israel*, Tel Aviv District Court (1 October 1998). Judge Talgam emphasized in the *Arad* case that the starting point must be the dignity of the patient, and not of the hesitant doctor.

4. See David Novak, *Jewish Social Ethics* (New York: Oxford University Press, 1992), 17; *Jewish-Christian Dialogue* (New York: Oxford University Press, 1989), 8, 142–151. For a contesting view, see Justice Elon in Civil Appeal 506/1988 *Yael Scheffer, through Talila Scheffer v. The State of Israel*, para. 20.

5. I thank Dr. Nachman Wilensky for showing Rabbi Lau's letter to me.

6. For an opposing stance, see Avraham Steinberg, "The Terminally Ill—Secular and Jewish Ethical Aspects," *Israel Journal of Medical Science* 30 (1) (January 1994): 134.

7. Haim H. Cohn, "On the Meaning of Human Dignity," *Israel Yearbook of Human Rights* 13 (1983): 246.

8. Cf. K. Higashi et al., "Five-Year Follow Up of Patients with Persistent Vegetative State," *Journal of Neurology, Neurosurgery and Psychiatry* 44 (1981): 552–554; and W. Arts et al., "Unexpected Improvement after Prolonged Post-traumatic Vegetative State," *Journal of Neurology, Neurosurgery, and Psychiatry* 48 (1985): 1300–1303. See also B. Steinbock, "Recovery from Persistent Vegetative State?: The Case of Carrie Coons," *Hastings Center Report* 19 (4) (1989): 14.

9. Will Gaylin et al., "Doctors Must Not Kill," *Journal of the American Medical Association* 259 (1988): 2139; Edmund D. Pellegrino, "Doctors Must Not Kill," in Robert I. Misbin (ed.), *Euthanasia: The Good of the Patient, the Good of Society* (Frederick, Md.: University Publishing Group, 1992), 27–41; Charles L. Sprung et al., "Is the Physician's Duty to the Individual Patient or to Society?," *Critical Care Medicine* 23 (4) (1995): 618–620. For a contrasting view, see Fredrick R. Abrams, "The Quality of Mercy: An Examination of The Proposition 'Doctors Must Not Kill,'" in Misbin, *Euthanasia: The Good of the Patient*, 43–51.

10. Charles Sprung, "Changing Attitudes and Practices in Forgoing Life-Sustaining Treatments," *Journal of the American Medical Association* 263 (16) (25 April 1990): 2214.

11. John Hardwig, "Dying at the Right Time," in *Is There a Duty to Die?* (New York and London: Routledge, 2000), 95. In the Netherlands, 91 percent of the physicians in the 1990 national study felt that only a physician may perform euthanasia. P. J. van der Maas et al., *Euthanasia and Other Medical Decisions Concerning the End of Life*, Health Policy Monographs (Amsterdam: Elsevier, 1992), 108. Faber-Langendoen and Karlawish argue that physician assistance in suicide might be necessary but that it is insufficient to ensure that assisted suicide is restricted to appropriate cases and occurs in an appropriate manner. The willingness of other health care professionals—nurses, social workers, and clergy—to participate and even take the lead in assisting suicides is critical, in their opinion, to meet society's interest that assisted suicide should be humane, effective, and confined to appropriate cases. They conclude that as long as legislation and guidelines focus exclusively on the physician's role, laws and regulations will fall short of meeting this assurance. Kathy Faber-Langendoen and Jason T. H. Karlawish, "Should Assisted Suicide Be Only Physician Assisted?," *Annals of Internal Medicine* 132 (21 March 2000): 482–487.

12. Civil Appeal 506/88 *Scheffer v. The State of Israel*, P.D. 48 (1) 87, 172–173.
13. Sprung et al. present data showing that doctors see CPR treatment as "useless" even when the patients' chances are 5 to 10 percent. They further note that the chances for giving such treatment drop when the patients are black and that many life-and-death decisions are made without the consent of the patients or their family members. See Charles L. Sprung et al., "Changes in Forgoing Life-Sustaining Treatments in the United States: Concern for the Future," *Mayo Clinics Proceedings* 71 (1996): 513–514.
14. Interviews with Dr. George Beausmans (Maastricht, 26 July 1999), and Dr. Gerrit K. Kimsma (Koog aan de Zaan, 28 July 1999).
15. Those opposed to my view will say that the Netherlands exemplifies a state in which the defining guiding lines for mercy killings are often crossed, resulting in many patients being killed against their will (see chapter 7). See also David Orentlicher, "The Legalization of Physician Assisted Suicide: A Very Modest Revolution," *Boston College Law Review* 38 (3) (May 1997): 459–462.
16. The anxiety over the slippery-slope syndrome was probably foremost in the minds of the participants of the Thirty-Ninth World Medical Assembly, held in Madrid in October 1987. In the World Medical Association Declaration on Euthanasia it was contended that euthanasia, "that is the act of deliberately ending the life of a patient, even at the patient's own request or at the request of close relatives, is unethical. This does not prevent the physician from respecting the desire of a patient to allow the natural process of death to follow its course in the terminal phase of sickness." For critical discussion of the slippery-slope syndrome, see R. G. Frey, "The Fear of a Slippery Slope," in Gerald Dworkin et al. (eds.), *Euthanasia and Physician-Assisted Suicide* (New York: Cambridge University Press, 1998), 43–63; Charles F. McKhann, *A Time to Die: The Place for Physician Assistance* (New Haven, Conn.: Yale University Press, 1999), 160–196; Ronald Dworkin, "When Is It Right to Die?," *New York Times*, 17 May 1994, A19; Bernard Williams, "Which Slopes Are Slippery," in Michael Lockwood (ed.), *Moral Dilemmas in Modern Medicine* (Oxford, U.K.: Oxford University Press, 1985), 126–137.
17. See, for example, Yale Kamisar, "Some Non-Religious Views Against Proposed 'Mercy Killing' Legislation," *Minnesota Law Review* 42 (6) (1958): 969–1042; Kamisar, "Against Assisted Suicide—Even a Very Limited Form," *University of Detroit Mercy Law Review* 72 (summer 1995): 736–769; Sissela Bok, "Death and Dying: Euthanasia and Sustaining Life: Ethical Views," in Warren T. Reich (ed.), *Encyclopedia of Bioethics* (New York: Free Press, 1978), vol. 1, 268–277; Bok, "Euthanasia," in Dworkin et al., *Euthanasia and Physician-Assisted Suicide*, 112–118; Peter A. Singer and Mark Siegler, "Euthanasia—A Critique," *New England Journal of Medicine* 322 (June 1990): 1881–1883; Charles J. Dougherty, "The Common Good, Terminal Illness, and Euthanasia," *Issues in Law and Medicine* 9 (2) (fall 1993): 151–166; Carl Elliot, "Philosopher Assisted Suicide and Euthanasia," *British Medical Journal* 313 (26 October 1996): 1088.
18. One of Swigart and colleagues' findings on the role of families in the critical care setting is that explanations should be made in language clearly understandable to family members. They note overuse of medical terms or presentations of medical minutiae that may be overwhelming and confusing for family members. Valerie Swigart et al., "Letting Go: Family Willingness to Forgo Life Support," *Heart and Lung* 25 (6) (1996): 492.
19. R. Anspach, *Deciding Who Lives* (Berkeley: University of California Press, 1993), 85–163. Quoted in Swigart et al., "Letting Go," 404.
20. Occasionally the media publish stories of alleged killings of patients by medical staff and of patients' deaths in questionable circumstances. "Police Ar-

rest 'Angel of Death' for L.A. Hospital Murders," Reuters, 9 January 2001; Lois Rogers, "Police Investigate Doctor over 50 Hospital Deaths," *The Times* (London), 15 October 2000, on the Internet at http://www.sunday-times.co.uk/news/pages/sti/2000/10/15/stinwenws01030.html; Joseph B. Frazier, "Grand Jury Refuses to Indict Nurse in Care Center Morphine Deaths," Associated Press, 13 September 2000; Roy Gibson and Hugh Martin, "Cancer Doctor on Murder Charge," *The Age*, 7 April 2000, on the Internet at http://www.theage.com.au/news/20000407/A54440–2000Apr7.html; "Report: Nurses Gave Too Much Morphine to at Least One Patient," Associated Press, 22 March 2000.

21. Occasionally the media publish stories of alleged killings of patients by family members or friends. David Reardon, "Family Denies Complicity in Death," *The Age*, 29 November 2000; Les Kennedy, "Two Accused of Wilful Murder for Sister's Hospice Death," *Sydney Morning Herald*, 13 April 2000, on the Internet at http://www.smh.com.au/news/0004/13/text/national06.html; "Elderly Man Charged in Wife's Death," Associated Press, 28 February 2000, on the Internet at http://www10.nytimes.com/aponline/a/AP-BRF-Mercy-Killing.html; Maxine Bernstein, "Man, 83, in Custody in Wife's Death," *The Oregonian* (Portland), 5 March 2000; David Reardon, "Family Questioned on Mercy Killing," *The Age*, 8 April 2000, on the Internet at http://www.theage.com.au/news/20000408/A56073–2000Apr7.html; Tracy Wilson, "Man Admits Killing His Ailing Spouse," *Los Angeles Times*, 15 March 2000, on the Internet at http://www.latimes.com/editions/valley/sfnews/20000315/t000024869.html.

22. In March 1998, Justice Antonin Scalia declared that Congress, not the Supreme Court, should decide such vexing questions as abortion rights, the death penalty, and physician-assisted suicide. Scalia said, "It is not supposed to be our judgment what the socially desirable answer to all of these questions is. That's supposed to be the judgment of Congress, and we do our job correctly when we apply what Congress has written as basically and honestly as possible." Glen Johnson, "Scalia: Let Congress, Not Court, Decide Abortion, Assisted Suicide," Associated Press, 9 March 1998.

23. Songs were written about Jack Kevorkian. For instance, Detroit rocker Mitch Ryder dedicated his song "Mercy" to Dr. Jack Kevorkian. Jack Kevorkian himself released a CD with twelve songs, eleven of which he wrote. The liner notes say that Kevorkian wants to be remembered as a doctor who helped relieve human suffering.

24. These are the documented cases. This information was obtained from http://www.finalexit.org/kevorkian.html. In December 1999, however, /kevorkian.html was no longer found on this server.

25. Cf. *People v. Kevorkian*, No. 90003196 (Oakland County, Mich., 14 December 1990); *People v. Kevorkian* No. 90–390963–A2 (Oakland County, Mich., 5 February 1991); Jim Persels, "Forcing the Issue of Physician-Assisted Suicide," *Journal of Legal Medicine* 14 (1993): 95–100.

26. Stephen Vicchio, "Death's Logic" (4 April 1999), on the Internet at http://www.sunspot.net.

27. *Jack Kevorkian and John Doe v. Arnett*, No. CV-94–6089 CBM (Kx), 939 F.Supp. 725 (11 September 1996), 351.

28. *State of Michigan v. Kevorkian*, Michigan CirCt (Oakland City), verdict 8 March 1996. On the Internet at http://www.courttv.com/verdicts/kevorkian.html.

29. Jack Kevorkian, *Prescription: Medicide* (New York: Prometheus Books, 1991), 222.

30. Ibid., 226.

31. Ibid., 227.

32. 2 April 1996: Pontiac, Mich: Kevorkian: Trial or Witch-Hunt?, from ERGO's electronic mailing list. E-Mail: ergo@efn.org.

33. Orlando Sentinel Online, "Kevorkian Responds to New Allegations," 31 December 1997; on the Internet at http://www.orlandosentinel.com/.

34. Brian Harmon, "Kevorkian: I'll Put Law On Trial. Suicide Advocate Says He'll Fight Attempts to Rein Him In," *Detroit News*, Metro, 1 January 1998, on the Internet at http://detnews.com.

35. Orlando Sentinel Online, "Kevorkian Responds."

36. Kevorkian explains his guiding rationale in his book *Prescription: Medicide*, especially in chapters 13 and 14.

37. Ibid., 223.

38. Ibid., 215.

39. Ibid.

40. Ibid., 225.

41. Ibid.

42. Compare Kevorkian's cold and detached descriptions to Quill's caring and humane train of thought in *Death and Dignity*, especially his depiction of the stories of Diane, Mark, Wendy, and Mrs. J. There are stark differences between the two. See Timothy E. Quill, *Death and Dignity* (New York: W. W. Norton, 1993), 9–16, 52–56, 84–91, 167–175, 177–179.

43. *The Detroit News*, Metro, 6 September 1997; on the Internet at http://detnews.com/1997/metro/9709/06/09060039.htm. For further discussion, see Woodman, *Last Rights*, 91–93.

44. Kevorkian had no training to detect or to treat depression. For further discussion, see Paul R. McHugh, "The Kevorkian Epidemic," *American Scholar* (winter 1997): 15–27.

45. "Coroner: Janet Good Would Have Lived More Than 6 Months," *Detroit News*, Metro, 6 September 1997; on the Internet at http://detnews.com/1997/metro/9709/06/09060039.htm.

46. Brian Harmon, "Critics: Kevorkian Taking All Comers. They Claim Terminal Illness No Longer Only Standard for Suicides," *Detroit News*, 1 March 1998; on the Internet at http://detnews.com; http://www.oregonian.com.

47. Woodman, *Last Rights*, 94–95.

48. Brian Harmon, "Paralyzed Man Fulfills Death Wish: Kevorkian Assists 21-Year-Old Hours After Leaving Hospital," *Detroit News*, 27 February 1998; "Kevorkian Speaks Out Against Police," Associated Press, 28 February 1998.

49. Brian Harmon, "Critics: Kevorkian Taking All Comers. They Claim Terminal Illness No Longer Only Standard for Suicides," *Detroit News*, 1 March 1998.

50. Ibid.

51. David Goodman, "Kevorkian Has Kidneys Available to Donate from Suicide," Associated Press, 7 June 1998. See also Joe Swickard and David Crumm, "Kevorkian Harvests Kidneys," *The Free Press*, 8 June 1998, on the Internet at http://www.freep.com/news/extra2/index.htm.

52. Chronology of events involving Kevorkian was available on the Internet at http://deathnews.com/TDNHOME/kevo. In March 2001, the Web site was no longer available.

53. OPINION Editorial, "Kevorkian's Needle," *Detroit News*, 22 November 1998.

54. Derek Humphry, 22 November 1998, on the Internet through ergo@efn.org.

55. CBS News, *60 Minutes*, "Death by Doctor," 22 November 1998.

56. Kevorkian *60 Minutes* poll results, 24 November 1998, on the Internet at http://www.freep.com/news/extra2/kevo_poll.htm. See also "Killing Not Murder, Most Say," on the Internet at http://www.freep.com/news/extra2/qpoll24.htm.
    For discussion on the ethics of showing Kevorkian's killing on televi-

sion, see Fritz Wenzel, "Media Are Ripped at U of M Forum on Assisted-Suicide Coverage," *Toledo Blade*, 23 February 1999; Brian Murphy, "Wallace Rethinks Suicide Episode," 23 February 1999, on the Internet at http://www.freep.com/news/metro/qdeath23.htm. See also http://www.freedom forum.org/professional/1998/12/3kevorkian.asp.

57. Ellen Goodman, "Kevorkian Has Punctured the Ethical Gray Zone Where Most of Us Live," *Boston Globe*, 3 December 1998; on the Internet at http://www.boston.com/dailyglobe2/337/oped/.

58. See Julie Grace, "Curtains for Dr. Death," *Time*, 5 April 1999, 50.

59. Associated Press report, "Kevorkian Gets 10 to 25 Years," Pontiac, Mich., 13 April 1999; *New York Times*, 14 April 1999, A23. For further discussion, see http://www.freep.com/news/extra2/index.htm; http://www.freep.com/news/extra2/qkevo14.htm.

60. "Scenes from 'Final Exit' Suicide Video," Associated Press, 3 February 2000.

61. Likewise, Barbara Coombs Lee, executive director of Compassion in Dying and a staunch supporter of Oregon's Death with Dignity Act, opposed the showing of the videotape. She called it "irresponsible": "The video's intended audience, terminally ill individuals, deserves better than hardware store paraphernalia and a secretive death with no family members present." Deborah Josefson, "Video Guide to Suicide Is Shown on Television," *British Medical Journal* 320 (12 February 2000): 398.

62. "Kevorkian Criticizes Suicide Video," Associated Press, 24 February 2000; e-mail sent by Kevorkian's friend to the Right to Die List, accessible at right_to_die@efn.org, 5 March 2000. See also letter, "'Final Exit' Aimed at Terminally Ill," *The Oregonian* (Portland), 4 January 2000.

63. Susan Kreifels, "An Oahu Man and Woman Both Choose Suffocation Just Days after the Station Aired 'Final Exit,'" *Honolulu Star Bulletin*, 7 March 2000. See also "Coalition Seeks to Stop Showing of Suicide Video Guide," Associated Press, 9 March 2000.

64. For further discussion, see R. Cohen-Almagor, *Speech, Media and Ethics* (Houndmills, U.K., and New York: Palgrave, 2001).

65. "Kevorkian Assistant Helps AIDS Patient Die," Reuters, 19 January 1998.

66. "Reding Believed Hiding in Europe," *Albuquerque Journal*, 26 January 2000.

67. Magnusson and Ballis published a research study they conducted into the practice of euthanasia among Australian health care professionals specializing in HIV/AIDS. Their study shows that illegal euthanasia is currently practiced by the medical profession and suggests that prohibition does not adequately resolve the agonizing dilemmas that health care workers face. They maintain that prohibitionism fails to take into account the reality of illegal euthanasia as it is practiced in an unregulated environment and that it is counterproductive because it does not assist in developing a social policy that reflects the reality of current practices while safeguarding patients. Roger S. Magnusson and Peter H. Ballis, "The Response of Health Care Workers to AIDS Patients' Requests for Euthanasia," *Journal of Sociology* 35 (3) (November 1999): 312–330.

68. Most bill proposals to legislate PAS in the United States specify that the consenting patient must be eighteen or older to qualify for the procedure. Russell Korobkin, "Physician-Assisted Suicide Legislation: Issues and Preliminary Responses," *Notre Dame Journal of Law, Ethics and Public Policy* 12 (2) (1998): 454.

69. See the Dutch requirements for careful practice, in John Griffiths et al., *Euthanasia and Law in the Netherlands* (Amsterdam: Amsterdam University Press, 1998), 66.

70. Many bill proposals for legislation authorizing PAS in the United States re-

quire a waiting period of fourteen or fifteen days. See Korobkin, "Physician-Assisted Suicide Legislation," 468.

71. Section 7, Rights of the Terminally Ill Act (1995) (NT).

72. In Australia, the law required a cooling-off period of nine days. In Oregon, the act requires a waiting period of fifteen days. I do not wish to suggest an arbitrary time period of waiting; instead, the patient should state his or her wish several times over a period of time. I concur with Miller and colleagues, who think that a fifteen-day waiting period may be highly burdensome for patients who are suffering intolerably and may preclude access to assisted death for those who request it just at the point of imminent death. Franklin G. Miller et al., "Can Physician-Assisted Suicide Be Regulated Effectively?," *Journal of Law, Medicine and Ethics* 24 (1996): 226. See also Oregon Death with Dignity Act, *Oregon Revised Statutes*, vol. 8 (1998 supplement), 982.

73. Griffiths et al., *Euthanasia and Law*, 66.

74. Oregon Death with Dignity Act, *Oregon Revised Statutes*, vol. 8 (1998 supplement), 980.

75. For a comparison of physicians' and patients' different conceptions of pain, see William Ruddick, "Do Doctors Undertreat Pain?," *Bioethics* 11 (3–4) (1997): 246–255.

76. Linda Ganzini et al., "Physicians' Experiences with the Oregon Death with Dignity Act," *New England Journal of Medicine* 342 (8) (24 February 2000): 563.

77. World Health Organization, *Cancer Pain Relief and Palliative Care: Report of a WHO Expert Committee* (Geneva, Switzerland: World Health Organization, 1990), 11.

78. Directive 7 in *The General Manager Circular*, Israel Ministry of Health, no. 2/96 (31 January 1996) holds: "Doctors must concentrate their efforts on easing the pain, torment, and suffering of the patient, a subject of highest priority in medical treatment, especially where terminal patients are concerned," 12 (Hebrew). For further deliberation on pain control mechanisms and their importance, see Timothy E. Quill et al., "Palliative Options of Last Resort," *Journal of the American Medical Association* 278 (23) (17 December 1997): 2099–2104; P. D. Doyle et al. (eds.), *Textbook of Palliative Medicine* (New York: Oxford University Press, 1998); Christine K. Cassel and Kathleen M. Foley, "Principles for Care of Patients at the End of Life: An Emerging Consensus Among the Specialties of Medicine," Milbank Memorial Fund Report (New York, 1999), reported by Vida Foubister, "Medical Experts Agree on Guide for End-of-Life Care," *American Medical News*, 7 February 2000, on the Internet at http://www.ama-assn.org/sci-pubs/amnews/pick_00/prsa0207.htm; Timothy E. Quill et al., "Palliative Treatments of Last Resort: Choosing the Least Harmful Alternative," *Annals of Internal Medicine* 132 (21 March 2000): 488–493. For further discussion on making palliative care decisions for incompetent patients, see Jason H. T. Karlawish et al., "A Consensus-Based Approach to Providing Palliative Care to Patients Who Lack Decision-Making Capacity," *Annals of Internal Medicine* 130 (18 May 1999): 835–840.

79. 13 Or. Rev. Stat. § 3.01 (1998).

80. Korobkin, "Physician-Assisted Suicide Legislation," 469.

81. Section 7, Rights of the Terminally Ill Act (1995) (NT).

82. On this issue, see Oregon Death with Dignity Act, Section 3, Attending physician responsibilities. Many bill proposals to legislate PAS in the United States specify certain information that must be communicated by the physician to the patient before honoring his or her request. See also Korobkin, "Physician-Assisted Suicide Legislation," 468. See also Section D: Consent to Medical Treatment of The Israel Patients' Rights Law, 1992, Law Proposal

2132 (16 March 1992); The Patients' Rights Law, 1996, *Israel Book of Laws*, 1591 (12 May 1996), 329–331; and *The General Manager Circular*, Ministry of Health, no. 2/96 (31 January 1996), 10–11 (all in Hebrew).

83. Most bill proposals to legislate PAS in the United States required that the treating physician refer the patient to a second consulting physician to verify the terminal nature of the disease. The Massachusetts bill required a third confirming opinion. Cf. Korobkin, "Physician-Assisted Suicide Legislation," 453. The first practical recommendation stated in *The General Manager Circular*, Israel Ministry of Health, no. 2/96 (31 January 1996), is that the diagnosis and evaluation that a patient's condition is "irreversible and terminal" should be made by two independent doctors. At least one of them is required to be a head of department, 9 (Hebrew).

84. Oregon Death with Dignity Act, *Oregon Revised Statutes*, vol. 8 (1998 supplement), 981–982.

85. Griffiths et al., *Euthanasia and Law*, 66, 104. The Dutch guidelines require the doctor to consult an independent colleague, not in order to advise the first doctor on medical treatment, but in order to verify whether the criteria of the guidelines have been satisfied. The consultation is about the patient's condition and life expectancy, the available alternatives and the adequacy of the request. Medical consultation in an earlier stage is part of normal practice. For instance, cancer patients who request euthanasia have invariably been treated in hospitals up to the point at which the doctors and the patient together decided to stop treatment.

86. Section 7, Rights of the Terminally Ill Act (1995) (NT).

87. Bregje Onwuteaka-Philipsen, *Consultation of Another Physician in Cases of Euthanasia and Physician-assisted Suicide* (Doctoral thesis. Amsterdam: Department of Social Medicine, Vrije Universiteit, 1999).

88. Proposals to legislate PAS in Illinois, Massachusetts, and Maine required that a patient seeking PAS obtain a consultation with a mental health professional in order to insure that the patient can pass the "impaired judgment" standard. Cf. Korobkin, "Physician-Assisted Suicide Legislation," 456. This guideline is somewhat similar to the guidelines of the Swiss EXIT protocol. See South Australian Voluntary Euthanasia Society, "DID YOU KNOW? Assisted Suicide in Switzerland," SAVES Fact Sheet No. 20, February 1997. SAVES, P.O. Box 2151, Kent Town, SA 5071, Australia—Fax 61 8 8265 2287. On the Internet at http://www.finalexit.org/.

89. Andrew L. Plattner, "Australia's Northern Territory: The First Jurisdiction to Legislate Voluntary Euthanasia, and the First to Repeal It," *DePaul Journal of Health Care Law* 1 (spring 1997): 648.

90. 13 Or. Rev. Stat. § 3.07 (1998).

91. In the Netherlands, physicians who intend to provide assisted suicide sometimes end up administering a lethal injection because of the patient's inability to take the medication. Cf. Johanna H. Groenewoud et al., "Clinical Problems with the Performance of Euthanasia and Physician-Assisted Suicide in the Netherlands," *New England Journal of Medicine* 342 (8) (2000): 551–556.

92. For further discussion, see the Dutch guidelines in Griffiths et al., *Euthanasia and Law*, 66; Oregon Death with Dignity Act, *Oregon Revised Statutes*, vol. 8 (1998 supplement), sec. 3, 983. Rebecca Cook pointed out to me that such a bureaucratic procedure might discriminate against minorities who will not find it easy to cope with the described demands. However, the demand for detailed documentation in my proposal is meant to prevent abuse, not to discourage people from getting the help they want. We should be sensitive to cultural differences and strive to meet special needs that arise from cultural norms but not at the expense of leaving the door open for "eliminating" unwanted people.

93. Directive 6 in *The General Manager Circular*, Israel Ministry of Health, no. 2/96 (31 January 1996) states: "The decision to respect a patient's objection to a life prolonging treatment shall be documented in the medical statutes, expressing maximum reasons for the decision and the discussions with the patient," 12 (Hebrew). See also Israel Patients' Rights Law (1996), 1591, Chapter E: medical documentation and medical information, 331.

94. Plattner, "Australia's Northern Territory," 648. The Illinois proposed bill to legislate PAS included a "Provider's Freedom of Conscience" clause, which explicitly said that physicians who object to the practice may not be required to participate or aid in PAS. Compare Korobkin, "Physician-Assisted Suicide Legislation," 464.

95. For further discussion, see Arthur L. Caplan et al., "The Role of Guidelines in the Practice of Physician-Assisted Suicide," *Annals of Internal Medicine* 132 (21 March 2000): 476–481.

96. 506/88 *Scheffer v. The State of Israel*, vol. 48 (1) 87, paragraph 65 of Justice Elon's opinion. For further discussion on incompetent patients and minors, see Edmund D. Pellegrino and David C. Thomasma, *For the Patient's Good* (New York: Oxford University Press, 1988), 148–161; Winifred J. Pinch and Margaret L. Spielman, "The Parents' Perspective: Ethical Decision-Making in Neonatal Intensive Care," *Journal of Advanced Nursing* 15 (1990): 712–719; American Academy of Pediatrics Committee on Bioethics, "Guidelines on Forgoing Life-Sustaining Medical Treatment," *Pediatrics* 93 (3) (March 1994): 532–536; S. Saigal et al., "Differences in Preferences for Neonatal Outcomes among Healthcare Professionals, Parents, and Adolescents," *Journal of the American Medical Association* 281 (21) (2 June 1999): 1991–1997; Norman Fost, "Decisions Regarding Treatment of Seriously Ill Newborns," *Journal of the American Medical Association* 281 (21) (2 June 1999): 2041–2043.

APPENDIX

1. Max Charlesworth, *Bioethics in a Liberal Society* (Cambridge, U.K.: Cambridge University Press, 1993), 108. For further discussion on the duties of the liberal state in maintaining the health of its citizens, see Troyen A. Brennan, *Just Doctoring* (Berkeley: University of California Press, 1991), ch. 3, 4, 8, 9.

2. Adopted by the International Health Conference held in New York from 19 June to 22 July 1946 and signed by the representatives of sixty-one states, in *The United Nations and Population: Major Resolutions and Instruments* (New York: Dobbs Ferry, 1974), 204.

3. See Daniel Callahan's writings: *The Troubled Dream of Life* (New York: Simon and Schuster, 1993); *What Kind of Life* (New York: Simon and Schuster, 1990); *Setting Limits* (New York: Simon and Schuster, 1987).

4. "Final Report from the Swedish Parliamentary Priorities Commission," 1995, 46.

5. On the Internet at http://medicare.hcfa.gov/stats/ombud.htm.

6. U.S. Bureau of Census, *Statistical Abstract of the United States: 1998*, 118th ed., National Data Book (Washington, D.C., 1998), 118.

7. Haavi E. Morreim, *Balancing Act: The New Medical Ethics of Medicine's New Economics* (Dordrecht, the Netherlands: Kluwer, 1991), 9.

8. Lakshmipathi Chelluri et al., "Intensive Care for Critically Ill Elderly: Mortality, Costs, and Quality of Life," *Archives of Internal Medicine* 155 (May 1995): 1013.

9. On the Internet at http://www.cdc.gov/nchswww/data/hus98.pdf.

10. On the Internet at http://www.cihi.ca/facts/nhex/1ju199.htm. See also Brennan, *Just Doctoring*, 178.

11. Robert J. Blendon et al., "Physicians' Perspectives on Caring for Patients in the United States, Canada, and West Germany," *New England Journal of Medicine* 328, (14) (1993): 1015.

12. Nancy Neveloff Dubler and David Nimmons, *Ethics on Call* (New York: Harmony Books, 1992), 328. For further discussion on the American health care system and its flaws, see James F. Childress, *Practical Reasoning in Bioethics* (Bloomington and Indianapolis: Indiana University Press, 1997): 237–262.

13. Jo Lenaghan, "Citizens' Rights to Health Care in the UK: Developing a National Framework of Entitlement," in Lenaghan (ed.), *Hard Choices in Health Care: Rights and Rationing in Europe* (London: BMJ Publishing Group, 1997), 69.

14. Memorandum by the Department of Health (20 April 1993), in House of Lords, *Select Committee on Medical Ethics*, session 1993–1994, vol. II, Minutes of Oral Evidence (London: HMSO, 1994), 14.

15. Rudolf Klein, *The New Politics of the NHS* (London and New York: Longman, 1995), 3rd ed., 98.

16. On the Internet at http://www.statistics.gov.uk/stats/ukinfigs/health.htm.

17. See Chelluri et al., "Intensive Care For Critically Ill Elderly," 1013–1022; Charles L. Sprung et al., "Is the Physician's Duty to the Individual Patient or to Society?," *Critical Care Medicine* 23 (4) (1995): 618–620; Helga Kuhse, "Quality of Life and the Death of 'Baby M,'" *Bioethics* 6 (3) (1992): 233–250; E. Haavi Morreim, "The Impossibility and the Necessity of Quality of Life Research," *Bioethics* 6 (3) (1992): 218–232; Rebecca S. Dresser and John A. Robertson, "Quality of Life and Non-Treatment Decisions for Incompetent Patients: A Critique of the Orthodox Approach," *Law, Medicine and Health Care* 17 (3) (fall 1989): 234–244.

18. See *Collected Works of John Locke* (London: Routledge, 1997), 9 vols. Some writings are available on the Internet at http://weber.ucsd.edu/~dmckiern/locke.htm. See also Martin Hailer and Dietrich Ritschel, "The General Notion of Human Dignity and the Specific Arguments in Medical Ethics," in K. Bayertz (ed.), *Sanctity of Life and Human Dignity* (Dordrecht, The Netherlands: Kluwer, 1996), 97.

19. H.F.F. Leenen, "Selection of Patients," *Journal of Medical Ethics* 8 (1) (March 1982): 33–36; Callahan, *Setting Limits*; Norman Daniels, *Just Health Care* (Cambridge, U.K.: Cambridge University Press, 1988); Norman Daniels, *Am I My Parents' Keeper?: An Essay on Justice between the Young and the Old* (New York: Oxford University Press, 1988); David M. Eddy, "Rationing by Patient Choice," *Journal of the American Medical Association* 265 (1) (2 January 1991): 105–108; Eike-Henner W. Kluge, "Medicine as a Service-Provider Monopoly: Implications for Equitable Access to Health Care," *Professional Ethics* 2 (3–4) (1993): 127–148; Tom L. Beauchamp and James F. Childress, *Principles of Biomedical Ethics* (New York: Oxford University Press, 1994) 326–394; Susan D. Goold, "Allocating Health Care: Cost-Utility Analysis, Informed Democratic Decision Making, or the Veil of Ignorance?" *Journal of Health Politics, Policy and Law* 21 (1) (spring 1996): 69–98; Len Doyal, "Rationing Within the NHS Should Be Explicit," *British Medical Journal* 314 (1997): 1114–1118; John Harris, "Justice and Equal Opportunities in Health Care," *Bioethics* 13 (5) (1999): 392–404.

20. Cf. Dubler and Nimmons, *Ethics on Call*, 329. Those who could afford private insurance will opt for that option. Thus, for instance, in the mid-1980s, an estimated 28 percent of hip replacement operations were conducted in the private sector (cf. Klein, *New Politics*, 156).

21. Klein (*New Politics*, 78) argues that in 1975 the number of patients being treated by dialysis (or with a functioning transplant) was 62 per 1,000,000 population in Britain, as against 136.1 in Switzerland, 132.4 in Denmark, 102.2 in France, 87.7 in Germany, and 85.4 in Sweden. In other words, Klein maintains that people in Great Britain are being turned away to die, whereas if those people lived elsewhere, they would be successfully treated.

22. Ibid., p. 179. For further discussion, see Darren Shickle, "Public Preferences for Health Care: Prioritisation in the United Kingdom," *Bioethics* 11, (3–4) (1997): 277–290.

23. Avraham Steinberg, "Limited Resources in Medicine—Moral Principles," *Medicine* 112 (10) (May 1987): 513 (Hebrew).

24. Cf. Klein, *New Politics*, 233–245; Doyal, "Rationing." For further discussion, see R. Klein et al., *Managing Scarcity: Priority Setting and Rationing in the National Health Service* (Buckingham, U.K.: Open University Press, 1996).

25. Cf. Klein, *New Politics*, 155; David J. Roy et al., *Bioethics in Canada* (Scarborough, Ontario: Prentice Hall, 1994), 101.

26. Cf. Klein, *New Politics*, 156.

27. Cf. Roy et al., *Bioethics in Canada*, 101.

28. Robert G. Evans, "'We'll Take Care of It for You,' Health Care in the Canadian Community," *Deadalus* 117 (4) (fall 1988): 167.

29. Cf. Kluge, "Medicine as a Service-Provider Monopoly," 135–136.

30. Cf. Roy et al., *Bioethics in Canada*, 95.

31. Ibid., 96.

32. For further discussion, see Lester C. Thurow, "Medicine versus Economics," *New England Journal of Medicine* 313 (10) (5 September 1985): 611–614.

33. For further deliberation on the contractarian approach, see John Rawls, *A Theory of Justice* (Oxford, U.K.: Oxford University Press, 1971); Rawls, *Political Liberalism* (New York: Columbia University Press, 1993).

34. Cf. R. Cohen-Almagor, *The Boundaries of Liberty and Tolerance* (Gainesville, Fla.: University Press of Florida, 1994), ch. 1, 3.

35. In Plato's eyes, the physician and the patient share the responsibility for treatment and its consequences equally. The therapeutic process is conceived as a common enterprise whose end and prospects of success are both based on the reciprocal relationship between the two parties under the extramedical and superindividual principles of social morality. Medical services should not be supplied to hypochondriacs or to those who neglect their health or indulge in harmful habits such as overeating, heavy drinking, and lack of physical activity. David Heyd, "The Medicalization of Health: Plato's Warning," *Revue Internationale de Philosophie* 3 (193) (1995): 390.

36. The discussion here concerns adults who supposedly are responsible for their own lives. The case is different when minors are involved, and certainly with infants who become addicted to drugs or alcohol while still in the womb.

37. Joseph M. Boyle, "The Concept of Health and the Right to Health Care," *Social Thought* (summer 1977): 5–17.

38. Another approach draws a distinction between discrimination among products and discrimination among people. While it is just to discriminate among products (such as cigarettes) by means of taxation, no discrimination among people should be made for the sole reason that they do not know how to preserve their health. See Evans, "'We'll Take Care of It,'" 163.

39. Professor Lehman-Wilzig writes in his comments that it is known that gobbling hamburgers is harmful to one's health and asks whether this logic applies to the regular clients of McDonald's. The answer is that an open

public discourse will determine the boundaries of responsibility. Today, a social agreement exists that the addiction of grown-ups to drugs or alcohol constitutes an abrogation of their responsibility for their own health. In the future, perhaps other actions will appear to constitute the relinquishing of this kind of responsibility.

40. Callahan, *Setting Limits*, 10.
41. Cf. Callahan, *What Kind of Life*, 152.
42. Callahan, *Troubled Dream*, 37.
43. *Judea, Samaria and the Gaza District Since 1967* (Jerusalem: Israel Information Center, 1986).
44. David C. Naylor et al., "Canadian Medicare: Prognosis Guarded," *Canadian Medical Association Journal* 153 (3) (1 August 1995): 286.
45. Callahan writes that the federal government defines a premature death as one that occurs before the age of sixty-five. He accepts this definition, arguing that there should be a reduction of funds for research to combat diseases of patients aged sixty-five or older. See his "Death and the Research Imperative," *New England Journal of Medicine* 342 (9) (2 March 2000); on the Internet at http://www.nejm.org/content/2000/0342/0009/0654.asp.
46. Callahan, *Troubled Dream*, 214.
47. Ibid., 213. Discussion with Dan Callahan, Hastings Center (18 March 1999).
48. Cf. Chelluri et al., "Intensive Care," 1014–1016.
49. The Swedish Support and Services Act that came into force on 1 January 1994 is equally problematic. It is an entitling act, implying positive discrimination of persons with severe functional impairments. Its aim is to facilitate full participation in the life of the community and, accordingly, equality of certain functionally impaired people. It does not apply, however, to persons over the age of sixty-five. "Final Report from the Swedish Parliamentary Priorities Commission," 1995, 16.
50. Cf. Callahan, *What Kind of Life*, 78–79.
51. *Sue Rodriguez v. The Attorney General of Canada*. File No. 23476 (September 1993).
52. 1141/90 *Benjamin Eyal v. The Lichtenshtedter Hospital* (Tel Aviv).
53. Callahan, *Setting Limits*, 116. See also Callahan, "Aging, Death, and Population Health," *Medical Student Journal of the American Medical Association* 282 (1 December 1999); on the Internet at http://www.ama/assn.org/sci-pubs/msjama/articles/vol_282/no_21/jms90040.htm.
54. Callahan, *Setting Limits*, 32.
55. For further criticism, see Shimon Glick, "Rationing and Priority Setting: Discussion," in Peter Allebeck and Bengt Jansson (eds.), *Ethics in Medicine* (New York: Raven Press, 1990), 77–87; and R.W. Hunt, "A Critique of Using Age to Ration Health Care," *Journal of Medical Ethics* 19 (1993): 19–23. On the virtues of longevity, see James Hillman, *The Force of Character* (New York: Random House, 1999), 25–28.
56. Discussion with Dan Callahan, Hastings Center (18 March 1999).
57. Interestingly, while discussing this essay, Callahan described himself as a communitarian when he explained the ideology underpinning his arguments. I said that his position sounded more like utilitarianism. Callahan was not happy with the description, but after some thought he conceded that it was unavoidable to be utilitarian if one was involved in policy matters. Discussion with Dan Callahan, Hastings Center (18 March 1999).
58. I do not claim that utilitarianism in itself is amoral. In certain circumstances utilitarianism could have positive moral consequences. In this particular matter I think that utilitarian results are amoral. For further discussion, see Daniels, *Just Health Care*; Shelly Kagan, *The Limits of Morality* (Oxford, U.K.:

Clarendon Press, 1989). For evaluation of utilitarian ethics, see Beauchamp and Childress, *Principles of Biomedical Ethics*, 47–55.

59. In 1994, during my first visit to the Hastings Center, I had some additional conversations with Callahan. In one of them I asked him whether he would have chosen the same assertive opinion if he had been dealing with his own parents. His reply was that it did not matter what the thoughts of Dan the person were, only the thoughts of Dan the citizen. The state cannot fulfil the wants of all. Its reasoning must be rational, not emotional, and therefore we require a calculated examination of the priorities in medicine. In 1999, Callahan reiterated the same line of reasoning while conceding that "I am not young anymore." Callahan, however, has private insurance and hence will not suffer the consequences of his suggested policy.

60. Cf. Cohen-Almagor, *Boundaries of Liberty and Tolerance*, ch. 1.

61. J. S. Mill, *Utilitarianism, Liberty, and Representative Government* (London: J. M. Dent. Everyman's edition, 1948), 151–152.

62. "Simpson Trial Cost More Than $9 Million, County Report Says," *Los Angeles Times*, 2 December 1995.

63. Capitalists would say that the judicial system must be controlled by the state, whereas the health care system could be held in private hands. I, on the other hand, do not see a replacement for the involvement of the state in medical affairs when individuals cannot pay for costly treatments. Furthermore, most people cannot pay for expensive transplant operations with personal funds, but only via private medical insurance. It might be the case that in the future we will hear more voices in the capitalist world calling for the privatization of the court system as well, out of materialistic-utilitarian considerations. In Israel, many economic disputes are resolved outside the courts, through mediation paid for by the sides to the dispute.

64. Cf. Callahan, *Troubled Dream*, 216.

65. Cf. A Letter from Dr. Keith Andrews, House of Lords, *Select Committee on Medical Ethics*, session 1993–94, vol. III, Minutes of Oral Evidence (London: HMSO, 1994): 221–224.

66. Eike-Henner W. Kluge, "Social Values, Socioeconomic Resources and Effectiveness Coefficients: An Ethical Model for Statistically Based Resource Allocation," in R. Cohen-Almagor (ed.), *Medical Ethics at the Dawn of the 21st Century* (New York: New York Academy of Sciences, 2000), 23–31.

67. Medicaid is a joint federal/state entitlement program that provides health insurance for certain low-income populations. It is administered at the state level, but responsibility for program funding and for setting program policy is shared by the federal and state governments. States receive a federal financial match for their Medicaid expenditures. See Shruti Rajan, "Publicly Subsidized Health Insurance: A Typology of State Approaches," *Health Affairs* 17 (3) (1998): 101–102.

68. John Elson, "Rationing Medical Care," *Time*, 15 May 1989.

69. See Senate Bill 27, 65th Oregon Legislative Assembly—1989 Regular Session. I acknowledge with gratitude the assistance of Monica Schreffler, Office of the Oregon Health Plan Administrator.

70. "The Oregon Health Plan: The Legal Framework." Material compiled by Monica Schreffler. See also Thomas Bodenheimer, "The Oregon Health Plan—Lessons for the Nation," part 2, *New England Journal of Medicine* 337 (10) (4 September 1997): 720–723.

71. Timothy Egan, "Oregon Lists Illness by Priority to See Who Gets Medicaid Care," *New York Times*, 2 May 1990: A1, A18.

72. David M. Eddy, "Oregon's Methods: Did Cost-Effectiveness Analysis Fail?," *Journal of the American Medical Association* 266 (15) (16 October 1991): 2135.

73. Merrill Matthews, Jr., "Would Physician-Assisted Suicide Save the Healthcare System Money?," in Margaret P. Battin et al. (eds.), *Physician Assisted Suicide* (New York and London: Routledge, 1998), 316.

74. David M. Eddy, "Oregon's Plan: Should It Be Approved?," *Journal of the American Medical Association* 266 (17) (6 November 1991): 2439; Thomas Bodenheimer, "The Oregon Health Plan—Lessons for the Nation," part 1, *New England Journal of Medicine* 337 (9) (28 August 1997): 651–652. See also "Oregon's Rationing Plan Isn't Denying Much Care, NEJM Report Says," *Medicine and Health* 51 (35) (8 September 1997).

75. Under Oregon's 1989 legislative package, the Medicaid portion of the Oregon Health Plan was only one of its two critical pieces. The other was the requirement that employers provide insurance to employees, with the prioritized list as the minimal benefit package. Small businesses lobbied for the repeal of this part of the legislation, and on 1 January 1996, the bill died. Gone was the hope of nearly universal health insurance in Oregon, with the prioritized list used for persons with incomes above the federal poverty level as well as Medicaid beneficiaries. See Bodenheimer, "The Oregon Health Plan," part 2, 720–723.

76. I prefer to use the term *services* and not *treatments* when assisted suicide is discussed. For further discussion, see Leonard M. Fleck, "Just Caring: Assisted Suicide and Health Care Rationing," *University of Detroit Mercy Law Review* 72 (1995): 901–926.

77. "The Oregon Health Plan: The Legal Framework." Material compiled by Monica Schreffler. See also M. R. Skeels, "The Oregon Health Plan and Public Health," *Journal of Health and Social Policy* 61 (1) (1994): 21–31.

78. Courtney S. Campbell, "Gridlock on the Oregon Trail," *Hastings Center Report* 23 (4) (July–August 1993): 6.

79. "The Oregon Health Plan," *Oregon Health Forum* (August 1995): 4.

80. Campbell, "Gridlock," 6; Chris Ham, "Retracting the Oregon Trail: The Experience of Rationing and the Oregon Health Plan," *British Medical Journal* 316 (27 June 1998): 1965.

81. Peter T. Kilborn, "Oregon Falters on a New Path to Health Care," *New York Times*, 3 January 1999, 1.

82. P. R. Sipes-Metzler, "Oregon Health Plan: Ration or Reason," *Journal of Medicine and Philosophy* 19 (4) (1994): 305–314. See also P. Southard, "The Oregon Health Plan," *Journal of Emergency Nursing* 18 (5) (October 1992): 471–473; Ralph Crawshaw, "Guide to the Oregon Trail," *Medical Audit News* 2 (7) (1992): 101–102.

83. Kristie Perry Dolan, "How's Oregon's Bold Rational Program Doing?," *Medical Economics* 74 (15) (28 July 1997): 44. See also "Outliers: Call It Coincidence, But Oregon Is Taking the Lead in Healthcare," *Modern Healthcare* (12 January 1998): 56.

84. Jim Montague, "Why Rationing Was Right for Oregon," *Hospitals and Health Networks* 71 (3) (5 February 1997): 64–65; "John Kitzhaber's Prescription," *Economist* (25 April 1998): 33–34.

85. Notes, "The Oregon Health Care Proposal and the Americans with Disabilities Act," *Harvard Law Review* 106 (1993): 1296–1313.

86. Joshua Wiener, "Rationing in America: Overt and Covert," in Martin A. Strosberg et al. (eds.), *Rationing America's Medical Care: The Oregon Plan and Beyond* (Washington, D.C.: Brookings Institution, 1992), 110.

87. Lawrence Jacobs et al., "The Oregon Health Plan and the Political Paradox of Rationing: What Advocates and Critics Have Claimed and What Oregon Did," *Journal of Health Politics, Policy and Law* 24 (1) (1999): 164–165.

88. Ibid., 165–166.

89. Ron L. Wyden, "Why I Support the Oregon Plan," in Strosberg et al., *Rationing America's Medical Care*, 115–118.
90. The symbiotic relationship between liberal ideology and the utilitarian approach is rooted in the nineteenth century, but bearing in mind the liberal principles that accentuate the principles of not harming others and respect for others, this may be seen as a historical accident.
91. Health authorities in Britain have been extremely reluctant to adopt policies of explicit rationing. Rather than following the Oregon model, and limiting the menu of services offered, they continue to leave decisions about which patients should be treated, and how, to clinicians. Rudolf Klein (*New Politics*, 245) argues that as a resource allocation strategy, the Oregon model is flawed. To exclude specific forms of treatment on the grounds that they are ineffective, or that the return on the money spent is low, is to ignore the fact that patients are heterogeneous. Even if nine out of ten patients do not benefit from a particular form of treatment, there may always be a tenth for whom it is cost-effective. Clinical judgment is therefore crucial in deciding which patients will respond to particular forms of treatment. Klein maintains that similarly, concentrating on rationing by exclusion risks ignoring the ability to better use resources in the management of patients: decisions about diagnostic tests, about preventive antibiotic therapy, about lengths of hospital stay, and so on. Implicit rationing by clinicians may therefore be more rational than rationing by explicit exclusion. For further criticism, see Sara Rosenbaum, "Poor Women, Poor Children, Poor Policy: The Oregon Medical Experiment," in Strosberg et al., *Rationing America's Medical Care*, 91–106.
92. David M. Eddy, "What's Going On in Oregon?," *Journal of the American Medical Association* 266 (3) (17 July 1991): 417.
93. Jacobs et al., "Oregon Health Plan and the Political Paradox," 167.
94. Bodenheimer, "Oregon Health Plan," part 1, 654–655. For further discussion, see Peter A. Glassman et al., "Medical Necessity and Defined Coverage Benefits in the Oregon Health Plan," *American Journal of Public Health* 87 (6) (1 June 1997): 1053.
95. For further information and discussion, see http://www.das.state.or.us/ohpa/ohpa.htm.
96. Montague, "Why Rationing Was Right," 64.
97. "John Kitzhaber's Prescription," *Economist* (25 April 1998): 33–34.
98. Peter T. Kilborn, "Oregon Falters on a New Path to Health Care," *New York Times*, 3 January 1998, 1. See also Jacobs et al., "Oregon Health Plan and the Political Paradox," 168.
99. Carole Pateman, *Participation and Democratic Theory* (Cambridge, U.K.: Cambridge University Press, 1979); Richard Dagger, *Civic Virtues* (New York: Oxford University Press, 1997).
100. Cf. Steinberg, "Limited Resources," 515.
101. A study about opinions of bereaved family members reports criticisms of physicians, including insensitive communication style, reluctance to use pain medication, and lack of time and attention to dying patients, especially those in nursing homes. Family members expressed their sense that dying patients had been abandoned. They also expressed a need for greater compassion and sensitivity in the physicians' style of communication. See Laura C. Hanson et al., "What Is Wrong with End-of-Life Care? Opinions of Bereaved Family Members," *Journal of American Geriatrics Society* 45 (1997): 1341–1343.
102. Cf. Cohen-Almagor, *Boundaries of Liberty and Tolerance*, ch. 1.
103. For further discussion, see David M. Eddy, "What Care Is 'Essential'? What

Services Are 'Basic'?," *Journal of the American Medical Association* 265 (6) (13 February 1991): 782–788; Eddy, "The Individual vs. Society—Is there a Conflict?," *Journal of the American Medical Association* 265 (11) (20 March 1991); Eddy, "The Individual vs. Society—Resolving the Conflict," *Journal of the American Medical Association* 265 (18) (8 May 1991): 2399–2406.

104. For further discussion, see Eike-Henner W. Kluge, "Designated Organ Donation: Private Choice in Social Context," *Hastings Center Report* (September/October 1989): 10–16; Raymond J. Devettere, *Practical Decision Making in Health Care Ethics* (Washington, D.C.: Georgetown University Press, 1995), 440–466.

Index

Index of Court Cases

About the Author

Raphael Cohen-Almagor received his doctorate from Oxford University and is a senior lecturer at the department of communication and chairperson of library and information studies at the University of Haifa, Israel. In 1999–2000 he was awarded the Fulbright–Yitzhak Rabin Award and was a visiting professor at the UCLA school of law and department of communication. He has published widely in the fields of medical ethics, philosophy, political science, law, media ethics, sociology, and history in English, French, Spanish, and Hebrew. He is the author of *The Boundaries of Liberty and Tolerance* (1994) and *Speech, Media and Ethics* (2001), and editor of *Basic Issues in Israeli Democracy* (1999, Hebrew), *Liberal Democracy and the Limits of Tolerance: Essays in Honor and Memory of Yitzhak Rabin* (2000), *Challenges to Democracy: Essays in Honour and Memory of Isaiah Berlin* (2000), *Medical Ethics at the Dawn of the 21st Century* (2000), and *Moral Dilemmas in Medicine* (2001, Hebrew). His book of poetry, *Middle Eastern Shores*, was published in 1993 (Hebrew). He is completing a book on the policy and practice of euthanasia in the Netherlands and is working on *The Struggle against Political Extremism in Israel*.